GO
TO A
WORLD
THAT IS
DYING

An orthopedic surgeon leaves modern medicine in the US to serve God for over twenty years in a primitive hospital in Bangladesh, accompanied by his wife, a professional artist.

JOHN E. BULLOCK

To my beloved Tense, my best friend and lifelong companion: You have selflessly loved and supported me through all the chapters of my life. I love sharing this life with you and serving our God together.

Go to a World that is Dying

Copyright © 2025 John E. Bullock

All Rights Reserved.

No part of this book shall be reproduced or transmitted in any form or by any means, electronic, magnetic, and photographic, including photocopying, recording or by any information storage and retrieval system, without prior written permission of the publisher.

No patent liability is assumed with respect to the use of the information contained herein. Although every precaution has been taken in the preparation of this book, the publisher and author assume no responsibility for errors or omissions. Neither is any liability assumed for damages resulting from the use of the information contained herein.

Unless otherwise indicated, all scripture quotations are taken from The Holy Bible: New King James Version (NKJV)® Copyright © 1982 by Thomas Nelson. Used by permission. All rights reserved.

Drawings by Hortense Bullock

Book cover design and interior layout by Jennie Miller.

ISBN: 979-8-3492-1920-7

Contents

Acknowledgments ix

Prologue xi

Turn Your Eyes Upon Jesus xiii

Part I: God Had a Plan (Ephesians 2:10)

1. Stranded! 3
2. Beginnings 7
3. Decisions 15
4. "Dr. Bullock" 23
5. Pursuit of Orthopedic Training 27
6. An Intriguing Challenge 33
7. The Brass Ring 37
8. Salvation and Surrender 41
9. Change of Command, Change of Course 45
10. Letting Go of the Brass Ring 51

11. The Assignment 59
12. Announcing Our Decision 63
13. Pre-Field Ministry 67
14. Hard Decisions and Saying Goodbye 73

Part II: Bangladesh at Last

15. On Wings of Eagles 81
16. Memorial Christian Hospital 87
17. Critical Time 97
18. Unexpected Changes 103
19. His Perfect Salvation to Tell 107
20. Working with an Interpreter 113
21. A New Medical World 119
22. Unexpected Responses to Medical Care 131
23. No Blood, No Admission 139
24. Learning Bengali 145
25. A New and Strange Culture 151
26. Family Reunion 159

Part III: Developing the Orthopedic Department

27. Working Full-time in the Hospital 165
28. Training Helpers 171
29. Indian Rope Trick 177
30. Provision and Protection 181
31. Return to Bangladesh 189

32. Hope for the Hopeless	197
33. Prosthetic Limbs	207
34. Every Life Matters	215
35. Equipment and Supply Challenges	225
36. God's Plan for Man	231
37. To Catch a Plane	237
38. Safe!	245
39. Improvisation	249
40. Typical Day in a Doctor's Life	257
41. Teaching Jungle Orthopedics	267
42. Challenging Cases	275
43. Grateful Patients	281
44. Teamwork	289
45. Seventeen Years!	297

Part IV: Reassignment

46. Life More Abundant	303

Conclusion: Only One Life	313
Photos	314
Notes	365
Bibliography	369
Glossary	371
Maps	374

Acknowledgments

We are truly thankful and deeply indebted to the great team of people who made it possible for us to serve God in Bangladesh at Memorial Christian Hospital (MCH) for more than twenty years. Those who supported us with letters of encouragement and news from home lifted our spirits. We consider each person who supported us financially and prayed for us to have had a significant part of God's work in Bangladesh, which has had an eternal impact on thousands of lives.

Tense and I are thankful for our ABWE teammates and coworkers and the national staff at MCH and in Chittagong whose faithful and dependable service enabled us to do the work that God had called us to do, in spite of NGO and national staff shortages, long working hours, and a multitude of patient and national crises. From our first arrival at MCH in 1974 until our last visit in 2015, I received excellent help from the US and Canadian nurses, whose work was essential to my survival at MCH. These were part of the team that not only gave physical care to the patients but also used every opportunity to share with them and their relatives the message of salvation and spiritual growth taught in the Holy Bible.

We are deeply indebted to Larry Golin, who developed and managed the Physical Therapy Department and the Limb and Brace Shop at MCH. His skill, foresight, and planning to set up the Limb and Brace Shop enabled us to transform the lives of amputee patients and reach them with the saving power of the gospel of salvation in Christ.

We are thankful for Dr. Steve Kelley, who quickly learned the principles of orthopedic surgery and continues this much-needed specialty at MCH. His sincere devotion to the mission of MCH and faithful service for many years testify to his compassionate desire to share the gospel with the people of Bangladesh.

We are grateful for John's cousin, Roy Chattin, who agreed to be responsible for John's mother's care when we left for Bangladesh in 1974 and to take care of her affairs when she died. His gracious help enabled us to go when we were desperately needed because of the acute doctor shortage.

We are extremely grateful to our daughters, Chrissa and Karen, who spent hundreds of hours sorting through over fifty years of correspondence, individual stories, notes, and photos and then typed and edited the manuscript to assemble and produce this book. We pray it will inspire those who read it to consider how they might serve God with their lives.

John and Hortense Bullock
March 2025

Prologue

*"You did not choose Me,
but I chose you and appointed you..."*
John 15:16

Through a series of extraordinary events, Tense and I found ourselves preparing to make a radical change in our lives and go to the mission field. We believed God had called us for full-time service at Memorial Christian Hospital in Bangladesh. I was a successful orthopedic surgeon, well-established in a multi-specialty clinic in San Luis Obispo, California. Tense was a professional artist who had her own studio and gallery. We were enjoying the good life after many years of hard work to get to that point. But God changed the course of our lives completely and changed us in the process. Tense and I were chosen by God, as a craftsman chooses his tools for a specific assignment.

This assignment was not possible to perform in our own strength without God's direct help. No amount of training could have prepared us for the challenges we faced. It was an exhausting task with multiple obstacles. I felt a heavy sense of responsibility to give the best care to my patients, even though I had limited resources or staff and no orthopedic consultants. Often, I was the only doctor. Yet, despite these challenges, knowing we were part of a team bringing spiritual hope and healing to the Bangladeshi people rather than seeking our own prestige and material profit made all of our efforts worthwhile.

Looking back, we realize that God was working in our lives from the time we were born, before we even realized He was there, training us in various skills and equipping us for the work He intended us to accomplish for Him. We learned that what may have seemed like failures to us along the way were part of God's plan to prepare us for the future. In His sovereignty, God knew everything that would happen. He had designed it for His purpose.

We gradually learned that He was in charge of our lives, and our accomplishments were with His strength and guidance. We came to expect His direction and enablement and were constantly aware of His protection over us. He provided the necessary equipment and help to accomplish this assignment at Memorial Christian Hospital in Bangladesh.

God can accomplish His will without help from anyone, but His plan is to work through men and women whom He chooses. We hope you will read the book carefully and with an open heart about how God might direct your life.

John and Hortense Bullock
March 2025

Turn Your Eyes Upon Jesus

O soul, are you weary and troubled?
No light in the darkness you see?
There's light for a look at the Savior
And life more abundant and free!

Through death into life everlasting
He passed, and we follow Him there;
Over us sin no more hath dominion—
For more than conq'rors we are!

His Word shall not fail you—He promised;
Believe Him, and all will be well:
Then go to a world that is dying,
His perfect salvation to tell!

Turn your eyes upon Jesus,
Look full in His wonderful face,
And the things of earth will grow strangely dim
In the light of His glory and grace.[1]

— Helen H. Lemel

PART ONE

God Had a Plan

"For we are His workmanship, created in Christ Jesus for good works, which God prepared beforehand that we should walk in them."

Ephesians 2:10

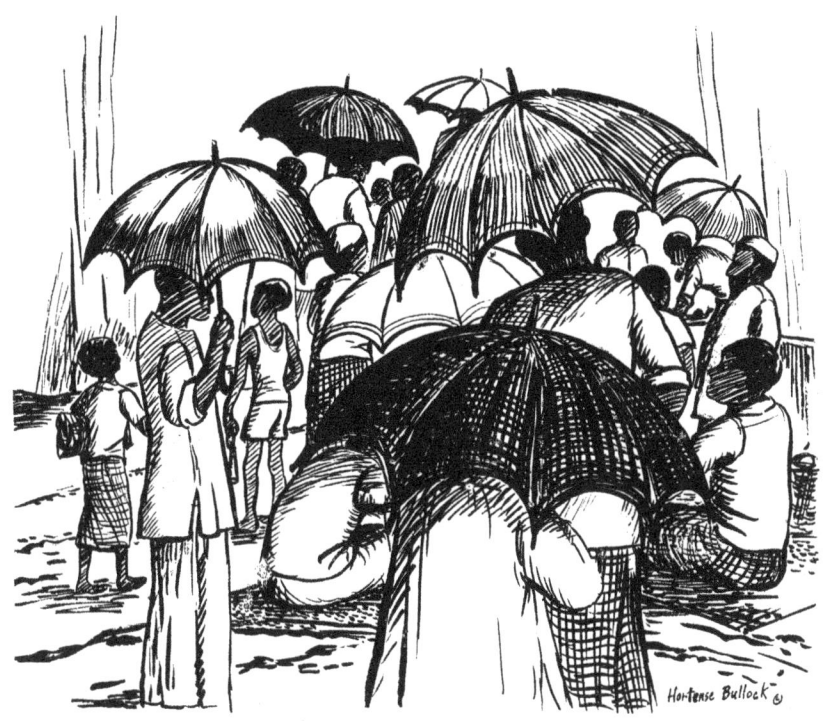

CHAPTER 1

Stranded!

A thin, wiry Bangladeshi man in a white tee shirt and black pants snatched up our suitcases, placed one on his head, and began weaving through the sea of travelers toward the door of the crowded train station. "Dad! Someone is trying to steal our luggage!" shouted David. The man gestured with his head for us to follow him, and we realized this must be the porter that the station master had promised to send. At the station master's direction, we had been waiting out of the weather in the first-class waiting room, which was considered "first-class" because it had a toilet. The station was crowded with Bangladeshi men and women in damp lungis, saris, and burkas. They stood silently at the window, watching the rain pouring down.

We leaped out of our seats to follow the porter and tried to keep him in sight. Through the open doorway, we caught a glimpse of the mail train covered with people clinging to the sides and roof, resembling a huge furry caterpillar as it rumbled into the station. It seemed hopeless to think that we and our belongings would ever be able to get onto that train. This unexpected change of course, caused by severe flooding, had stranded us at this remote location in Bangladesh, and we realized we could be in grave danger. We had no way to communicate with our co-workers or other Americans who could help us.

We were going to Dhaka to take our son David to the airport to return to college in the US. We also planned to meet a short-term medical intern and his family to escort them back to Memorial Christian Hospital. David, Tense, and I were traveling with two Bangladeshi nationals who spoke English and had been incredibly helpful. What usually would have been a routine trip to the city had turned into a life-threatening situation. Our bus had to stop because of deep flood waters from the torrential rains descending on Bangladesh. We were making a last-ditch effort to catch the mail train to Feni, where the higher roads might provide safer travel options.

To our surprise, the porter with our luggage led us toward the locomotive. There, he began handing our suitcases to someone in the cab. He indicated that we should climb the ladder to the cab. Wearing our bright orange ponchos, we managed to climb up the tall, slippery ladder attached to the side of the cab, pulling and pushing each other. We reached the top and stepped into the cab. We were surprised to find that there were other passengers in the cab with the engineer. About a dozen of us and our luggage were crammed into that tiny space. I squeezed into the corner beside a side window and straddled a suitcase. Through the three-foot-square window in the back of the cab, we could see hundreds of other passengers clutching the sides and top of the "furry" train. Through the small front cab windows, we could see the tracks ahead leading to the river.

Finally, the engineer grabbed the whistle rope above his head and gave a sharp pull, producing a shrill whistle. He pushed the throttle to start the train moving forward, and it crept toward the swollen river. As we continued at a snail's pace, an uneasy silence reigned in the cab, where we stood anxiously watching the soggy scenery slide by. Suddenly, the train stopped with no station in sight, and we all stared in shock at the flooded river ahead, which had risen high above the banks. Muddy water churned and swirled around floating trees and other debris the river had swallowed on its journey. From my vantage point behind the engineer, I could see through the front locomotive window a man up ahead waving a red flag at the beginning of what was supposed to be a railroad bridge now submerged under the swirling water.

The engineer climbed down the ladder on the side of the locomotive and slogged through deep puddles to talk with the flagman. We watched them through the narrow window at the side of the cab. The two men looked at the raging torrent while gesturing and talking, and then the man holding the red flag shrugged his shoulders and looked down. The bridge across the river was invisible. We hoped the steel girders supporting the bridge remained intact and supported by the brick pylon in the center. The location of the rail was marked only by a slight ripple in the raging waters. We had no assurance that the whole bridge was still there or that it was strong enough to support the weight of the heavily loaded train.

The engineer waded back to the locomotive and scrambled back up into the cab. He gripped the throttle, pushing it forward to start the train in motion. Once more, the man waved the red flag back and forth, alerting the engineer. Again, the engineer pulled back the throttle to stop the train and climbed down to talk with the flagman. Finally, the flagman turned his palms upward and shrugged his shoulders helplessly.

The engineer climbed up into the cab again, where he sat surveying the situation. We watched, barely breathing. Then he made his decision. Releasing the brake and moving the throttle forward a little, he eased the locomotive onto the bridge. The train lumbered forward and crawled slowly onto the bridge. The bridge was only about 100 feet long, but it seemed like it was taking an eternity to cross it. There was silence in the cab as every person held his breath and thought how quickly that heavy locomotive would sink if the bridge collapsed.

"This mighty engine has great power to pull this huge load," Tense thought, "but our God has far greater power, and He is in control."

As David studied the small window at the rear of the cab, he wondered how he would get his parents out that window when the train plunged into the water.

I looked back through that window and saw the silent passengers hanging out the doors and windows and clinging all over the outside of the train, fearfully looking down at the raging torrent. Then, I looked at my wife and son, all of us like prisoners in that cab. I began to think over my life, remembering how God had revealed His extraordinary plan for my wife and me, prepared us both for the work we had been doing here in Bangladesh, provided everything we needed to serve Him, and protected us thus far.

I wondered if this was to be the end of our time in Bangladesh and on Earth.

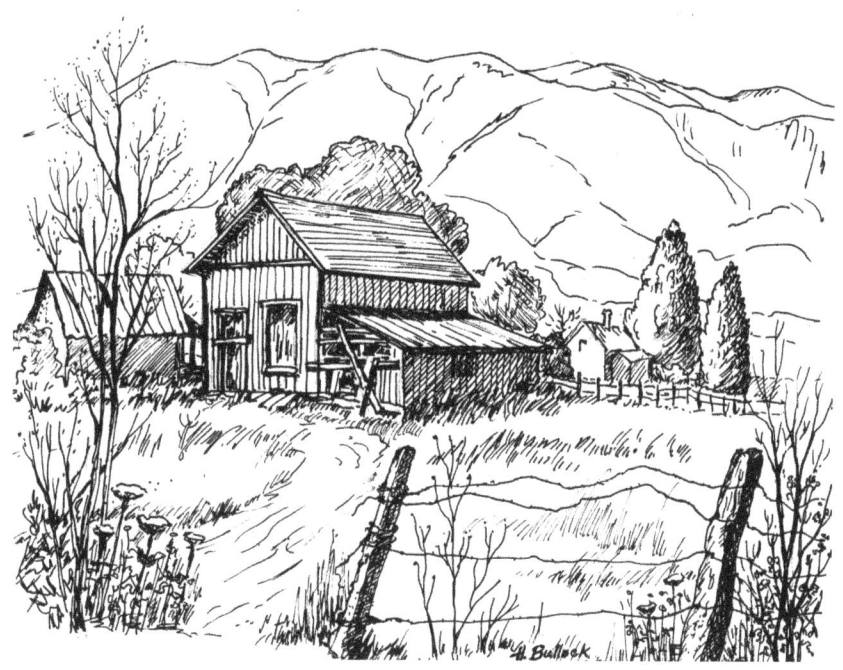

CHAPTER 2

Beginnings

God Had a Plan for a Boy

God had a plan for a boy to be born in Montana in 1927, the second child of Lynnie and Fred Bullock. Their first child, Freddie, died of pneumonia at age four. The doctor advised Lynnie not to have any more children because of complications with Freddie's birth, but she did not want to remain childless. So, ignoring the doctor's advice, she gave birth to me about two years after Freddie died.

We soon moved to Lewistown, Montana. Those were the years of the Great Depression, and we were poor. Money was scarce for everyone, and there were few frills. We had a garden, and my mother did a lot of canning. We had rutabagas, potatoes, and onions stored in the cellar. At Christmas, I would get an orange in my stocking—a real treat.

Next, we moved to Bozeman and then Helena, Montana, as my father changed jobs. He had a degree in agronomy from Montana State College in Bozeman and went on to work in various wheat-related jobs. He eventually became Montana's chief grain inspector. I got used to moving and changing schools and had no problem making new friends each time.

My mother graduated from college with a degree in home economics and worked as a teacher in a one-room schoolhouse near her father's sheep ranch. Many of her students were from Norwegian families who helped on the ranch during sheep-shearing and docking. Mother was a meticulous housekeeper and taught me manners and discipline. At her insistence, I took nine years of piano lessons and learned to play classical music. She also made sure I learned to be self-sufficient by teaching me how to cook and bake.

When I was a child, my family attended a Presbyterian church where my father was a deacon. My parents took me to Sunday school now and then, where I heard Bible stories but never really could put it all together. Our church attendance was sporadic, and I lived my adolescent years with little or no spiritual emphasis. God was not often mentioned in our daily routine, nor do I remember hearing the good news about salvation. I did know the name of Jesus Christ, even though I was not exactly sure who He was, and later, I wondered why people seemed to worship Him rather than God.

My father owned a 12-gauge Browning pump-action shotgun, which he used for hunting wildfowl. I can still remember the first time I ever shot that gun. He had me stand on a stump about two feet high; then he loaded and cocked the gun and had me hold it and pull the trigger. It knocked me off the stump, and I was extremely impressed! Later, I learned to shoot high-flying geese and ducks with the gun. My father gave me a single-shot .22 rifle. I was disappointed that it was not a multi-shot gun with a magazine, but he told me that bullets were not cheap, and I had to make sure each shot counted. He told me that God's creatures, such as songbirds, were not meant for targets and that I should shoot only what I planned to eat. I had no idea that learning to shoot a gun would one day save the life of one of my teammates on the other side of the world.

My mother's parents lived on a 160-acre ranch high in the Crazy Mountains above Big Timber, Montana, where they raised sheep and had a large garden. I enjoyed visiting my grandparents on the ranch despite the primitive conditions of no electricity or running water. Grandpa was a carpenter and built all the buildings on the ranch with his hand tools. I loved to spend time in Grandpa's workshop, examining and playing with his tools. He had a large grinding wheel, which I loved to pedal and spin. The ranch was a fascinating place for me, and each time we visited it, I learned many things about tools, animals, and gardening. All this was part of my training for eventual service in a primitive situation.

Move to San Luis Obispo

My father had been in the Army in World War I and remained active in the Army Reserve and the National Guard. As World War II started, he was called back into active duty and was stationed in San Luis Obispo, California, where he was in the Finance Officers Training School at Camp San Luis Obispo. He eventually became a full colonel.

On December 7, 1941, we went on a family outing to gather mistletoe from oak trees for Christmas decorations. When we returned home, we learned that the Japanese had attacked the US Navy ships in Pearl Harbor. The US officially entered the conflict with Japan the next day. The war had suddenly come uncomfortably close. After the Pearl Harbor attack, Japanese submarines attacked several ships off the coast of California. The Civil Defense program required us to cover our windows every night to maintain black-out conditions. This was to prevent any lights that might silhouette our offshore ships, which could be in danger from enemy submarines.

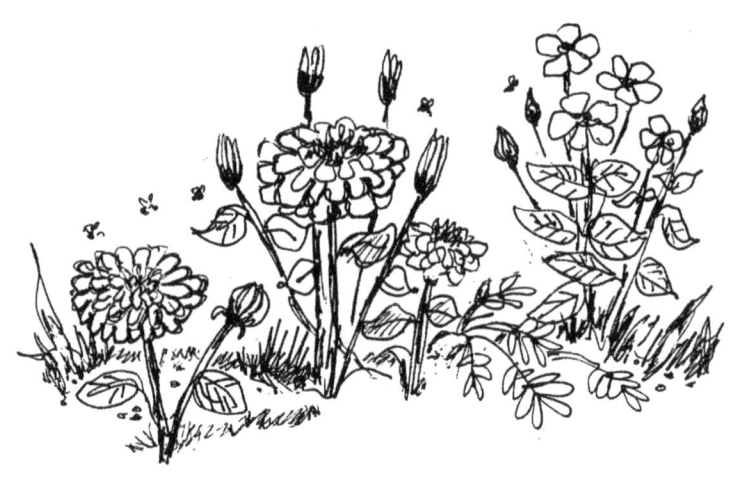

God Had a Plan for a Girl

God also had a plan for a girl to be born in Missouri to an osteopathic medical student, George Jennings, and his wife, Hortense, just ten days after I was born in 1927. She was named "Hortense" after her mother but nicknamed "Tense" to avoid confusion. When Tense was a little girl, she went to Sunday School and church in Kansas with her parents and grandmothers and heard many Bible stories.

Move to Medford

In 1936, after practicing medicine for a few years in a small general practice in Kansas, Tense's father moved his family out of the Dust Bowl to Medford, Oregon, where he could enjoy the fishing and hunting he loved. They became actively involved in a Presbyterian church and attended regularly. Tense loved to sing hymns. Her favorites were "In the Garden" and "When Morning Gilds the Skies."

Tense loved art. She especially enjoyed the coloring time when she started school and won a first-grade coloring contest. In fourth grade, Tense's favorite part of school was leisure arts, such as making baskets, wood puzzles, scrapbooks, and other projects. As a young teenager, Tense found a book at the library about how to make marionettes. Following the directions in the book, she cut out the fabric and sewed the bodies for the marionettes. In the garage, she found sticks she could use to make the cross-brace controls. At first, Tense and her sisters just played with the marionettes, but later, she made marionettes of Bible characters and used them to give plays for children's church and Christmas programs.

Tense loved her Sunday School class teacher, who was very sweet and took an interest in the girls. She let Tense help her tell the Christmas story using her marionettes. The year Tense was 14, her Sunday School teacher encouraged her class to attend a Christian camp. Some of Tense's school classmates were in her Sunday School class, so they went to the Christian camp together.

Each of the campers received a small booklet of Bible study lessons. The lesson that impacted Tense was from Luke 5:32 (King James Version), where Jesus said, "I came not to call the righteous, but sinners to repentance." In discussing it with the teacher, Tense understood she was a sinner and needed her sins forgiven. The teacher explained to Tense that Jesus died on the cross to pay the penalty for her sins. That day, Tense bowed her head in prayer and thanked Jesus for dying for her sins. She asked him to forgive her and to become her Savior.

On the last night of camp, they had a bonfire and gave testimonies. Tense threw a stick in the fire and shared how she had received Christ as her Savior and made a commitment to live for Jesus. Of course, she didn't know just what that would mean.

On December 7, 1941, Tense's family heard over the kitchen radio the news about the bombing of Pearl Harbor and America's entry into World War II. The War affected all of us in many ways. There was gas rationing, but Tense's dad had a "C" card because, as a doctor, he needed the gas to get to his office and the hospital. Children and adults were cautioned, "Loose talk can cost lives." We were told not to mention any news about the War in case we knew where troops would be sent or some matter that a spy might hear. We saved our tin cans, took off the lids, smashed them, and turned them in to recycle the metal for use in building military supplies.

Tense continued to develop her art skills in high school. Her art teacher gave the students projects in watercolor and design and taught them about famous artists. She was an ideal art teacher who gave Tense a lot of encouragement. Tense made float decorations for school parades, designed stage scenery for drama club performances, and painted signs for other school activities. At Christmas during the War, Tense's art class painted snowy Christmas scenes with poster paint on the large windows of the USO building downtown. She did the same at home on her family's large living room window. Tense loved art so much that she dreamed of studying art in college and someday having her own art studio.

Meeting Tense

Although we were born 1,000 miles apart when people did not move often or travel regularly, God had a plan to bring Tense and me together in Medford, Oregon, partially through world events. After the attack on Pearl Harbor, my father was transferred to Medford. There, he served as the Finance Officer for Camp White, where troops were trained for the War. I began attending Medford High School in tenth grade and was in classes with Tense. There were several new students at Medford High whose families were in the military, but Tense took special note of the new boy, "Johnny," with blonde hair and hazel eyes, whom she thought was "quite handsome." My family attended the same church as Tense's family, and our mothers were active in the ladies' group and helped with dinners and other events.

In our junior year of high school, Tense and I were both on a committee to make decorations for the Junior-Senior Prom. I liked to do carpentry and art, so I became her co-chairman. Tense was the most interesting girl I had ever met! We became friends and grew increasingly interested in each other. We loved to talk about practically everything. She had long, wavy, dark brown hair, a beautiful smile, and deep brown, twinkling eyes. Her bubbly personality swept me off my feet. Eventually, we started going together as boyfriend and girlfriend and spent many hours talking, riding bicycles, swimming, and going on picnics. I knew I had met the girl who would become my wife, the love of my life, my best friend, and my life-long traveling companion.

That year, I was nominated for the office of Student Body President. I wasn't particularly interested in that position, but Tense made some

"Elect John E. Bullock" signs, and, amazingly, I was elected. This, too, was part of God's plan to direct the course of my life.

I was finishing my junior year of high school when my father was transferred to Vancouver, Washington. We were going to move again. However, my parents knew I had a girlfriend whom I cared for deeply and that I had been elected student body president. They decided that it was important for me to spend my senior year at Medford High School, and so they arranged for me to board in the home of one of my friends. My father bought a 1929 Ford Model A coupe for my transportation because the place where I was to live was more than a mile from the school.

Tense and I dated for about a year before graduating from high school. By April of 1945, we had become so interested in each other that I asked her if she would marry me someday.

"Yes!" she cried without hesitation.

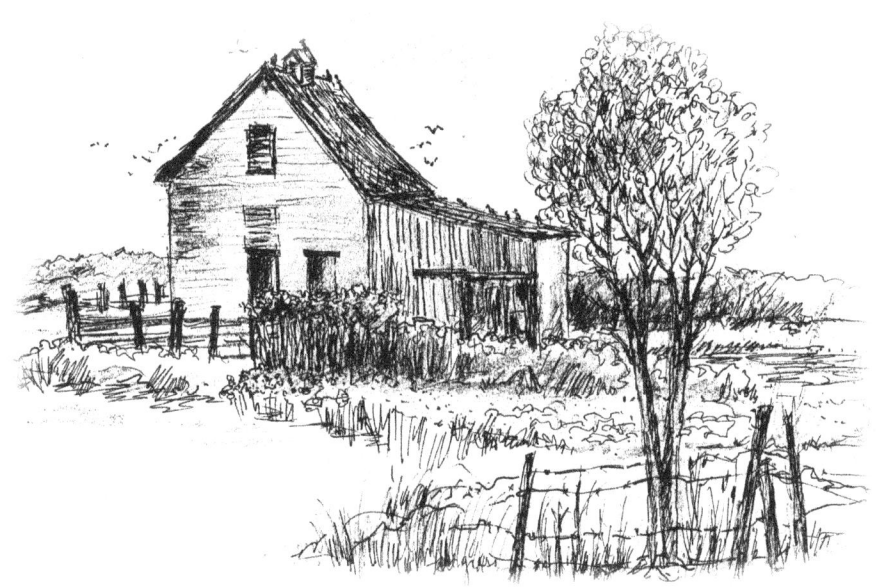

CHAPTER 3

Decisions

The Navy

World War II continued, and while still in high school, I was recruited to join the Naval Reserve and signed up. Upon graduating from high school in 1945, I traveled to Vancouver to visit my parents and say goodbye before leaving for boot camp.

"Well, Son," my dad spoke as we said goodbye, "I have tried to teach you the difference between right and wrong. Now, it is up to you to decide what you will do." I remember him demonstrating honesty often, such as telling a clerk when he received too much change. "Honesty is like pregnancy," he told me. "Either you are, or you aren't. It is an absolute." I will never forget that illustration and the other things he taught me.

I was sent to the Electronic Technician Training School in Gulfport, Mississippi, and later to Corpus Christi, Texas. Many years later, I used the electronics training I learned in the Navy while working in the Audiovisual Department at Memorial Christian Hospital (MCH) in Bangladesh. This was just one of many examples of how God prepared me for a job he had for me to do in the future. While I was in the Navy, Tense went to the University of Oregon in Eugene, Oregon, and majored in art. She was a talented artist.

After I had been in the Navy for thirteen months, the war ended, and I received an honorable discharge. It had been a long thirteen months of separation for Tense and me, and it seemed more like thirteen years. However, in God's plan, those thirteen months in the Navy qualified me for three years of the GI Bill education benefits for veterans, which was especially important because my parents did not have the resources to send me to college.

College in Montana

After the war ended, my parents moved to Bozeman, Montana. I joined them to start my education at Montana State College because I qualified for resident tuition. Tense persuaded her parents to let her transfer to Montana State College so we could be near each other, and she continued to study art during her sophomore year.

When I entered college, the Veterans Administration (VA) required veterans to take a vocational interest and aptitude test to identify a career goal and choose the right educational program to reach that goal. I expressed my desire to become a medical doctor, but they advised me to pursue engineering because my test results suggested that engineering aligned better with my interests. I took this advice and enrolled in a combined five-year Mechanical and Chemical Engineering program.

Marriage

During my first year of college, my parents accepted employment with the VA in Seattle, Washington. This required them to move to Seattle, and I remained in Bozeman to finish my first year at Montana State College. I moved into a friend's basement and cooked meals for myself. I ate dinner at the fraternity house on Sundays and washed dishes to pay for my meals.

My parents bought a house in Seattle and established their residency in Washington, which would allow me to attend the University of Washington as a resident. I had planned to move there in the summer to live with them, but Tense and I decided that our summer break would be a good time for us to marry. My parents suggested we live with them in Seattle after our wedding to save money while I attended the University.

Our wedding was simple, as were most weddings during the post-war era. On June 28, 1947, we were married in Tense's parents' front yard in Medford, surrounded by our high school friends and families.

Change of Course–Engineering to Premed

Shortly after our wedding, Tense's father persuaded me to transfer from engineering to premed and become an osteopathic physician like him. He felt that there would be too many engineers after the war, and he thought I would have a better earning potential as a doctor than an engineer. He encouraged me to apply to the Kansas City College of Osteopathy and Surgery, where he had trained. I did not realize that osteopathic doctors had a different approach to medicine and that there was a strong separation between osteopathic medicine and allopathic medicine. But I respected Dr. Jennings and decided to accept his advice.

College in Seattle

We made our first home in the attic of my parents' house in Seattle. We built inexpensive furniture using creative ideas and made our attic home as comfortable as possible. Tense decided to put her college plans on hold and instead found a typist job in downtown Seattle to help pay bills. She rode the bus to work while I began my second year of college. We attended a Presbyterian Church after we were married.

Medical School in Kansas City

After completing my premed, I applied to the Kansas City College of Osteopathy and Surgery and was accepted. We took a Greyhound bus to Kansas City, where we moved into a basement apartment in the same building as other medical students. Coming from a more rural, western upbringing, it took time for us to adjust to living in a large midwestern city. Tense worked at various secretarial jobs to provide us with an income, and my parents were able to help with a modest sum. I concentrated on my studies during the school year, but in the summer, I worked as a door-to-door salesman selling hospital insurance. I also worked in a factory that made tank trucks. All that and my GI Bill got me through four years of medical school. Growing up during the Depression, Tense and I learned to live frugally and make the most of limited resources.

Our first daughter, Chrissa, was born in November 1951, during my last year of medical school. Tense stayed home to care for her and babysat to earn a little money.

Osteopathic Medicine

As I began medical school, I learned that doctors of osteopathic medicine (DOs) have a holistic approach to medicine. They treat the entire person rather than merely the symptoms of the disease. They also emphasize preventative health care and wellness.

The philosophy of osteopathic medicine was developed in 1874 by Andrew Taylor Still, MD, a doctor in rural Kansas. Dr. Still had become disillusioned with traditional medical practices and believed that many of the medicines and treatments of that day were dangerous to patients. One medical commentator has observed, "Some of the medicines commonly given to patients during this time were arsenic, castor oil, whiskey, and opium. In addition, unsanitary surgical practices often resulted in more deaths than cures."[2] In 1864, three of his children died from spinal meningitis. None of the medications in use at that time were sufficient to save the lives of his children.[3]

Full of grief after the death of his children, Dr. Still devoted his life to studying the human body to find better ways to treat illness than the current traditional practice of medicine.[4] "He was one of the first in his time to study the attributes of good health so that he could better understand disease."[5]

Dr. Still studied the teachings of Hippocrates, the "Father of Medicine," which helped him understand that the body functions as one unit, with each part working together. Dr. Still believed that the musculoskeletal system governed the nervous and circulatory systems and many body functions and was an essential factor in the health of the body. Through a comprehensive study of the anatomy of the human body, he "observed that abnormal blood and nerve supplies to the body (caused by some dysfunction or change in the musculoskeletal system) often were found in diseased or abnormal tissues or organs."[6] He was convinced that osteopathic manipulative treatment to massage the connective tissues, especially along the spine, would improve circulation and activate the body's healing forces "to cure and prevent disease and chronic pain."[7] The result was so effective that people flocked to him for this new treatment.

Dr. Still established the American School of Osteopathy in 1892 in Kirksville, Missouri, to train doctors in this new concept of osteopathic medicine.[8] Its graduates were given the Doctor of Osteopathy (DO) degree. At that time, the traditional school of medicine was allopathic medicine, and its graduates were granted a Doctor of Medicine (MD) degree. The allopathic school of medicine strongly resisted any changes in medical care and contested this new philosophy of medicine. MDs considered DOs to be inferior, substandard doctors and were forbidden to associate with them. DOs could not use the same hospitals as MDs in many states.

However, things slowly changed over time. "Since osteopathic medicine in the U.S. began more than a century ago, its principles and practitioners have become part of the medical mainstream." [9]

In November 2020, the American Osteopathic Association (AOA) and the American Medical Association (AMA) issued a joint statement in a press release.

> Misrepresentation of osteopathic medicine harms the credibility of the 121,000 osteopathic physicians who care for our nation's sick and injured. The American Osteopathic Association (AOA) and the American Medical Association (AMA) stand united in an effort to combat the mischaracterization of doctors of osteopathic medicine by media, celebrities and companies.
>
> Osteopathic physicians, also known as doctors of osteopathic medicine (DOs), are fully licensed physicians who practice in every specialty area. Doctors of medicine (MDs) and DOs have equivalent training and practice rights.
>
> DOs account for approximately 11% of all physicians in the United States. They are pediatricians, ob-gyns, internists, anesthesiologists, psychiatrists, oncologists, family medicine physicians, emergency medicine physicians, dermatologists, plastic surgeons, ophthalmologists, cardiothoracic surgeons, and more.

* * *

> Like MDs, DOs complete four years of education at accredited medical schools, which includes two years of clinical sciences followed by two years of clinical rotations. DOs and MDs pass comprehensive national licensing exams and then train side-by-side in residency and fellowship programs for three to eleven years, depending on specialty. Upon completion of their training, the only two types of fully licensed physicians, DOs and MDs, work side-by-side in equivalent roles in hospitals, clinics, laboratories, research facilities and more.
>
> DOs receive additional training in osteopathic manipulative medicine (OMM), which is the therapeutic application of manual techniques (i.e. stretching, gentle pressure and resistance) to diagnose, treat and prevent illness or injury. OMM can be used

to treat arthritis, stress injuries, sports injuries, headaches, and pain in areas such as the lower back, neck, shoulders, and knees. For some patients, it serves as an alternative to opioids or other pharmaceutical treatments.[10]

Today, many DOs and MDs work alongside each other in hospitals and clinics throughout the United States. "The majority of DOs are family-oriented primary care physicians. Many DOs practice in small towns and rural areas, where they often care for entire families and communities."[11]

Rural Medicine

I graduated from the Kansas City College of Osteopathy in May of 1952. I had plans to spend the next year as an intern at the Kansas City Osteopathic Hospital, but I would have to wait three months for the previous class to finish before beginning my program. At about that time, an osteopathic physician from Elmo, Missouri, came to the college to recruit a recent graduate to work for three months in his six-bed osteopathic hospital and clinic. I eagerly accepted this opportunity and worked with him until my internship could begin. He taught me much about rural osteopathic family practice and working in a small hospital. I learned more practical tips about practicing medicine during that busy summer than in the following year of my internship. That was another instance of God's provision and preparation for my future work in a small hospital in Bangladesh.

CHAPTER 4

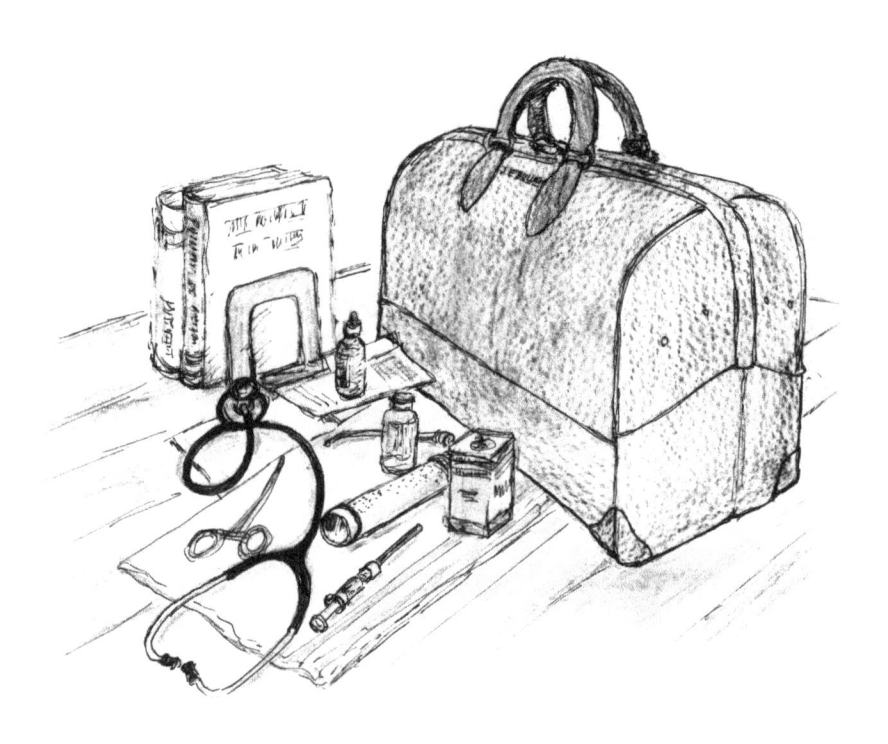

"Dr. Bullock"

Return to Medford

   Tense's father, Dr. Jennings, had invited me to return to Medford after my internship to join him in his practice. I accepted his offer, and Tense and I moved to Medford with baby Chrissa after graduation and internship. I began working with Dr. Jennings in his office on the fourth floor of a downtown building. In 1954, our first son, Peter, was born while we lived in Medford. At that time, my parents had moved to Medford for retirement. My father's health was deteriorating, and he had suffered a heart attack.

California Medical License

I also wanted to obtain a medical license in Washington and California to keep future career options open. Washington allowed reciprocity with Missouri, but I needed to take the California Osteopathic Medical Board examination to obtain a California osteopathic physician's license.

In July 1955, during my second year in Medford, I took the examination. In September 1955, I received notice that I had passed and was awarded a Physician's and Surgeon's Certificate by the Board of Osteopathic Examiners of the State of California, allowing me to practice osteopathic medicine in California. Although I did not plan to move to California then, knowing I had that option, if needed, was reassuring. I had no idea how important that certificate would become.

General practice as an osteopathic physician in Oregon at that time was a challenge for me since the American Medical Association ethics committee prevented MDs from associating with DOs. Since DOs could not use regular allopathic hospitals in Oregon, one osteopathic physician in Medford had converted an old house into a small hospital. That was where I could admit my patients in need of major surgery, but I had to guarantee the patient's hospital bill.

I stayed with Dr. Jennings for two years but did not feel like I was practicing as a fully-trained doctor. My practice was slow and seemed to be limited to chronic complaints, mostly manipulation of the spine. I trained as a general practice physician and wanted to start my own medical practice to apply my skills. While in Medford, I met an osteopathic general surgeon. He encouraged me to start a general practice in a small town near the hospital he used in Albany.

Scio – Rural General Practice

During my three-month experience at the small hospital and clinic in Missouri, I became familiar with rural general practice, which appealed to me more than city practice. I worked on improving my medical skills by taking continuing education courses at nearby medical colleges. Eventually, I relocated to Scio, Oregon, a small town with 250 people.

There, I established a general practice in an office on Main Street. I had a laboratory for limited lab work and a small operating room for minor surgeries. I used the Albany Osteopathic Hospital to admit patients, but it was eighteen miles away. Because of the distance, I had to purchase an X-ray machine for my office in Scio and take my own X-rays for my patients.

Our second daughter, Karen, was born in 1956 at the Albany Hospital. Our little family was growing. Tense stayed busy raising our three young children and participating in church activities, including helping with arts and crafts at Vacation Bible School.

As I worked with the general surgeon at the Albany Osteopathic Hospital, he taught me general and spinal anesthesia, which allowed me to practice what I had learned in one of the post-graduate courses I had recently completed. I received excellent training in primary skills that prepared me for the primitive situation I encountered years later in Bangladesh when I was the only doctor at Memorial Christian Hospital for months.

Milwaukie – Partnership

After I practiced for two years in Scio, the Albany hospital closed. So, the osteopathic general surgeon and I decided to become partners, and we opened a new osteopathic clinic in Milwaukie, Oregon. There, I could use the Portland Osteopathic Hospital. Our fourth child, David, was born at this hospital in 1959.

Tense and I had a house built in Milwaukie near the hospital in a neighborhood with other young families. We occasionally attended a Presbyterian church, but I got nothing from the sermons.

"I could better spend my time staying home and reading the Reader's Digest," I told Tense one Sunday after hearing another boring sermon.

During that time, our two oldest children were invited by a neighbor girl to attend a Vacation Bible School in a Baptist church in Milwaukie. They each heard and believed the gospel message of salvation.

CHAPTER 5

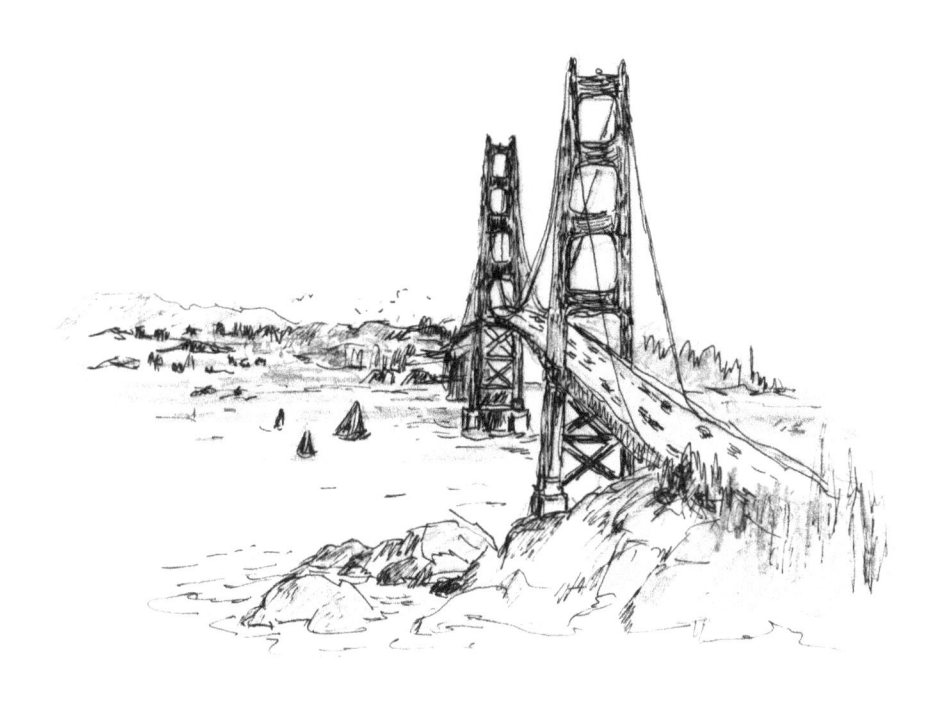

Pursuit of Orthopedic Training

My partner and I had a well-developed general practice in Milwaukee. However, after seven years of general practice, I still did not have the expertise to perform advanced procedures. I wanted to specialize, but deciding which specialty to pursue was difficult, as I was interested in everything. I considered orthopedics because I had some mechanical skills, which are required when working with skeletal structures, and I enjoyed working with tools. Although I knew getting orthopedic training in osteopathic medicine would be difficult, I decided to pursue this specialty.

Orthopedic Preceptorship in Oregon

About that time, an osteopathic orthopedic surgeon moved to Oregon and began using the Portland Osteopathic Hospital. I asked him to set up a preceptorship program for me in orthopedics. This method was like an apprenticeship and was one way of obtaining specialty training. He agreed to do this, and we applied for and received approval from the American Osteopathic Association. The preceptorship was to last for three years.

During the preceptorship, I realized I was only being taught what that doctor had been trained to do. I wanted to learn and practice other procedures with which he was not familiar. So, I realized I needed to pursue a different course to get more orthopedic training. At that time, only a few osteopathic hospitals had orthopedic residencies. I applied to several of them for orthopedic residency training but was not accepted. They told me they preferred to take recent graduates from their internship programs for residency training.

I tried to gain acceptance to formal residency programs in allopathic (MD) hospitals but was turned down because of my DO degree and the separation between MDs and DOs. It looked like the doors were closed for me to get the additional training I wanted. Frustrated by the limited options of continuing as a general practitioner or settling for a subpar preceptorship program, I contemplated leaving the medical profession altogether if I couldn't secure a suitable residency.

California Merger—DO to MD

Then, a remarkable thing happened that suddenly changed the course of my life. In 1961, the California Medical Association merged with the California Osteopathic Association. As part of this merger, the College of Osteopathic Physicians and Surgeons in Los Angeles was renamed the California College of Medicine (CCM) and became an MD-granting medical school. DOs with a California license could acquire an MD degree from the California College of Medicine by submitting their transcripts, attending a training class, and paying a small fee.[12] This merger opened the possibility of specialty training in regular allopathic

(MD) hospitals. I was eligible for this program because I had already taken and passed the examination for a California license to practice osteopathic medicine.

In 1962, I applied for the MD degree from the California College of Medicine in hopes that it might open the doors for me to get further training in a large allopathic (MD) hospital residency program. That decision was risky because I knew the American Osteopathic Association (AOA) would reject my membership if I applied for the MD degree. Little did I realize the magnitude of that pivotal decision and its effect on my future ability to practice medicine in Bangladesh.

As I expected, the AOA did not approve of my decision to apply for the MD degree, so my membership was terminated. It was a difficult decision, but I was determined to stick with it to get the orthopedic training I wanted.

French Hospital—General Surgical Training

I had learned that orthopedic residencies required one preliminary year of general surgery, so I applied for a one-year general surgery residency at several hospitals in San Francisco. Upon acceptance from French Hospital, I moved my family from Oregon to the San Francisco Bay Area. General surgery residency was an interesting experience. Much of my time was spent observing doctors in surgery and assisting them in the operating room. I learned operating room protocol and surgery skills I would need in my future overseas assignment. The hardest part about my time at French Hospital was going down to the level of a resident when I had been in a decision-making status as a doctor in my own practice for many years. It was like going back to junior high school after being in college.

Application for MD Residency

That year, I applied for an orthopedic residency in various allopathic (MD) training programs in California. However, many California MDs initially hesitated to accept the new merger or to invite a former

DO into their program. The Chief of the Orthopedic Department at the University of California in San Francisco asked me whether the American Board of Orthopedic Surgery would allow me to take the certifying examination upon completion of an orthopedic residency. I had to answer that I did not know. "If they won't let you get certified, then we will not give you the training," he said. Again, it looked like the door was closed.

Orthopedic Residency—San Francisco

Realizing that I might not be able to get into an orthopedic residency, I applied to various medical groups for employment as a general practitioner. I was accepted at one group in northern California and had a contract on my desk ready to sign when the phone rang. It was Dr. S.H., the head orthopedic doctor at St. Joseph's Hospital in San Francisco. That hospital was one of the seven hospitals that were part of The San Francisco Combined Program for Orthopedic Residency Training, headquartered at St. Mary's Hospital in San Francisco.

"Dr. Bullock," he said. "We are trying to figure out this merger. We don't quite know how to deal with doctors like you, since we have limited knowledge about your training. Would you be willing to come for six months on probation, so we can evaluate you before deciding to let you come on as a full-term resident?"

I immediately told him I would be happy to accept his offer. Thrilled at this new opportunity, I started my residency at St. Joseph's Hospital in San Francisco and continued rotating through five other hospitals in the San Francisco Combined Program. I worked with several dozen orthopedic surgeons who had trained in multiple disciplines. Finally, I was getting the broad range of orthopedic training I wanted.

Six months passed without Dr. S.H. questioning my qualifications, and I slid into the regular residency program. In 1964, I researched and wrote "Arthrography of the Adult Hip," which was entered into a resident training contest and was accepted for presentation at the Western Orthopedic Association (WOA) meeting in Las Vegas. I received a Resident Award from the WOA for this research, and Tense and I were treated as special guests and provided lodging in a nice hotel.

Tense Teaches Art Classes

While I worked as a general practice doctor in Oregon, Tense was busy raising our four children and managing our home. She had started a fine arts correspondence course to complete her art training.

When we moved to San Francisco, we placed David in a co-op nursery school, where each mother was required to help in class one day a week and attend an evening education class. Tense volunteered to paint murals and decorative designs on the school walls and trim. One evening a week, she taught an oil painting class to some of the preschoolers' mothers. One of the mothers suggested Tense could teach adult education art classes through the school district.

With great interest in this new job opportunity to teach art, Tense contacted the school district office and applied for her teaching credential. Upon receiving a Lifetime Teaching Credential to teach watercolor and oil painting, she taught an evening adult education art class at the local high school. Tense continued to teach adult education art classes during my residency training.

CHAPTER 6

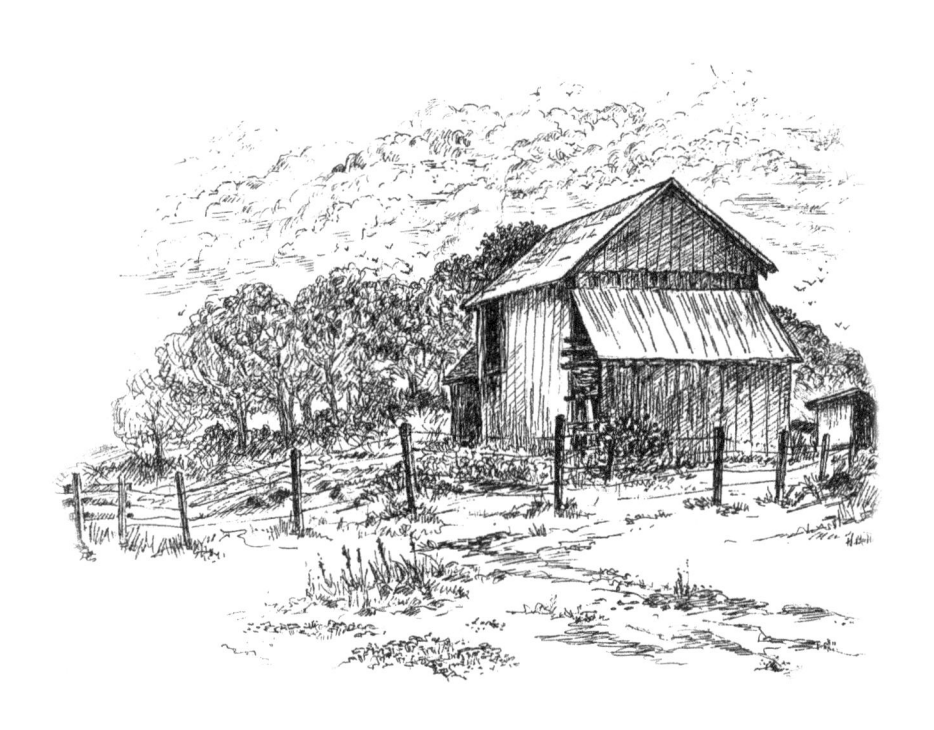

An Intriguing Challenge

Move to Walnut Creek

The area where we lived in San Francisco was foggy and chilly, so we decided to move out of the city and across the bay to warm and sunny Walnut Creek. We purchased an old farmhouse at a reasonable price, which was a much better place for our family to live while I continued my residency training. Our children enjoyed living in a rural neighborhood with empty fields for exploring, a creek where they could wade and fish, and a swim club a few blocks from our house. My commute was long and tiresome, but the benefit to my family was worth it. I continued with my rotations through the various hospitals in the program and was often gone for several days each week. During this time, Tense taught daytime and evening adult education art classes at several locations in the Walnut Creek area.

The Real Reason

Unknown to us, there was another important reason we made that move. I had only occasionally attended church when we were living in San Francisco, but after our move, we decided to attend a small Swedish Baptist Church in Walnut Creek. There, I received an intriguing challenge. It was the beginning of a major change in my life.

One Sunday, the pastor said from the pulpit, "This morning, there are many professional people sitting in this congregation—doctors, lawyers, teachers, engineers, scientists. You have studied thick textbooks and memorized great portions of them to get where you are today. But my challenge to you is this: Have you given the same diligent study to the most important book of all, the Holy Bible, in the same exhaustive way you have studied your professional textbooks?"

Wow! It was as if he had spoken directly to me! I knew little about the Bible and what it taught. I had never read the entire Bible. Sitting there, I resolved to read and study the Bible, as the pastor had suggested. I drove my family to a peaceful location on a rural road and parked the car. I informed them about my choice to read and learn from the Bible and expressed my desire to attend church regularly.

Returning home, I picked up the King James Version of the Bible and tried to speed-read it as I had learned to read my textbooks in medical school. However, I struggled to speed-read the King James Version. I looked at several versions in modern language and found them easier to understand. Finally, I picked up one called *The New Testament in Modern English*, translated by J. B. Philips.[13] At last, here was a version that I could speed read. During my San Francisco-based residency, I spent part of each week away from home at my rotation hospital in Sacramento. I began reading and studying the Philips translation during my nights away from home.

Years earlier, I had heard a minister say from the pulpit that "the Bible was never intended to be taken literally. It is an allegory, a collection of fables or stories made up to illustrate fundamental principles." Over the next few weeks, I found some verses that contradicted that line of thinking. They changed my life. As I read in the book of 2 Peter, I found these remarkable statements:

> We were not following a cleverly written-up story when we told you about the power and coming of our Lord Jesus Christ—we actually saw his majesty with our own eyes. He received honor and glory from God the Father himself when that voice said to him, out of the sublime glory of Heaven, 'This is my beloved Son, in whom I am well pleased.' We actually heard that voice speaking from Heaven while we were with him on the sacred mountain. The word of prophecy was fulfilled in our hearing! You should give that word your closest attention, for it shines like a lamp amidst all the dirt and darkness of the world, until the day dawns, and the morning star rises in your hearts. (2 Peter 1:16-19, J.B. Phillips Translation, 1963).[14]

Here was someone named Peter saying he had been an eyewitness to a particular event. Certainly, these things were neither fables nor allegorical portrayals. According to the testimony of eyewitnesses, they were the truth. Turning back a few pages to Chapter One of the Book of John, I found another eyewitness account from a man named John.

> At the beginning God expressed himself. That personal expression, that word, was with God, and was God, and he existed with God from the beginning. All creation took place through him, and none took place without him. In him appeared life and this life was the light of mankind. The light still shines in the darkness, and the darkness has never put it out. (John 1:1-5).[15]

I recalled reading a few days earlier in Acts chapter four about Peter and John, whom Jewish leaders arrested for preaching and teaching about Jesus Christ. They were told that they must stop talking and teaching about Jesus.

> So they called them in and ordered them bluntly not to speak or teach a single further word about the name of Jesus. But Peter and

John gave them this reply: "Whether it is right in the eyes of God for us to listen to what you say rather than to what he says, you must decide; for we cannot help speaking about what we have actually seen and heard!" (Acts 4:18-20).[16]

These men had personally witnessed a miraculous event, and no one could make them stop talking about it, even at the risk of their own lives. They knew how important it was to know about this event and this person, Jesus Christ.

At that moment, I realized that the Bible is the truth. I suddenly wanted to know more about its truth and resolved to begin studying it diligently. I could hardly wait to get home and share with Tense how God had revealed to me that the Bible is true!

CHAPTER 7

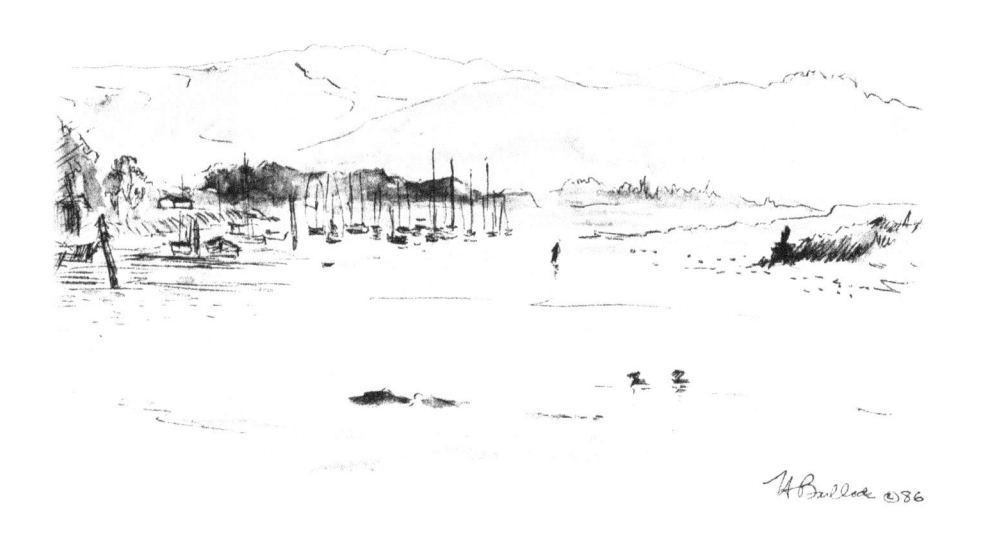

The Brass Ring

Application to the ABOS

In preparation for completing my orthopedic residency program and deciding where to practice, I applied to the American Board of Orthopedic Surgery (ABOS) for permission to take the certifying exam. "We do not know enough about doctors like you to decide," they replied. "We are studying the problem and will let you know. In the meantime, we advise you to go into practice with a group."

I discussed the advice of the ABOS with Dr. S.H., and he gave me several suggestions for orthopedic practices he knew about that might interest me. He then invited me to join him in his practice in San Francisco. I did not want to work and live in San Francisco, so I applied to the San Luis Medical Clinic, a multi-specialty medical group in San Luis Obispo, California, where my family had lived for one year while my father was in the Finance Officers Training School. San Luis Obispo was a small college town near the coast. Tense and I thought it would be a wonderful area to raise our family.

San Luis Medical Clinic

I was thrilled to receive the news that I was accepted into the San Luis Medical Clinic. My family and I started planning and imagining our new life in the charming town of San Luis Obispo and the nearby seaside town of Morro Bay. For a long time, I had been dreaming of owning a boat and exploring the beautiful California coast with my family. I couldn't wait to go fishing and snorkeling with them. We moved our family to San Luis Obispo in November 1966. I returned to Sacramento to complete my residency before officially starting at the San Luis Medical Clinic in January 1967.

Tense's Art Studio

After I had completed my orthopedic training and began working at the Clinic, Tense could finally pursue her ambition of having her own art studio. She joined the San Luis Obispo Art Association and had a one-person show of her art. She became friends with another artist in the Association. They shared an art studio located above the shops in downtown San Luis Obispo. They often enjoyed painting in various outdoor locations.

Tense later rented a studio and small gallery downtown, where she taught oil painting and watercolor classes. Her dream had become a reality. This allowed Tense to develop her ability as a teacher, giving her insight into how to work with different age groups. She enjoyed teaching and helping others develop their skills.

Board Certified

Three years after the end of my orthopedic residency, I received a letter from the American Board of Orthopedic Surgery informing me that I would finally be allowed to take the certification examination. I was concerned that I had forgotten many details in the three years I had been out of my residency. I discussed this with my colleagues, who agreed to let me take mornings off to study. After two months of reviewing, I went to Chicago to take the exam in January 1970.

Three months later, I received a letter stating that I had passed the examination and was now a Diplomate of the American Board of Orthopedic Surgery. I was ecstatic! Subsequently, I was admitted to the American Academy of Orthopedic Surgeons and the Western Orthopedic Association in 1970. I had finally achieved my goal of becoming a Board-Certified Orthopedic Surgeon.

During our childhood years, carousels were popular rides at county fairs. Many of them had a brass ring hanging on a peg at one end of a wooden arm that was suspended above the riders, barely out of reach. As the carousel circled round and round, riders would reach out to attempt to grab the ring. If a person could catch hold of that brass ring, he or she would be rewarded with a prize. Reaching for the ring was risky and required leaning out with the possibility of falling. It required strong motivation.

After twenty-five years of hard work, I felt like I had finally caught that brass ring.

CHAPTER 8

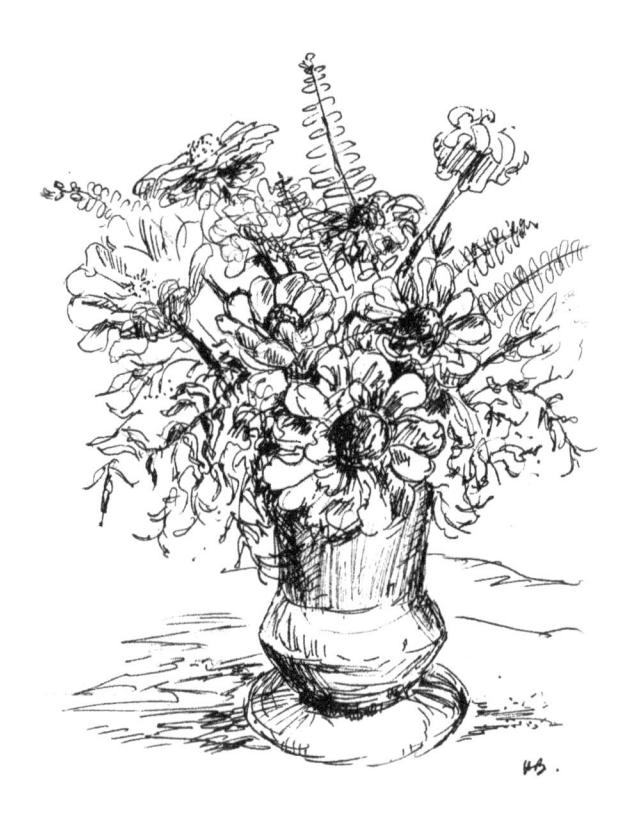

Salvation and Surrender

Salvation

When we moved to the beautiful little town of San Luis Obispo, California, we thought we finally had found our permanent home and could begin living our dream. We first lived in two rental houses before purchasing a comfortable home in a nicer neighborhood where other doctors resided. Soon, our family began attending Calvary Baptist Church, which was close to our neighborhood. One morning, the pastor preached a message on salvation from a series of verses called the "Romans Road" found in the Epistle to the Romans.

> As it is written: "There is none righteous, no, not one; (Romans 3:10, New King James Version).
>
> For all have sinned and fall short of the glory of God (Romans 3:23).
>
> But God demonstrates His own love to us, in that while we were still sinners, Christ died for us. (Romans 5:8).
>
> For the wages of sin is death, but the gift of God is eternal life in Christ Jesus our Lord. (Romans 6:23).
>
> That if you confess with your mouth the Lord Jesus and believe in your heart that God has raised Him from the dead, you will be saved. For with the heart one believes unto righteousness, and with the mouth confession is made unto salvation. For "whoever calls on the name of the LORD shall be saved." (Romans 10:9-10, 13).

This was the first time I could remember hearing that I was estranged from God because of my sin, that Jesus Christ had taken the penalty for my sin on himself, and that He had died on the cross in my place. Sitting in the church pew that day, I prayed silently, confessing my sin to God. I told Him that I believed Jesus had paid the penalty for my sin, and I wanted to accept His gift of salvation. By faith, I received Christ as my Savior that day.

Surgery for Tense

Not long after buying our new house, Tense began to have medical problems. She eventually found herself in the hospital, facing serious surgery. She wondered if she would leave the hospital alive. Lying there, she had time to think about her life in the light of eternity. "If I died," she thought, "would I be ashamed to face God? Would the things I had done here on earth be temporary and worthless like wood, hay, and straw, as the Bible describes in I Corinthians 3:11-14? Or would they have an eternal significance?"

> For no other foundation can anyone lay than that which is laid, which is Jesus Christ. Now if anyone builds on this foundation with gold, silver, precious stones, wood, hay, straw, each one's work will become clear; for the Day will declare it, because it will be revealed by fire; and the fire will test each one's work, of what sort it is. If anyone's work which he has built on it endures, he will receive a reward. (I Cor. 3:11-14).

"Yes," she thought, "they probably would not be worth eternal value. I want my life to count for eternal things."

During her recovery, Tense began to read and study the Bible diligently. She studied books about Christian growth and living and attended a Bible study on the Book of Romans. Tense began to get involved with our church's active women's ministry group and used her art skills to help with our college outreach. The women's group asked her to contact Marjorie Beals and inquire how our group could assist with their needs in East Pakistan. Mel and Marjorie Beals, who served with The Association of Baptists for World Evangelism (ABWE), had recently visited our church to report about their work in East Pakistan. Marjorie shared with Tense some ways we could help, and we gladly gathered men's clothing and household goods for the Beals to take to East Pakistan for relief work. Tense and Marjorie became friends and began writing letters to each other. Tense and I had started teaching a junior high class at our church on Sunday nights. We had our students write letters to the Beals to learn more about their work in East Pakistan. We also started receiving *The Message* magazine produced by ABWE, eagerly reading about their global ministry activities.

Surrender and Dedication

One Sunday, after Tense recovered from surgery, she sat in the evening church service and listened as the pastor began to preach from Romans chapter twelve.

> I beseech you therefore, brethren, by the mercies of God, that you present your bodies a living sacrifice, holy, acceptable to God, which is your reasonable service.

And do not be conformed to this world, but be transformed by the renewing of your mind, that you may prove what is that good and acceptable and perfect will of God. (Rom. 12:1-2).

As she listened to this challenge from the scripture, Tense reflected on her recent hospital experience and how it had changed her thinking about her activities and goals. That night, Tense decided to fully surrender her life to God so that her focus would be on what truly matters for eternity. She told God she would serve Him wherever He wanted her to go.

CHAPTER 9

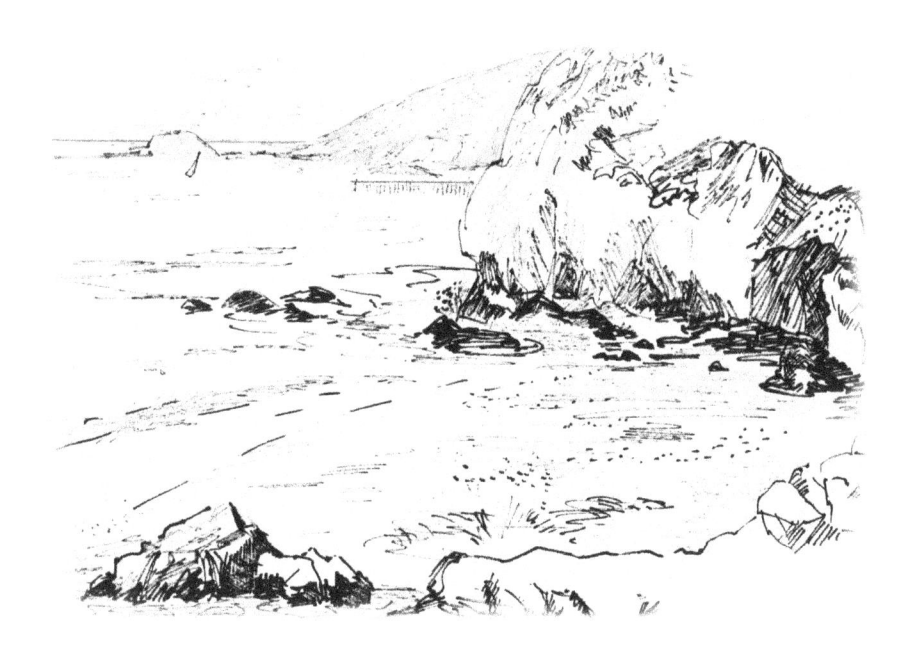

Change of Command, Change of Course

Trip to Boston

In November 1970, Tense and I visited Boston for an orthopedic meeting. We had planned to stay a few days longer after the meeting for a short vacation, but we received an urgent phone call informing us that a critical situation had developed. We canceled the rest of our trip and started home immediately.

As we walked up the ramp to board the plane, I felt anxious about the situation and did not know what to do. Tense slipped into my hand a small booklet that she just happened to have in her purse. It was called *Christian at Ease!*[17] I opened the booklet and read:

> Be careful for nothing, but in everything by prayer and supplication, with thanksgiving, let your requests be made known unto God. And the peace of God, which passeth all understanding, shall keep your hearts and minds through Christ Jesus (Phil. 4:6-7, King James Version).

"In everything?" I thought, "Even in something like this?" Everything means exactly that, even something like this. We settled into our seats and then prayed together on the plane. By the time we arrived back home, I felt that "peace of God which passeth all understanding" and was able to function smoothly through the problem at hand. Later, as I reflected on these events, I was amazed that Tense had that particular booklet in her purse at that precise time.

My Divine Appointment

The timing of this early return was critical. I had an important divine appointment—I just didn't know about it. I did not know that an evangelist, Dr. Phil Shuler, had been scheduled to have a week of meetings at our church, starting with the Sunday services. Usually, I could not attend mid-week services because of my medical responsibilities with my hospital patients. However, because of our early return, I still had a week of vacation. It seemed that we had been directed to return from our vacation early so that we might attend the week of meetings. Those meetings were about to change the course of our lives. Dr. Shuler got my attention quickly when he announced he would present three questions during the week and explain the answers as the week progressed.

"What is life?" Dr. Shuler asked. This first question immediately caught my attention. He explained that we are now experiencing a phenomenon that we have chosen to call "life." But what is it? He said that life is present in other forms, such as trees and plants, insects, birds, animals, and fish, but not inanimate things like rocks and metal. That caused me to think deeply about this until the next meeting.

"**Why are we alive?**" Dr. Shuler asked the second question at the next meeting, as I was still pondering how to answer his first question. "Are we like leaves on the trees that appear every year only to drop off and die in the fall, or are we like the grass and flowers that grow, bloom, and die? Or is there a purpose for our lives?" he continued, giving me more things to ponder.

Near the end of the week, Dr. Shuler asked the third question, which was the most important. **"When you are no longer alive,"** he asked, **"will it have made any *eternal* difference that you lived? Or will you simply leave this world?"** He pointed out that we could accumulate great wealth, prestige, or notoriety during our lifetime, but these things have no eternal value. Only things that are done for God will have eternal value.

During that week, Dr. Shuler preached from chapter two of Ephesians. Ephesians 2:1-3 accurately described my life before I trusted Christ for my salvation. I was spiritually dead because of my sin and had been living for my selfish desires and ambitions.

> And you He made alive, who were dead in trespasses and sins, in which you once walked according to the course of this world, according to the prince of the power of the air, the spirit who now works in the sons of disobedience, among whom also we all once conducted ourselves in the lusts of our flesh, fulfilling the desires of the flesh and of the mind, and were by nature children of wrath, just as the others. (Eph. 2:1-3, New King James Version).

Dr. Shuler explained that we deserve neither God's love nor His forgiveness, yet he loves us in spite of our sins. When, by faith, I believed in Jesus' sacrifice for me and humbly accepted his salvation, that was a gift I could never have earned by any good works.

> But God, who is rich in mercy, because of His great love with which He loved us, even when we were dead in trespasses, made us alive together with Christ (by grace you have been saved), . . . For by grace you have been saved through faith, and that not of yourselves; it is the gift of God, not of works, lest anyone should boast. (Eph. 2:4-5,8-9).

Dr. Shuler then explained that verse ten teaches us that once a person is made alive in Christ, he is to be full of good works for God. I had been dimly aware of God's presence since I trusted Christ as my Savior, but He was not in my every thought and action. I was still focused on my own goals and ambitions. As Dr. Shuler expounded on verse ten, he explained that God had a plan for our lives even before we were born. He said God has chosen to use people as His tools to carry out His plan. He prepares us to do this work by equipping us with spiritual gifts. Through the power of His Holy Spirit in us, God directs and guides our service for Him.

> For we are His workmanship, created in Christ Jesus for good works, which God prepared beforehand that we should walk in them. (Eph. 2:10).

Dr. Shuler gave an example of the potter and the clay to explain how God chooses and prepares a person to work for Him. I listened attentively as he described how the potter selects a piece of clay and adds just enough water to make it the right consistency that will allow it to be molded into a useful vessel. It can't be too hot or too cold. Everything must be just right for the potter to be able to shape the clay, or it will be useless and thrown into the fragment pile. As the potter begins to mold and shape the clay with his hands, he determines how it will be shaped for his desired purpose. The clay does nothing to shape itself or choose its final form or purpose. The potter is the one who shapes the clay for the purpose he has chosen.

> But now, O Lord, You are our Father; We are the clay, and You our potter; And all we are the work of Your hand. (Isaiah 64:8).

He further explained that God may not always let us know what that plan is until we are willing to follow Him. When, where, what, and how He wanted to use me were up to Him. Dr. Shuler gave a familiar example. When one person asks another, "Will you do me a favor?" the second person usually responds with a question: "What is it? Tell me what you want me to do, and I will decide if I will do it or not." That is not what God wants to hear when He asks us if we are willing to follow His plan. He wants to hear, "Yes, God, whatever you tell me to do, I will do to the best of my ability—no strings attached."

I thought about my life and considered that I was reasonably happy with my situation. After many years of hard work, I finally obtained certification from the American Board of Orthopedic Surgery. I was a partner in a prestigious multiple-specialty medical clinic in San Luis Obispo. I had a wonderful wife and four children. We lived in a comfortable home with a swimming pool. My 24-foot ocean-going fishing boat was moored thirteen miles to the west in Morro Bay. My wife had finally achieved her dream of becoming a professional artist and art teacher and had her own art studio and gallery in downtown San Luis Obispo. Everything seemed on track for a pleasant, purposeful life. I was like the psalmist, David, who said in Psalm 30:6, "Now in my prosperity I said, 'I shall never be moved.'" I had an attitude of self-sufficiency.

But complications were developing in my life for which I had no solutions. I was facing professional problems at the clinic and hospital, and it was becoming difficult to make correct decisions regarding these problems. I was like a boat in shallow waters, frequently scraping the rocky bottom, and I was ready for help and guidance in my life.

Dr. Shuler pointed out that if I asked God to take control of my life and use me according to His purposes, He had promised He would guide me to make the correct choices to handle the situations I faced. No longer living for my selfish desires and ambitions, my life's work would have eternal significance.

> Therefore submit to God. Resist the devil and he will flee from you. Draw near to God and He will draw near to you. (James 4:7-8a).

At the end of the service, Dr. Shuler invited anyone willing to let God have control of his or her life to respond by standing up and walking down the church aisle to the front to signify that he or she had made that decision.

In the Navy, we had an effective communication method. First, the shrill "too-wee" sound of the Boatswain's whistle penetrated all other sounds and caught our attention. Then came the harsh command, "NOW HEAR THIS!" We snapped to attention and listened intently to the announcement that followed because it might change our course of action. It might be a mundane announcement such as "Smoking lamp is on (or off)," or it could be a crucial message like "CHANGE OF COMMAND, CHANGE OF COURSE!" which required immediate action on our part.

As Dr. Shuler spoke, I felt like I was hearing the message "CHANGE OF COMMAND, CHANGE OF COURSE!" I was sitting near the aisle in the center of the church. It seemed as though invisible hands caused me to leap out of my seat and propelled me down that aisle to the front of the church.

In the counseling room, I tearfully asked God to take control of my life and use me as His tool. I told Him I was ready to turn my life over to His direction and live according to His plan, whatever that might be. I admitted that I had not done well in managing the affairs of my life—not by His standards. There had been many failures. I realized that God had been working in my life in many ways, just as the potter shapes the clay, preparing me for that day. I told Him I would leave my medical work and get other training if He chose. However, I was certain I was giving God control of my life and was willing to do whatever He told me to do.

I had no idea what was going to happen next. But what did happen was totally beyond my imagination. I had no idea I would end up moving to the other side of the planet to a world vastly different from the one I was familiar with and that I would face challenges beyond description.

CHAPTER 10

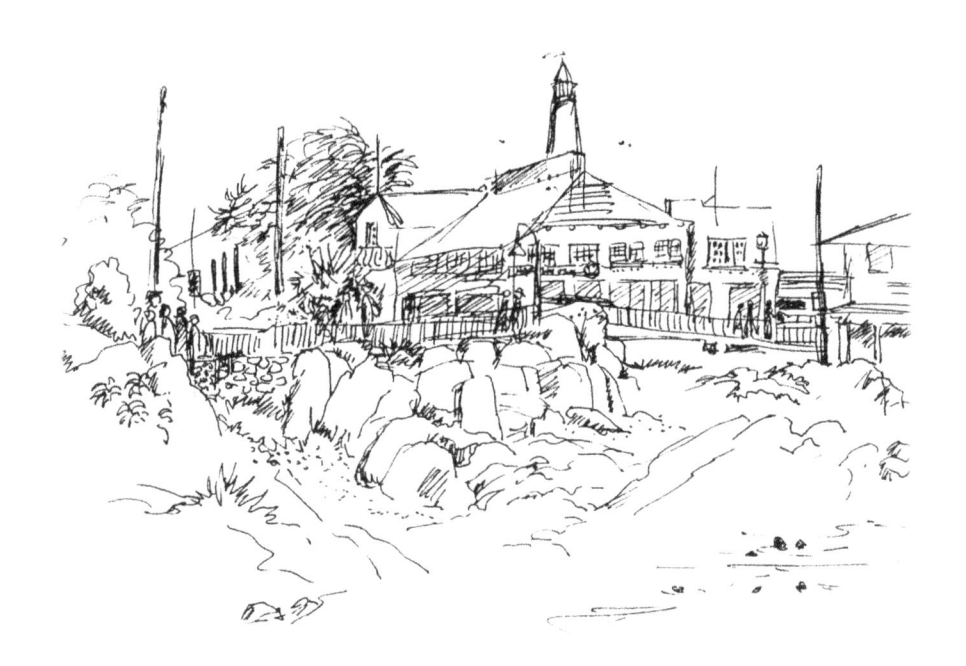

Letting Go of the Brass Ring

The Message

In the 1971 November/December issue of *The Message*,[18] Tense noticed an obituary of Rose Marie Durham. Like Tense, she was also born in 1927. Rose ministered in the Philippines until 1971 with her husband, the Director of the Baptist Bible Seminary and Institute. Rose served as the Dean of Women and a teacher in the Bible Institute, taught children's Bible classes, and was active in a variety of responsibilities with the mission while raising their three children.

Tense thought about how Rose had been serving God with her life. At that time, Tense was a busy mother of four children, a professional artist, and an art teacher.

"The contrast between Rose's life and mine impacted me," Tense told me after reading the obituary of Rose Durham. "I wonder how God might use me to do something for Him."

Divine Appointments

Soon after I had committed to serve God in whatever he wanted me to do and wherever He wanted me to go, He began to reveal His will for me through successive divine appointments. He brought people into our lives who were serving in various parts of the world. They shared with us the incredible need for people with training like mine in their fields of ministry.

A retired ABWE missionary named John Schlener came to speak at our church. Mr. Schlener, his brother Paul, and their wives had been missionaries in Brazil for many years and established "The Port of Two Brothers" mission station on the Amazon River, far upstream from the ocean. He told us about his amazing medical experiences in Brazil. None of his team had any medical training other than first aid, but they had been forced to deal with horrendous medical problems. The nationals came to them for help with medical conditions, often traveling long distances by canoe. Mr. Schlener told us about unbelievable cases, and I listened with rapt attention. The Schleners did the best they could with their meager supplies of medicines and bandages. While helping the national Indians who lived along the river with their medical needs, the Schleners shared the gospel with them.

We invited Mr. Schlener to have dinner at our home so we could learn more about his work in Brazil. He explained that he had retired from the foreign field but had been appointed the West Coast Representative of ABWE. I told him that it was obvious that someone with medical skills could make a huge contribution to God's work anywhere. "I could be interested in doing something like that after my house is paid for, my children are educated, and my investments are complete," I told Mr.

Schlener. I also told him that I might be too highly trained to be of use to God as a medical missionary in a jungle. As an orthopedic surgeon, I needed a well-equipped hospital, an operating room, x-ray facilities, and a laboratory to practice as I had been trained. I didn't think God had any such hospitals, and I was pretty sure he didn't want me to waste the skills He had given me to be content with bush surgery. However, I assured Mr. Schlener that, eventually, I would be willing to devote a few years to medical missions if there was somewhere I could fit in.

Mr. Schlener smiled and then went right to work as the West Coast Representative of ABWE. That evening, he called Dr. Lincoln Nelson, a medical missionary serving in the Philippines with ABWE. Dr. Nelson had established a small hospital on the island of Mindanao. The Nelsons just happened to be home on furlough and were living only a few hours from us in Santa Barbara. "Linc," he asked Dr. Nelson, "Could you use an orthopedic surgeon in your hospital?"

Amazed, Dr. Nelson replied, "We have just now been praying that the Lord would send an orthopedic surgeon to help us!" Dr. Nelson then called and invited us to visit him in Santa Barbara. He said he had a 16mm movie film about the hospital that he could send us. I told him I would like to see it, so he sent it to us immediately.

Most people did not have a 16mm movie projector in their home, but we just happened to have one. Our television had stopped working, and the repair shop said it would take several weeks to get the part needed from Japan to repair it. Our children were missing their television shows. I knew the public library had a collection of 16mm educational films we could borrow, so I went to a camera shop and asked if I could rent or buy a 16mm projector. I was amazed when the owner told me that two used 16mm projectors had just been brought in and were for sale. I bought one, and my children were pleased to have library movies to watch while the television was in the repair shop. Even the neighbor children enjoyed watching movies on the projector at our house.

When Dr. Nelson's film arrived, we immediately watched it using our new projector. I saw a collection of orthopedic problems for which I had the necessary training. What I saw captivated me. After watching the film, I told Tense we should drive to Santa Barbara to return it and meet the Nelson family. We drove to Santa Barbara the next weekend and spent Sunday afternoon with them, learning about the clinic in the Philippines and their need for an orthopedic surgeon.

Turn Your Eyes Upon Jesus

As we drove home from visiting the Nelsons, we listened to recorded music on our car stereo. I listened intently to the music and heard these words:

> Turn your eyes upon Jesus,
> Look full in His wonderful face,
> And the things of Earth will grow strangely dim
> In the light of His glory and grace.[19]

I may have heard that song before, but the words had not penetrated my mind and heart. That day, God spoke to me through those words. After years of privation and struggle, we were beginning to enjoy the affluence of our life after medical training. I had worked long and hard to get to this place in life. But my life of beginning affluence suddenly lost its attractiveness. As I listened to the words of that song, I realized that the orthopedic practice I had worked so hard to achieve, the nice house, my boat, our swimming pool—all those things suddenly seemed unimportant as I considered the challenge that was presented to me as we talked with Dr. Nelson about the need for an orthopedic surgeon in the Philippines.

I felt strongly drawn to commit my skills and life to serving God at a hospital on the mission field. I realized that just as a carpenter or mechanic selects his tools and sharpens them for the work ahead, God had already been preparing us for a special job He had for us. It seemed that God might be directing us to work with Dr. Nelson in the Philippines.

I thought about everything that had happened in my heart and life over the past few months, and willingly, I let go of the brass ring.

"Get Ready to Go"

"I think God may be telling us He wants to use us when we are young and not tired rather than when we are old and retired," I told Tense. "How would you feel about going now?"

I was not quite prepared for her answer.

"Yes, I am ready to go," she said. Then she told me this story about what she had heard when she was in her art studio with a fellow artist: "One day, we were in the studio getting ready to sketch a little girl who was modeling for us. As I was looking at the paintings and empty canvases around me, I heard in my heart this message: 'GET READY TO GO.' I didn't know what that meant. But as I pondered this strange message, I wondered if the Holy Spirit was speaking to me."

Although Tense was uncertain where she was to go, she was convinced she should stop renting the downtown studio and stop teaching art. After packing up her studio and taking her art supplies home, Tense had more time to be involved with various ministries of our church. Tense joined other ladies in our church to teach children's Bible clubs called "Joy Clubs." She attended a Child Evangelism Fellowship training program and met with the other teachers on Monday mornings to pray for the clubs and study the weekly lessons. Tense was thrilled to be part of this ministry and see children come to know Christ as their Savior through the ministry of the Joy Clubs.

Mr. Amstutz

Soon after we returned home from our visit with the Nelsons, we received a call from Mr. Amstutz, the candidate secretary for ABWE. He said Mr. Schlener had told him we were interested in serving God as medical missionaries. He asked if we had had any Bible school training. Our answer was, "No, other than what we had received at church and through Tense's training to teach Joy Clubs."

"Would you be willing to get some training?" he asked.

"How can we do that?" I asked. "I can't just stop my medical practice and go to Bible school."

"How about a correspondence school?" Mr. Amstutz asked. "Moody Bible Institute has one called The Scofield Bible Correspondence Course." It was a course that normally took three years to accomplish. We were interested in getting more Bible training, so we agreed to take the Bible Correspondence course.

Mr. Amstutz told us about the ABWE Candidate Class held in July at Baptist Bible College in Clarks Summit, Pennsylvania. He recommended that we attend. It was a four-week session that would introduce us to ABWE and its work in foreign countries. If we attended the Candidate Class, ABWE could evaluate our suitability to work with them. After his phone call, we received a formal invitation to come to the Candidate Class along with applications and other forms to complete.

There was also an information letter that said the applicants would have the opportunity to tell the ABWE board about their experiences sharing the gospel. That concerned me, so I went to my pastor to discuss this.

"I plan to go as a medical missionary," I told him. "Surely, they don't expect me to be involved in sharing the gospel. I have not had any experience in that direction."

"John, they will want you to be involved in sharing the gospel," my pastor replied. "If you are unwilling or unable, perhaps you are not the person they are looking for."

Later, I discussed with my wife how I could get experience sharing the gospel. She suggested I purchase small booklets of a modern English version of the Book of John and give them to my patients. I thought that sounded like a good idea, so we ordered some. I determined I would present one to every patient I put into the hospital.

Handing out those booklets was one of the scariest things I had ever attempted to do. I made up a little speech that went like this: "You are going to be in the hospital for a while and might like to have something to read. I want to give you this little booklet and invite you to read it. If you have any questions, I will gladly discuss them with you." I could say that in about thirty seconds, put the booklet on their nightstand and get out of there. Well, that turned out to be a real adventure. They did read the booklet. They did want to talk about it. That led to some opportunities for spiritual discussions about what they had read. For example, I had admitted a rough-looking, grumpy man to the male four-bed ward. I was sure he would not be interested in my little booklet, so I did not give him one. I went downstairs to sign out on the in-out board. As I reached up to turn the switch to "out," a voice seemed to speak to me.

"You said everyone. Did you really mean everyone?" Pausing, I could not bring myself to turn the switch to "out." Instead, I went back upstairs and into the ward, put a booklet on his stand, said my little speech, and left quickly. Only then could I sign out on the board.

The next morning, I went to the hospital to make rounds and went to that ward. The man greeted me with a surly expression.

"You remember that booklet you gave me?" he growled.

"Yes," I said and waited for what I thought would be his negative response.

Instead, he said, "Well, we were up half the night talking about that book." One of the hospital's male nursing assistants was in the room and told me he had been in on the discussion. He said he was a Christian and that he had been able to answer a lot of the man's questions. I had not known until then that this nursing assistant was a Christian. It was an exciting development.

Passing out that booklet and getting the patient's response became one of the highlights of putting a patient into the hospital. Some of the nurses asked me if they could also have a booklet. I was learning that medical work could open opportunities for spiritual teaching. I never got a negative response, and many of my patients responded gratefully to the booklet. Now, I had something positive to tell the mission board about my experiences sharing the gospel.

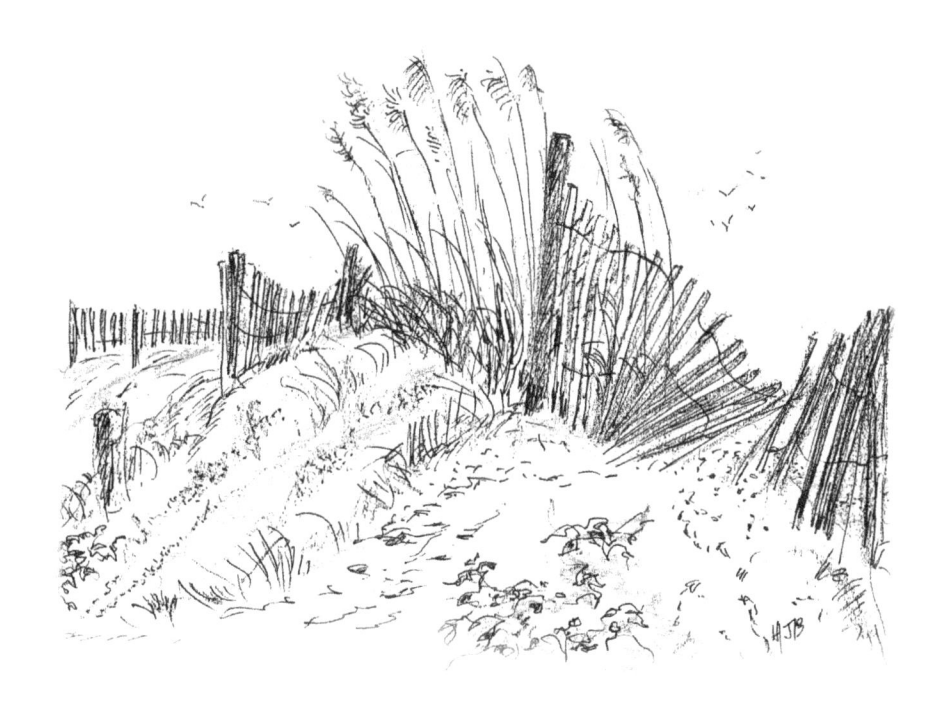

CHAPTER 11

The Assignment

Meeting Dr. Viggo Olsen

Before leaving for Candidate Class, we received a phone call from Dr. Viggo Olsen, a general surgeon serving with ABWE in Bangladesh at Memorial Christian Hospital (MCH), which he founded in 1966. The goal of this hospital was not just to provide medical care but to use medicine as a tool to bring people to a place where they would have an opportunity to learn of the gospel of salvation as taught in the Holy Bible and receive spiritual healing.

Dr. Olsen had learned that we were interested in medical missions. He was home on furlough and wanted to meet with us to discuss the need for an orthopedic surgeon at MCH. He informed us he was scheduled to speak at the General Association of Regular Baptists Churches meeting in San Diego and invited us to attend. We decided to drive down to San Diego to hear his report and meet him, as I thought our paths might cross someday. It was also our twenty-fifth wedding anniversary, so we considered it an anniversary trip.

At the conference in San Diego, we sat spellbound as Dr. Olsen talked about the fierce, nine-month-long Liberation War between East Pakistan and West Pakistan, which were geographically separated by India. Both countries had previously been part of India. He told of the daring escape of thirteen expatriates and their twenty-one children through the jungles of Burma when the hospital compound was in danger from raiding troops. The details of these accounts are told in Dr. Olsen's book *Daktar: Diplomat in Bangladesh*.[20] When the war ended in December 1971, East Pakistan became the new nation of Bangladesh. However, the war had taken a drastic toll on the struggling new nation, leaving it nearly destitute. As the West Pakistani troops withdrew from East Pakistan, they slaughtered thousands of professionals and intellectuals, leaving only a few trained doctors for the country of approximately 75 million people. Several million Bangladeshis were killed, leaving many widows. Millions of people were displaced. Medical care was nearly non-existent in most areas.

After the meeting, we introduced ourselves to Dr. Olsen and arranged to meet with him and his family the next day to learn more about MCH. The next morning, we joined them for breakfast in a restaurant and listened with rapt attention. Dr. Olsen told us how God had called him and his wife, Joan, to the country of East Pakistan to establish a hospital in the southern portion, where there was no medical facility. ABWE leased 25 acres of land from the government to build the hospital complex. This area, called Malumghat, was sixty miles south of Chittagong and thirty miles north of Cox's Bazar. A team of medical personnel was assembled, and the hospital officially opened in 1966. It had only been in existence for six years. MCH had one obstetrician/gynecologist surgeon (OB/GYN), two general surgeons, and one national doctor. They also had a physical therapist, a lab technician, two nurse anesthetists, and several registered nurses. Additional nurses and an X-ray technician were joining soon.

I asked specific questions about the facilities at MCH. Dr. Olsen said it was a fifty-bed modern hospital serving as the major medical center for an area of approximately ten million people. It had a reasonable X-ray department, a physical therapy department, and a well-equipped laboratory, all necessary for orthopedic surgeries. There had never been a full-term orthopedic surgeon serving at that hospital, but they had many patients with orthopedic problems. The only American orthopedic surgeon in Bangladesh at that time was Dr. Ronald Garst, who came to Bangladesh from India to treat the thousands of amputees resulting from the war. Dr. Garst was working in Dhaka, about 240 miles north of MCH.

I was overwhelmed by the enormous need for an orthopedic surgeon in Bangladesh. I didn't know a hospital like this existed on a mission field. If I went to Bangladesh, my practice would be mainly orthopedic. It seemed to me that the equipment and facilities at MCH were suitable for my orthopedic work. However, I assumed that in the Philippines, I would do mostly general practice at the small, clinic-like hospitals because they had limited X-ray and lab facilities and were not set up to handle orthopedic cases.

I reasoned that God had allowed me to get orthopedic training for a special purpose. It seemed that He was directing me to Bangladesh. When we left San Diego after talking with Dr. Olsen, we were convinced we should offer to serve at MCH in Bangladesh instead of going to the Philippines. As we drove home, we reflected on the stepping stones God had placed before us to bring us to this point.

Candidate Class

We joined approximately forty other missionary candidates when we arrived for the four-week ABWE Candidate Class in July 1972. We listened to daily presentations describing the various locations where ABWE missionaries served worldwide. We also learned detailed information about their policies and practices. We participated in active sports in the afternoons, such as badminton, soccer, and basketball.

During these four weeks, the Candidate Class Committee carefully observed us in our interpersonal relationships and our ability to work together as a team. In the last week of Candidate Classes, we had to appear before the ABWE Board and answer questions about our doctrinal beliefs and goals.

On August 16, 1972, we were officially appointed to serve with ABWE at Memorial Christian Hospital in Bangladesh. Dr. Dick Stagg and his wife, Carol, and Alice Payne, RN, were also in that Candidate Class with us and were appointed to Bangladesh. We chose I Peter 4:2 as our goal and decided to spend the rest of our lives serving God and not living for the temporary pleasures of this world. We were privileged to work together as "soldiers of the cross," seeing God's plan unfold.

> That he no longer should live the rest of his time in the flesh for the lusts of men, but for the will of God. (I Peter 4:2).

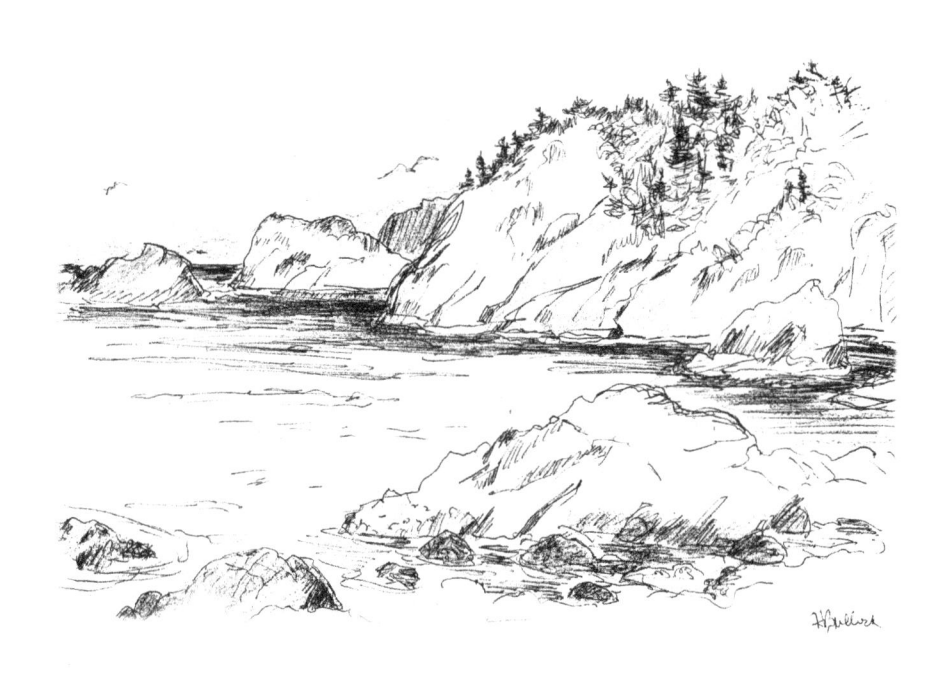

CHAPTER 12

Announcing our Decision

Chrissa's wedding

We returned home just a few days before our daughter Chrissa's wedding in August 1972. Chrissa and Karen had worked hard to prepare for the wedding while we were away in Candidate Class. With so many changes happening simultaneously, life seemed to be moving quickly.

Telling Tense's Family

As soon as we made the decision to serve in a foreign medical situation, we let Tense's parents and siblings know of God's plan for our lives and our decision to go to Bangladesh. Her parents were thrilled and encouraged us greatly by immediately pledging to support us financially each month with a small gift and to pray for us. While we were concerned Tense's parents might need assistance as they aged, we were comforted that Tense's brother and sister lived nearby and could be responsible for their care. We planned to visit them between terms when we were back in the US for furlough.

Telling My Mother

The situation was a little different with my mother. I was an only child, and there was no one else to take care of her. I prayed for wisdom about the best way to break the news to her. She was active and enjoyed living in the Seal Beach Leisure World, where she had moved following my father's death in 1960. Moving to Leisure World had given her a group of friends in a safe and pleasant environment, even though she had suffered a heart attack and was taking blood pressure medicine.

The events of one particular day in the fall of 1972 illustrated how God was directing us. On my return trip home from a meeting in Southern California, I drove northward on the Ventura freeway. I decided to take the opportunity to stop at my mother's apartment at Leisure World in Seal Beach to tell her about the momentous decision that I had made. When I arrived at her house, she was having a bridge party with friends, and they were all having a great time. It did not seem like the proper time to discuss this decision with Mother, so I told her I would return. As I drove in the heavy traffic on the freeway, I was suddenly overcome with intense fatigue and drowsiness. The feeling was so strong I was certain I would fall asleep in the middle of the freeway. Exiting at the next offramp, I returned to my mother's apartment. The party was nearly over, so I told Mother I wanted to rest and went to her bedroom, where I quickly fell asleep.

When I awoke sometime later, the party was over, and Mother was waiting for me expectantly. We sat at the kitchen table and talked. Before

I could say anything about my decision, she opened the conversation by telling me about a special function held at their clubhouse. Her words are etched on my memory.

"I want to tell you about the wonderful program we had at the clubhouse a few days ago," she said. A man spoke to us about India and showed us slides as well. He told about the people and their needs." She went on, "Those people have so many needs. Wouldn't using your life to help people like that be wonderful?"

I was dumbfounded. What an opening! I knew this was the correct time to tell her about my big decision.

"Mother," I said, "there is something I must tell you about. I have decided to give up my medical practice in San Luis Obispo and pursue medical missions. We will work with a mission organization called the Association of Baptists for World Evangelism and head for Bangladesh as soon as we raise our support."

Her next statement also surprised me. "I'm not surprised," she said. You always were interested in Albert Schweitzer and his work."

After I told her it would take a while to raise our support, she made the first negative comment after considering the matter for a moment.

"When you do leave for Bangladesh, that will mean I will never see you again," she said. She knew that four years, until our first furlough, would be a long time to wait and that she might not live that long. I had no answer except to assure her we would see her often before we left.

Telling My Colleagues

In September 1972, I sent a letter to my medical colleagues and friends announcing that I planned to give up my orthopedic practice at the San Luis Medical Clinic and go to Bangladesh to work with a mission hospital. In my letter, I stated, "A missionary call is a conviction that becomes a compulsion." I explained that this summed up what led Tense and me to apply to ABWE to go to Bangladesh and work at Memorial Christian Hospital. I told them that this small but modern hospital of only fifty beds had only been in operation for six years and served an area of about ten million people. The war between East and West Pakistan had left the country nearly destitute, with little medical care in many areas. I described the staff situation and told them I would be the first and only full-time orthopedic surgeon at the hospital.

The response to my letter was varied. Some of my colleagues thought I was crazy. Others implied they would be interested in doing something like that if their spouses would accompany them. I told my colleagues I would remain at the clinic until my replacement could be found. Within one month, an orthopedic surgeon coming out of the military applied to the clinic and was chosen to take my place.

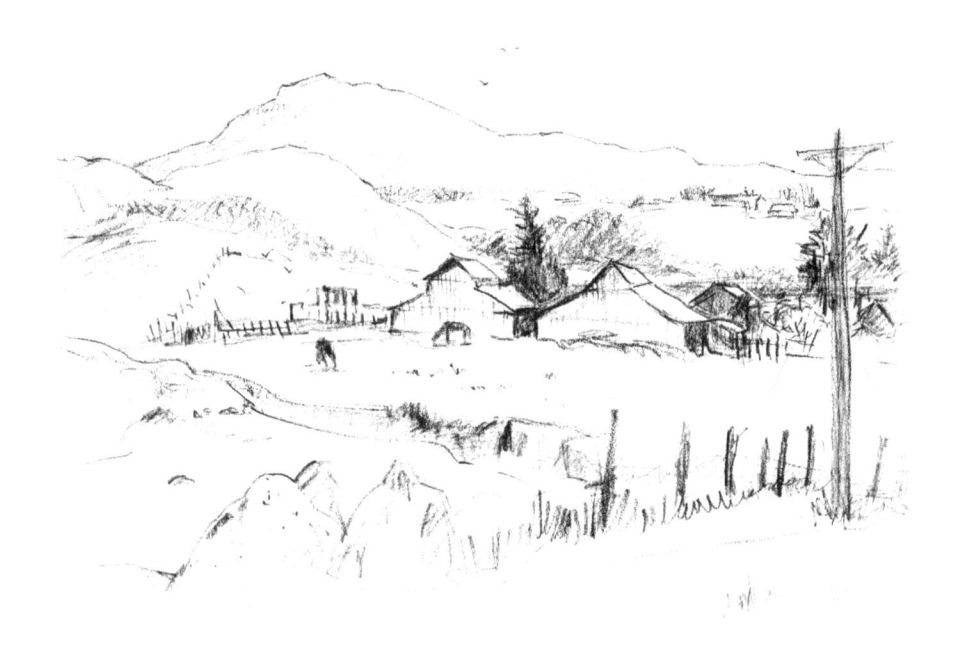

CHAPTER 13

Pre-Field Ministry

Learning to Depend on God

After Chrissa's wedding, our next step was to begin our pre-field ministry. God had some lessons to teach us through pre-field ministry. We needed to learn to depend fully on God and to allow Him to direct our path. ABWE was a faith mission, which meant they did not pay a salary to missionaries. We had to raise our financial support by visiting local churches and introducing them to the field where we would work.

During these presentations, we gave them an overview of our future ministry, and the churches would then decide whether to give us monthly financial support, prayer support, or any other form of assistance. Women's missionary groups rolled strips of sheets into bandages and gathered donated medical supplies and eyeglasses. Several individuals also made commitments for financial and prayer support. One couple volunteered to mail our prayer letters to supporting churches and individuals several times yearly. We were required to have 100 percent of our pledged support before we could leave for the field.

Travel and Packing Barrels

I left my practice in San Luis Obispo on November 30, 1972. We sold our home and moved into a rental house until Karen and David finished their school year in San Luis Obispo. When school was out, we moved to Martinez, California, where they could attend a Christian school the following year. Then, we began to gather the equipment and personal effects we would need in Bangladesh for the next four years. We knew many items would be unavailable in the country after the recent war, so we had to take everything we thought we might need. We packed and shipped more than forty steel drums and several crates to Bangladesh with the assistance of a Christian packing and shipping ministry in Oakland called Home of Peace.

We started our pre-field ministry travels by visiting churches on the weekends to raise the required support. During the next eighteen months, we visited over 100 churches in five Western states. Whenever possible, we visited my mother and Tense's parents.

Getting invitations to speak to churches was a formidable assignment. We had arranged a few meetings with local churches in our area but had limited contact with other churches and pastors. Most churches on the West Coast were small, and other missionary candidates were also seeking support from these churches.

John speaks at Asilomar

The pastor of our home church said he would send letters to pastors he knew, asking them to allow us to speak to their congregations. To help me connect with churches, he invited me to attend the California Regular Baptist Churches meeting at Asilomar, California, near Monterey. Many West Coast pastors attended that meeting, and I was able to speak to the whole group. That was a huge assignment for me. I had never spoken to a large group of pastors like that. It was intimidating. What should I tell them? I had little time to prepare any message, so it would have to be spontaneous. That was scary.

After arriving at Asilomar and getting settled in our cabin, I drove to a parking lot overlooking the ocean. As I watched the waves crashing onto the rocks, I prayed. The coast at Asilomar is rugged, with rocks and trees and a roaring surf. The power of the surf was impressive. As I watched the surf, these verses in Psalm 8 came to my mind.

> When I consider Your heavens, the work of Your fingers, The moon and the stars, which You have ordained, What is man that You are mindful of him, And the son of man that You visit him? (Psalm 8:3-4).

I was encouraged as I realized that God had brought me here, and I trusted He would give me the words to speak to the pastors. When my turn came to speak the next day, I went to the speaker's podium and looked out at the intimidating sea of pastors. I was confident, not nervous. But they had already heard many messages from missionary candidates, so what could I tell them that was new?

"I have never spoken to a group of pastors before," I told them. "I am not a pastor, have never been to Bible college, and am not ordained. I realize your spiritual knowledge is greater than mine, but I will try to explain my calling to you." I read to them the verses in 1 Corinthians Chapter 12, which used the illustration of many parts of the human body. It demonstrates the variety of abilities and gifts of the believers in the church, including the "gift of healing."

> For as the body is one and has many members, but all the members of that one body, being many, are one body, so also

is Christ . . . Now you are the body of Christ, and members individually. And God has appointed these in the church: first apostles, second prophets, third teachers, after that, miracles, then gifts of healings. (I Corinthians 12:12, 27-28).

"God has allowed me to become reasonably proficient in an area different from every one of you. I believe God can use my skills as an orthopedic surgeon as a powerful tool in reaching the nationals of Bangladesh and visitors who might come there. The little hospital where I will be working is the only well-equipped general hospital for an area of about ten million people who have nowhere else to turn for good medical care. There is an enormous need for an orthopedic surgeon to work at that hospital, and I believe that God has called me to be that orthopedic surgeon. The Bangladeshi people will come to our hospital for medical treatment and will be able to hear the good news of the gospel of salvation from the Holy Bible while they are there for treatment and recovery."

The pastors listened respectfully and intently, and then, immediately after the meeting, invitations began to come in from churches for us to present our future ministry in Bangladesh. After visiting churches for several months, we saw only a trickle of support coming in. Frankly, we were discouraged. I felt we might not have been "His chosen" after all. Then, when we returned home after being on the road for several more weeks, we were astonished to see letters of commitment for support from five churches! It was as if God was saying, "Don't be discouraged. You are being used to make churches aware of the need in that remote part of the world." It was also an opportunity to recruit others for missions and to come to MCH in Bangladesh. Several of the pastors of the churches we visited eventually also went into full-time missions.

Provision of Orthopedic Equipment

Orthopedic treatment requires special instruments and medical supplies. I had to know what equipment was already present at Memorial Christian Hospital and what I would need to procure and bring with me or have sent. The general surgeons at MCH had done some orthopedic procedures, such as treating fractures of long bones and hips, plus some neurosurgical procedures. However, I did not know how diversified their equipment supply might be. I contacted the current doctors at MCH and asked them to tell me what surgical instruments they had on hand. They replied that the instruments they had were old and in bad condition. "Bring as much as you can of things you think you will need," they instructed.

I reasoned that since God had shown me where to go, He would supply whatever I might need to use once I got there. I made up a list of basic tools I would need and then checked prices in instrument catalogs. The total very quickly came to more than $10,000. The floodgates opened when we notified our supporting churches of the hospital's need for orthopedic equipment and supplies! Sunday School classes often donated to purchase specific instruments. One little boy gave his birthday money to buy a metal pin cutter that cost over $90.

An orthopedic surgeon donated his personal surgical instruments when the hospital where he worked purchased new equipment and requested that doctors remove their instruments. He also gave me his collection of orthopedic instructional books and journals dating back to the original issues. A pastor friend gave me an annual Journal of Bone and Joint Surgery subscription. Their support was encouraging. I also obtained a large supply of new-quality instruments donated by the manufacturer. During our two years of pre-field ministry, God provided many donated items of surgical equipment, which I estimated were worth hundreds of thousands of dollars. We arranged to have these items shipped to the field before our arrival.

Ready to Go

"Do you still have your medical practice in San Luis Obispo?" someone asked at one of the churches we visited. "No," we told them. "We have sold our house and many of our possessions. We are ready to go when we get the required support." After eighteen months, we finally reached the required level of financial support and received permission from ABWE to travel to Bangladesh. Many churches and individuals promised varying amounts of financial support. Most importantly, they also committed to praying for us and the work God had prepared us to do in Bangladesh. We especially needed their prayer.

During our pre-field ministry, we learned valuable lessons about patience and perseverance. We were being trained, like tools being sharpened for a task. We learned that the timing of when we would be allowed to go to Bangladesh was up to God. We learned that we could trust God for everything and lean on the Holy Spirit to guide us, which gave us the confidence that He would guide and direct us when we reached Bangladesh.

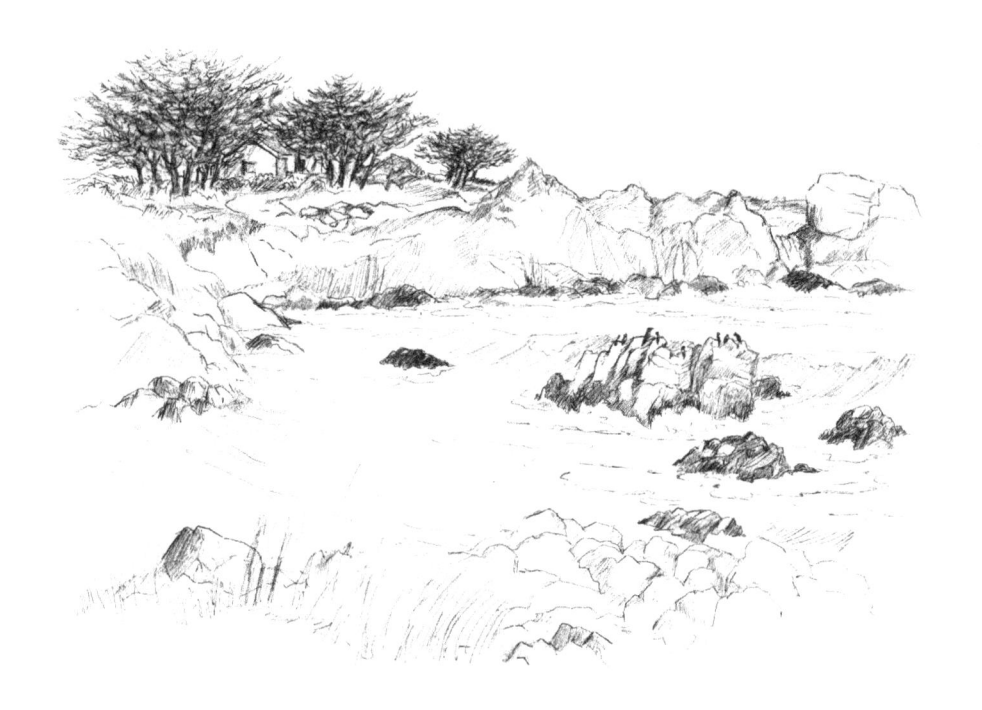

CHAPTER 14

Hard Decisions and Saying Goodbye

Tense's Father Dies

On December 6, 1973, Tense's mother called to say that Tense's father was having a lot of heart trouble, and his lungs were filling up with water. Medical tests showed an enlarged heart. Tense's mother said they planned to travel to California to see a specialist. A week later, Tense's father passed away from a heart attack. Tense traveled to Medford to help her mother and be with the family. I joined her there after I finished meetings in Washington. At a time like this, we were thankful that Tense's brother, George, also lived in Medford and would care for their mother while we were in Bangladesh.

Mother's Stroke

One day in August 1973, I received a phone call from my mother telling me that her left arm was numb and she was having difficulty talking. I suspected that she had suffered a stroke and told her to call an ambulance immediately. I took the first flight I could get to Los Angeles and met her at the hospital. When I arrived, her neurosurgeon was preparing to do a cerebral arteriogram and allowed me to go into the X-ray room while that procedure was performed. Afterward, he told me the procedure revealed that surgery would not help her, so he recommended she be put on conservative management. My tiny 4'11" mother seemed so frail as I looked down at her in that hospital bed, and I struggled with what to do about her care.

Tense and I returned a few days later when my mother had improved enough to be released. She could read, write, talk, and get about without assistance but was still somewhat confused. We took her home with us and placed her in a nursing home close by in Pleasant Hill until we could make a decision about her care. We realized she could not continue to live alone in her Leisure World apartment. She would have to live in an assisted living facility because we had no room for her in our small rental home. If she came to live with us, we would need to rent or buy a larger house. Should I forget about going to Bangladesh and remain in the US until Mother died? I did not know how long she would live. I reasoned that she could live for many years without further trouble. But there was the possibility that she would have another stroke and become permanently paralyzed or die. We knew we were desperately needed at MCH. Was this development a ploy of Satan to prevent me from going?

This was a huge dilemma, and I agonized over this decision night and day. I carefully studied what the Bible teaches regarding the care and treatment of our family members. Exodus 20:12 commands us to "honor your father and your mother." I Timothy 5:8 makes it clear that everyone is responsible for his father's and mother's welfare. "But if anyone does not provide for his own, and especially for those of his household, he has denied the faith and is worse than an unbeliever." (I Timothy 5:8). I also considered this verse in the book of Matthew that says, "He who loves father or mother more than Me is not worthy of Me. And he who loves son or daughter more than me is not worthy of Me." (Matthew 10:37).

I considered all my options. I could postpone going to Bangladesh and return to medical practice in the US to take care of my mother. I would have to take a leave of absence from the mission and find a medical group that would take me temporarily, which might be difficult and would mean a substantial financial commitment. However, we had raised nearly all our support and travel expenses and were just about ready to go overseas. Putting all that on hold and preparing to go to Bangladesh later would be difficult if I was caught up in starting a new medical practice.

My other option was to trust God and go to Bangladesh as planned, leaving Mother as well cared for as possible. I asked my cousin, Roy Chattin, who lived in northern California, if he would manage my mother's finances if we went to Bangladesh. He agreed. Roy was the closest thing I had to a brother. Without his help, I would never have felt I could go to Bangladesh while Mother was still alive.

I believed that God had clearly called us to Bangladesh, had assisted us in getting ready to go, and had prepared us for this task. I concluded that He did not want us to divert from our assignment. Having done everything I could to make every possible arrangement for my mother's care, I trusted God to take care of her in His perfect plan.

We asked Mother where she would like to live, and she said she wanted to return to the Los Angeles area to be closer to her friends in Seal Beach. We found an attractive, well-managed assisted living community that she could afford in a quiet neighborhood near Seal Beach and her friends. We drove her to her new home, unpacked her things, and helped her settle into her room. I built a wooden flower box for her on the patio outside her window and planted flowers. Her little flower garden was an immediate success. Several other residents admired it and asked if they could help her take care of it.

We arranged for her to receive medical care in a nearby clinic and helped her make funeral arrangements, leaving the documents with the manager of the facility. I reviewed her finances in detail with Roy and set up a bank account and checkbook for her. She seemed well situated, with a nurse to help with medications, a pleasant place to live, and all her needs met, except for our being able to see her often. We visited her as often as possible in the remaining months before we left the country, and she seemed reasonably content but still slightly confused.

I told Mother we would try to bring her to visit us in Bangladesh after we settled and her health improved. She was on anticoagulants, but she could have her blood clotting tests done at our hospital in Bangladesh. We would arrange to have her travel with one of the returning expatriate teammates, or I would make a special trip home to take her back with me. This was all possible, and I had every intention of doing it. We prepared for our departure and made one last trip to see Mother before leaving the US. This was a tearful time for her and for us, as we all realized the possibilities of seeing one another again in this life were slim.

Delayed Departure

Finally, we were ready to go. Only David was going with us, as Peter and Karen were starting college and Chrissa was married and expecting her first baby. Our drums and crates were ready for shipment at Home of Peace in Oakland. We sent our passports and visa applications to the Bangladesh Embassy in Washington, DC, and purchased our plane tickets. When we did not receive our passports with our visas by the date we needed them, I called the Bangladesh embassy. I was told, "They were mailed yesterday. " Since we had to wait for the passports to arrive, we postponed our departure for a week.

One More Visit

Because of the unexpected delay in our departure, I returned alone to see my mother again. I stayed with her for two days, spending the night in her little apartment. We had a wonderful visit, and she seemed quite cheerful. She seemed eager to hear about our forthcoming "adventure."

As I prepared to leave, I told her, "Mother, I don't know whether I will see you again here on earth, but I am confident I will see you in Heaven." She agreed, and we parted with a kiss.

PART TWO

Bangladesh At Last

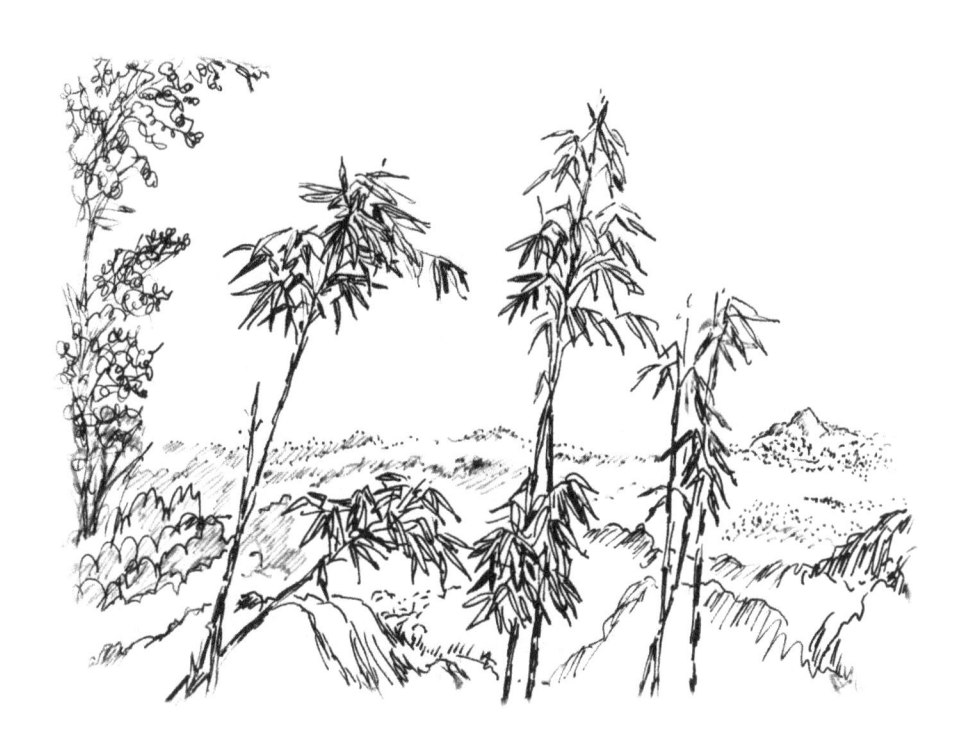

CHAPTER 15

On Wings of Eagles

Provision of Flight Companions

When the visas finally arrived after several days, we noticed they had been postmarked the day after my phone call to the Embassy. Although this delay was disappointing, we soon discovered it was God's plan. A group of friends from Bethany Baptist Church in Martinez took us to the airport to send us off. As we boarded the plane, we struggled with all our luggage and equipment, including a tripod, cameras, and multiple carry-on bags. We settled into our seats across the aisle from a lady traveling with six teenagers. David began conversing with the teens and asked them where they were going. "Manila in the Philippines," they told him.

When David told them he was going to Bangladesh, the teens' mother turned to me and asked, "Where are you going in Bangladesh?"

"Memorial Christian Hospital," I replied.

Her eyes widened, and she said, "I am Nancy Ebersole, formerly Nancy Goehring, who used to live at Hebron, the ABWE station in the Chittagong Hill Tracts in Bangladesh." Nancy told us that their original flight had been canceled due to a mechanical error, so they returned to New Jersey for the night. Her husband had rescheduled them on this direct flight to Manilla. We were excited as we realized God had changed our schedules to put us together on this flight.

As we flew across the Pacific Ocean, we shared our story with Nancy of how God had called us to serve at MCH in Bangladesh. Then Nancy told us how she and her husband, Harry, had worked with the Tipperah tribal people at the Hebron station. Harry died only two years after they had arrived in Bangladesh. His grave was located on the MCH hospital compound. Nancy and her children returned to the US to live with her mother in Indiana. Four years later, Nancy married Russ Ebersole, an ABWE teammate stationed in the Philippines. Russ's wife had died from cancer the same year Harry had died. Harry and Russ had been good friends, and Nancy had met Russ in Candidate Class. After Nancy and Russ were married, they returned to Manila to serve together in the Philippines.[21]

We landed in Manila and walked out of the airport into a huge crowd of dark-haired people waiting for passengers in the arrival area. A small group of people from the crowd stepped forward to greet Nancy and her family and take them home. No one from the ABWE office was there to meet us, as they had not received our telegram informing them of our arrival time in Manila. Nancy arranged for the van to take us with them to the ABWE headquarters and then to the guest house. That night, we attended a station meeting at the Ebersoles' home and met the other ABWE teammates in Manila, many of whom became our long-term friends. We rejoiced in God's protection and provision as

He arranged our meeting with the Ebersoles on our flight and friends to welcome us along the way.

We continued to Mindanao, where we met with Lowell and Virginia Edwards, our daughter Chrissa's in-laws. Lowell had taken an early retirement to go to the Philippines on a short-term aviation assignment with ABWE. Lowell flew us in the mission plane to Malaybalay to see Bethel Baptist Hospital, where we had considered going before being appointed to Bangladesh. We met with Dr. Linc Nelson and his wife, Lenore, and visited there for a few days to become familiar with the work for a possible future working relationship.

After leaving the Philippines to continue our journey to Bangladesh, we stopped in Hong Kong and Singapore. In those cities, we gathered the information we needed for future purchases of hospital equipment and other items we might need that we could not obtain in Bangladesh. We joined Dr. Vic Olsen and his wife, Joan, on their way back to Bangladesh, flying together to Dhaka.

Dhaka

We arrived in Dhaka on July 26, 1974. Upon arrival, we experienced a sudden culture shock when we realized that the world we had entered was significantly different from the one we left behind. The two weeks of travel through several countries on our journey to Bangladesh allowed us to slowly get used to different cultures, customs, time zones, and scenery. We were thankful to be traveling with Vic and Joan as we entered Dhaka's arrival lounge and approached the passport control desk. The Olsens helped us with the bewildering paperwork required since we were applying for residency and would be importing household goods. They also helped us get our permanent visas to stay in the country and arranged housing for us in Dhaka at the home of Dr. Mark and Ida Tucker. Dr. Tucker was the head of the Cholera Research Lab in Dhaka.

When we finally cleared the customs counter and stepped outside the airport, poverty was evident everywhere. Suddenly, we were surrounded by begging children with outstretched hands crying, "Baksheesh," as they jostled each other to get close to us. As we stood there in shock, overcome with the plight of these children, we heard people shouting,

"Nomoshkar!" This Christian Bengali greeting from friends waiting to take us to the Tuckers' home was the first word we learned in Bengali.

As we traveled through the heavily congested city traffic, it appeared that we were driving on the wrong side of the road. Bicycle rickshaws and "baby taxis" (three-wheeled motorbikes with a two-seater cab at the back) wove in and out of the traffic, and cows and dogs wandered the streets among the crowds.

On Sunday morning, we attended the international church with the Olsens and met Dr. and Mrs. Ron Garst. He invited me to tour Sher-E-Bangla Hospital, where he treated war veterans.

Dr. Garst had many years of experience working in India and gave me valuable advice regarding equipment, procedures, and orthopedic practices in Southeast Asia. He had to manufacture many of the rods and pins he needed for orthopedic treatment. He imported different sizes of type 316L alloy stainless steel rods and wires from the US. They came in three to six-foot lengths and had to be cut into the sizes he needed. When we returned to the US for furlough, I ordered a supply of these rods and pins to use at MCH for my orthopedic work.

Dr. Garst also taught me how to make plaster cast rolls because they were unavailable in Bangladesh. We continued to have contact with Dr. Garst for many years and became life-long friends.

Chittagong

We said goodbye to the Olsens after spending a few days together in Dhaka. Vic had to stay in the city for several weeks to negotiate with the Bangladesh National Board of Revenue (NBR) to obtain duty-free status for MCH. The Chittagong Customs officials had been holding hospital shipments in their warehouses and were asking for thousands of dollars in duty and sales tax. Dr. Olsen had experience negotiating with government officials and had personal connections in high government offices. [22]

Tense, David, and I flew south to Chittagong and were met at the airport by the Stagg family, who had been in Candidate Class with us. They took us to the guest house in the ABWE mission van. As we traveled alongside the river toward the city, we saw badly damaged hulks of large ships in the water. These remnants of the war that West Pakistan waged on East Pakistan just three years before our arrival were a sobering reminder of the devastation this country had endured. Jeannie Lockerbie described the history of that event in the book *On Duty in Bangladesh*.[23]

The port city of Chittagong was built on the banks of the Karnaphuli River and sat between the Chittagong Hill Tracts and the Bay of Bengal. It was a much more picturesque city than Dhaka. We saw large government buildings constructed by the British in the 1800s. In stark contrast to the orderly brick buildings, a tangled web of haphazard electric wiring was strung along poles and attached to buildings in messy clumps with no visible pattern. The streets were crowded, extremely narrow, and occupied with hordes of people, along with honking cars, trucks, and buses. To add to the confusion, ox carts and push carts struggled to navigate the endless sea of motorcycles, bicycles, rickshaws, and baby taxis. As we had seen in Dhaka, mangy dogs and little scrawny cows wandered through the streets. The noise of the continuous horn honking was deafening.

There didn't seem to be any organized traffic plan or traffic lights. Traffic jams were frequent, some lasting an hour or more. When obstructed by such a jam, it was not unusual to have pedestrians climb over the cars to get from one side of the street to the other. Policemen were scarce. At some intersections, we could see a policeman standing on a pedestal, waving his arms, seemingly not impacting the traffic movement. The chaotic flow of the masses of people and vehicles reminded me of the swirling Brownian motion of small, fast-moving particles observed under a microscope in a drop of pond water.

In later years, we usually avoided driving in this hazardous traffic and instead rode in the hospital van with an experienced driver. We also discovered that it was dangerous to leave a car unattended. The wheels could have been stolen while we were away. The mission van driver stayed with the van to guard it while we shopped. Going to a bank to get money was also dangerous. Bandits watched for people coming out of a bank with a package that might contain money. Our driver would let us off at the door and then return to the door to pick us up.

After getting us settled at the guest house, Dick Stagg took us to meet some of our teammates. It was a great relief to be off those noisy, crowded streets. We received a joyous welcome from our future coworkers as they sang, "There's a Christian Welcome Here." It sounded beautiful after the long wait for our visa and the journey halfway around the world. Our teammates in Bangladesh formed a close-knit family community and, on special occasions, often filled the place of our extended family.

Medical License in Bangladesh

While in Chittagong, I applied for my medical license to practice in Bangladesh. I learned that the medical schools there were still following the British system, and graduates of their medical colleges received a Bachelor of Medicine, Bachelor of Surgery degree (MBBS). The Bangladesh Medical and Dental Council did not recognize the Doctor of Osteopathic Medicine degree (DO). They assumed DO meant Doctor of Ophthalmology. I might not have been given my full Bangladesh medical licensure if I had applied as a DO rather than an MD. The MD degree I obtained from California College of Medicine proved essential to get my medical licensure in Bangladesh. This was another confirmation of God's preparation for our assignment in Bangladesh.

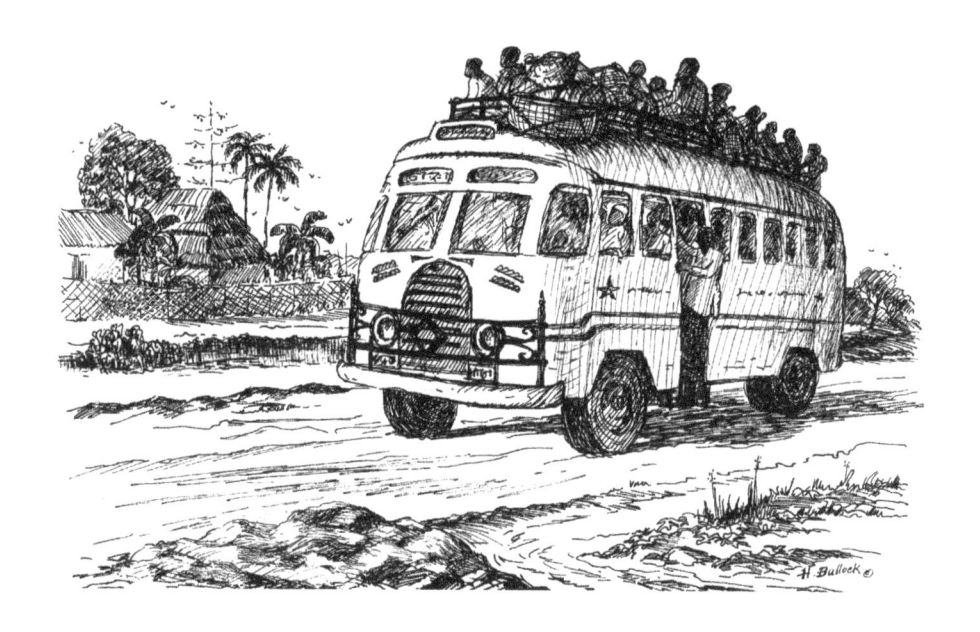

CHAPTER 16

Memorial Christian Hospital

Road to Memorial Christian Hospital

After we finished our business in Chittagong, we traveled to MCH in the hospital van. Our driver was experienced and familiar with the treacherous one-lane road from Chittagong to Malumghat, which crossed over about 100 rivers, creeks, culverts, and bridges. When we came to a bridge, the first vehicle to enter the bridge had priority. No other vehicle could cross the bridge while a bus was on it. If two drivers came onto the bridge and neither wanted to yield, they would come to a full stop and wait until one of them relented and backed off the bridge. This caused delays, especially when other drivers were waiting to cross the bridge. Persistent horn honking encouraged vehicles to get out of the way. One bridge was shared with a train, which definitely had the right of way.

When approached by a bus, our driver quickly moved onto the shoulder of the road to let the bus pass because larger vehicles like trucks or buses had the right of way. The buses were homemade, constructed out of wood, covered with thin metal sheeting, and painted with brightly colored designs. The result was a flimsy structure that could travel on the highway but was mechanically unstable and unreliable. We avoided riding on those country buses if possible.

Another peril on the road to Malumghat was the ditches on the sides of roads, which could be quite deep, even up to eight feet. During heavy rain, these ditches would fill with water, and the ditch would no longer be visible. Often, the road itself became indiscernible when covered with water. Unfortunately, this would often result in car and bus accidents, both on the road and in the ditches.

Once we left the heavy traffic, we thought we could sit back and relax. However, we soon came to a village bazaar along the sides of the road that was thronged with people, animals, and push carts overflowing onto the highway. Our driver drove slowly and honked the horn constantly. As we approached, the crowd reluctantly separated just enough to let our vehicle through. On each side of the road, the open-front stalls, called dokans, were piled high with a varied collection of multicolored vegetables, fruit, rice, and spices. Large chunks of meat hung from hooks in front of the butcher shops, and we saw little black goats tied up for slaughter. Some dokans sold plastic and wooden furniture, metal pots and pans, and hardware tools. Further down the road toward the hospital, the distance between villages and bazaars increased, and the countryside was dotted with beautiful lime-green rice paddies on both sides of the road. Near the end of our thrill-packed journey on the narrow road from Chittagong to Malumghat, we drove through a beautiful forest of teak trees.

Arrival at Malumghat

When we finally approached the hospital, it was night. The hospital lights shone brightly on the right side of the road. A small white building sat back from the road, nestled among tall Gurjan trees. On the front of the building were the words "Memorial Christian Hospital" written in large letters in Bengali and English. On the other side of the road, a row of dokans sat in darkness. We could see the silhouette of a village and rice paddies reflecting the moonlight.

We turned off the highway onto a brick road leading up to the hospital gate. As we drove toward the hospital, the front gate darwan (guard) recognized our van and opened the gate. We were there!

Guest House

Mel and Marjorie Beals welcomed us to Malumghat and helped us settle into our rooms at the Guest House, where we were assigned to stay while our permanent housing was being constructed. We looked forward to serving alongside the Beals at MCH. They had advised us on what to bring and how to ship it to Bangladesh. The Guest House had four motel-like rooms, a large meeting room, and a dining room where we ate our daily meals prepared by the Bangladeshi kitchen staff. We lived in two rooms at the Guest House for over a year, storing our extra belongings in steel drums on a large veranda at the back of the building.

Tik-tiki House Lizards

It didn't take long to discover that we were not the only occupants of our room. Small lizards, known as "tiktikis," lived on walls and ceilings, hunting mosquitoes and insects. They chirped a "tiktiki" sound from time to time, which is where they got their name. They were harmless to humans, but sometimes when we opened a dresser drawer, we would find tiny tiktiki eggs in a corner.

A local belief was that if a tiktiki chirped before someone left their house, they had to wait until it chirped again to leave safely. This, of course, was superstition, but it was ingrained into the minds of the nationals. Even if the person summoned was a midwife being called to assist in delivery, she dared not leave her house to perform her duty if the tiktiki chirped just before she was ready to leave her house.

Hospital Compound

The next morning, as we went to the hospital to meet our teammates and survey our surroundings, we could see that we were in a beautiful park-like setting with many flowers, neat brick and cement houses, and trim yards. The hospital compound was located on a 19-acre property leased from the Bangladesh Forestry Department.

Behind the hospital compound stretched a large khal that was a busy cargo port with many kinds of boats coming and going every day. The boats carried lumber, animals, bricks, straw, firewood, and people and was a constantly changing show. Some boats were large, made of hardwood lumber several inches thick, and covered with tar and pitch.

Brick cobblestone roads led to the back of the compound where the expatriate family housing was located along with the MK children's school, a tennis court, the single women nurses' residences, and the Guest House. These brick buildings were built to survive typhoons. Between the family homes and the hospital were the national school, the soccer field, and staff housing for the national employees. This would be our home and place of service for the next 18 years, and we were excited to be there.

Meeting the Doctors, Nurses, and Staff

We were eager to meet each doctor, nurse, and staff member and tour the hospital. After being introduced to our teammates at the morning chapel, I gave my testimony and told how God had called Tense and me to Bangladesh. It was exciting to meet Dr. Peter MacField and his wife, Reba, Bangladeshi doctors who joined the MCH staff in 1972. I had learned Peter was interested in having me train him in orthopedic surgery. I had brought the orthopedic books and instructional teaching materials given to me during our pre-field ministry, which I could use in training him.

During the war, Peter and Reba had barely escaped from the West Pakistan Army. They briefly hid at Malumghat and then fled to Burma with some of our Bangladeshi staff to take refuge there until the war ended. There, Peter had the opportunity to learn of God's love for him, and he believed in Jesus for salvation. After the war, they returned to Chittagong, where Reba finished her medical training. Following her graduation, Dr. Peter and Dr. Reba came back to MCH to be part of our medical team.[24]

Tour of the Hospital

After chapel, one of the expatriate nurses took me on a hospital tour. As we walked through the halls, she told me that the patients had come to them in buses, rickshaws, or on foot, often from more than 100 miles away. I looked out at the crowd of several hundred new arrivals and returning patients who had assembled at the front gate—men dressed in white Punjabis and white caps, other men in tee shirts and lungis, women in saris holding young children and babies, pregnant women, and people with crutches. They all hoped to be admitted to the Outpatient Department (OPD) and possibly the hospital for surgical, medical, or obstetric care. Our national medical staff would triage them, and then a decision would be made to either accept them for treatment or turn them away.

As we toured the hospital, I was struck by how dreary and crowded everything seemed. There was little of the polish and shine of the usual medical facilities that I was accustomed to in the US. The male and female wards were constructed of bamboo upper walls and ceilings, painted concrete stem walls, and bare cement floors. I noticed black mold growing on the exterior walls of the buildings because of the humid tropical climate. There were electric ceiling fans and windows with screens but no air conditioning.

The floors seemed relatively clean. I watched a Bangladeshi man with a broom made from grass and twigs bustling around, sweeping up trash.

"Our sweepers wash the floors daily with an antiseptic solution," the nurse told me as we walked through the wards. "Our infection rate is quite low in spite of the primitive conditions."

The hospital hallways were filled with nurses and staff carrying out their duties. The nurses looked tidy and professional in their white uniforms. The x-ray technicians and the operating room personnel wore green or brown scrubs. As we walked past the nurses' station and entered the wards, I noticed at least one person in each bed and other family members and visitors around it. The nurses informed me that additional patients would be put onto gurneys, cots, or the floor when these beds were full. As I smiled and greeted the patients as we walked through the ward, I wondered how long it would be before I could talk to them in their language and tell them of the spiritual healing of salvation which is taught in the Holy Bible.

Underneath each bed, there were pots and pans and sometimes even people. My guide explained that each patient was supposed to be accompanied by an attendant called a "sangi" (shongee), who would stay at his or her bedside to help with personal care and to provide food. She said that because we dealt with at least three major religious communities, each having their dietary restrictions, we did not provide food for the patients. Behind the hospital was a Bangladeshi-style kitchen in a shed with multiple cooking areas on the ground. The sangis brought the necessary cooking pots and pans and prepared meals for the patients and themselves in that kitchen. After the meals, the pots and pans were stored under the patient's bed. If a patient had no sangi to help them, prepared meals could be purchased from a restaurant across the road from the hospital and brought to the patient. Typically, the sangi would sleep on a floor mat beside the bed. However, there were occasions when the sangi would sleep in the bed with the patient, or the patient would choose to sleep on the floor to allow the sangi to have the bed. During my rounds to visit patients in the wards, it was essential to clearly identify who the patient was. Children were usually put into the female ward with their mothers.

I noticed that the beds in the wards were a mixture of various models. Some could be cranked into different positions and had a head and footboard to attach overhead frames, all made of wood and bamboo. God provided a remarkable variety of orthopedic equipment that I collected during my pre-field travels, which would be available when the hospital shipment arrived. Amazingly, this included metal over-bed frames to replace the wooden and bamboo bed frames that were currently in use.

Also included were the multiple side arms, trapezes, and pulleys to make the overbed equipment functional. I was relieved to discover that some hospital beds in the wards were modern enough to accommodate this equipment. Along with these important pieces, I brought an orthopedic surgical table with all the accessories for my use during surgery.

Across the hall from the male nurses' station was a small Emergency Room, which also served as a room for minor surgery. It was about eight feet by ten feet, with an examining table, an overhead light, and a refrigerator for medication storage. If the application of a cast was necessary, it was done in the OPD or the operating room. Sadly, I could see that there was no area designated for orthopedics.

To the right of the Emergency Room were the doors to the clean hall leading to the two Operating Rooms and a delivery room/obstetrical operating room. We walked past several women in labor lying on gurneys in the hall, waiting their turn to deliver their babies.

We also toured the Intensive Care room. What made it "intensive" was that it was near the nurse's station and had blood pressure monitors attached to the wall beside each bed. It doubled as a post-anesthesia recovery room. Behind the male nurses' station were a few private and semi-private rooms. Two portable X-ray machines were positioned in the hallway, ready to be relocated to any department in the hospital as needed. The X-ray films were processed in the darkroom. The Central Supply Room (CSR) was located next to the X-ray room and held medical supplies and the autoclave for sterilizing instruments.

Behind the hospital was the workshop, where the mechanics maintained our vehicles, repaired and assembled equipment, and maintained the hospital facilities. Next to the workshop was a "godown," a storage room for hospital supplies. The hospital business office and post office were across the driveway from the main entrance to the hospital. I knew Tense would eagerly check our mailbox there every day for letters from home.

The nurse who gave me the tour told me that usually, there was at least one general surgeon on duty at the hospital, in addition to a family practice doctor and an OB/GYN. There was also a staff of three or more expatriate nurses from the US and Canada, along with national nurses.

She mentioned that the number of doctors could be severely limited for various periods of time. It was not unusual for them to be absent for furloughs, medical care, or government or family matters. This was not what I had expected. Suddenly, I realized that I could be the only physician at the hospital for months at a time.

I could see that the hospital was functional but very primitive by US standards. I thought I was prepared for that but had not realized how primitive it was. Much of my medical training had been in modern hospitals. I knew I would see things I had not even read about. At that time, there was no one with whom I could consult and no internet or even telephones at the hospital. I would have to rely heavily on the old books in the medical library. I was encouraged when I remembered the extensive collection of orthopedic journals and textbooks that had been donated and were on their way.

Reflections

At the end of my hospital tour, the nurse showing me around turned to me. "What do you think?" she asked.

Reflecting on my background and experience, I could see God had prepared me to serve in such a facility. The skills I had gained in a small country practice where I had to do everything myself, including X-rays and some lab tests, would be invaluable in this setting. I could improve and upgrade the X-ray department, which was vital to my work as an orthopedic surgeon. My seven years of general practice, my experience with obstetrics, and my training in general surgery had prepared me for the times when I would be the only doctor at MCH.

"I'm impressed," I told her. "I can see that much thought and preparation has gone into the hospital's planning. I am certain I will be able to function here." She seemed pleased with my answer.

During the tour, though, I realized that I would need to make some necessary changes at the hospital to render good care to my orthopedic patients. I would need a designated orthopedic space because some procedures must be done on tables with special equipment. I needed to set up an orthopedic department with a cast room. I also needed to train some of the staff as orthopedic technicians to assist me in orthopedic procedures and aftercare. However, all that had to wait as my first assignment was two years of learning the Bangladeshi language. During that time, I was not supposed to become involved with patient care, devoting all my time and energy to learning the difficult language.

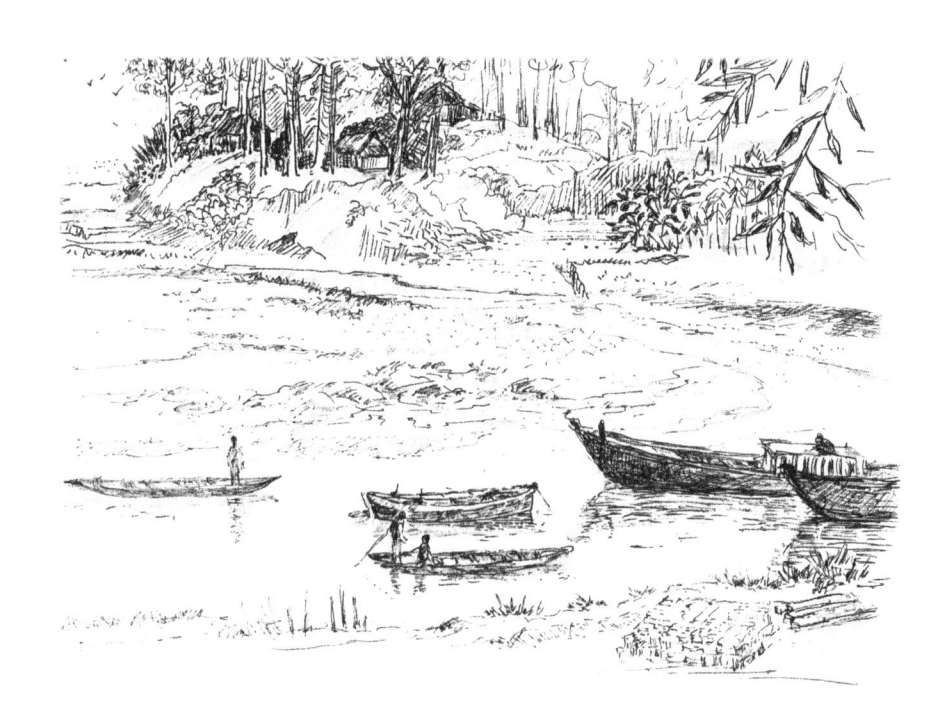

CHAPTER 17

Critical Time

We were eager to begin our study of Bengali and hoped to become sufficiently fluent to converse with our Bangladeshi friends and patients. Language study had previously been held in Chittagong and was a two-year program. This year, the class was to be held at the hospital compound at Malumghat since Tense and I and two nurses, Karen and Alice, would all be working there. None of the language teachers were available immediately, so the class was postponed until December.

Our arrival was at a critical time. The short-term surgeon filling in for the summer had just left, and Dr. Olsen was still in Dhaka working on administrative matters. Since there was a severe doctor shortage with only one other surgeon on duty, the Medical Committee asked if I could begin work at the hospital with a translator until our language class began. I happily agreed to do this, but I told my coworkers that the patients would assume that I could speak or understand Bengali. They told me I should tell my patients I could not speak Bengali by saying, "Ahmi Bangla jahni na," which translates to "I don't know Bengali." The confusing part was that I told them in Bengali that I didn't know Bengali.

Doctor Shoppers

One group of patients, whom we called the "doctor shoppers," were an annoyance to the medical staff. In Bangladesh, doctor's offices did not keep the patient's medical records (except for MCH). Instead of doctors and hospitals holding medical records, patients were given their records to carry with them. Occasionally, when dealing with persistent shoppers, the documentation tended to become rather extensive. We called these people "thick chart patients." It was annoying because it took a lot of time to review the records to determine the patient's problem and discover what diagnostic work and treatment had already been done. We also realized that we would not be the final doctor for this type of patient. He would soon be on his way with our recommendations in his hands to give to the next doctor.

One day, as I was leaving the post office in front of the hospital, I was approached by one of these "thick chart patients" holding his sheaf of documents. He began speaking to me, and I politely replied, "Ahmi Bangla jahni na." He looked surprised but began speaking again, this time in a louder voice. Again, I told him in Bengali that I did not understand Bengali. With an even more surprised look, he spoke again, louder and with a bit more urgency in his voice. For the third time, I told him, "Ahmi Bangla jahni na."

Exasperated, he burst out, "Sahib, I am speaking English." His accent was so thick that it sounded like Bengali, but he was speaking English.

Help Arrives

Steve Morris, a senior medical student who later became a plastic surgeon, had just arrived, increasing our doctor coverage. I began doing surgeries immediately, assisted by Steve Morris and Dr. Peter MacField. Dr. Peter helped get me oriented at the hospital, and I learned much from him. One evening, the MacFields joined us for dinner at the guesthouse, and Dr. Peter and I discussed my plans for his orthopedic training.

I saw some spectacular orthopedic cases and challenges in the first two weeks. One patient was a woman whose hip had been dislocated for four months before she came to the hospital. Another was a girl whose hip had been fractured for two months. We also handled cases of severe osteomyelitis, several tumors, a hand tendon transplant, and a tetanus case. All these cases required long-term follow-up care, which gave the patients time to hear the good news of salvation as taught in the Holy Bible. On my third day of working in the hospital, we were suddenly inundated with emergency patients from a bus accident caused by a head-on collision. There were many orthopedic trauma cases. I was just six years out of my orthopedic residency, and I was seeing things I had only read about. This was my first indication of how challenging my work would be in my new assignment at MCH.

News from Home

We received a telegram in early August about the birth of our first grandchild, Rachel. It had been difficult to go to Bangladesh before she was born. Chrissa's letter with details about Rachel's birth arrived two weeks later. We did not meet our new granddaughter until our first furlough three years later.

Soon after arriving at Malumghat, we began receiving letters from my mother in the US. It was comforting to know she was well cared for in her new senior retirement home, enjoying church activities and making new friends. In her letter, she mentioned she was reading her Bible, praying every morning after breakfast, and planning to speak to her pastor about getting baptized. She was also looking forward to her sister's upcoming visit. She sounded so happy, and I was encouraged by her cheerful letter.

Heart House

As I began working at the hospital, Tense assisted with the behind-the-scenes work, helped unpack shipping drums, and sorted and organized medicines. She also helped with the Heart House ministry. Heart House was a rehabilitation support ministry on the MCH compound created after the war for Bangladeshi widows and disabled women. At Heart House, these women were taught to make handicrafts to sell to support their families. They made a variety of handicrafts, including Bengali cultural dolls dressed in colorful costumes, beautifully embroidered fans, table runners, and bags made from woven tribal cloth.

Doctor Olsen and Dr. DeCook Return

On August 16, Dr. Olsen arrived from Dhaka and gave our team the wonderful news that he had been able to negotiate "Duty-free and Privileged Person" status with the Bangladesh government for our team and the hospital. That would allow duty-free entry of goods and supplies sent to the hospital. It would also allow our NGO staff to import vehicles and household goods duty-free. Our being at MCH to handle the patient load had enabled Dr. Olsen to spend the necessary time in Dhaka to work on this important matter. Dr. Joe DeCook, an OB/GYN, returned to Malumghat with his family on August 20th, shortly after Dr. Olsen returned to the hospital.

Physical Therapy Department

Patients who came to MCH often required more than quick medical or surgical treatment. They needed many hours of careful, compassionate physical therapy to improve or restore function to disabled limbs and backs. This was something for which the doctors and nurses had neither the time nor the expertise. In 1970, God brought a well-trained physical therapist named Larry Golin to the hospital. He immediately began to assemble a Physical Therapy (PT) Department. Larry trained men and women nurses to be his PT Department staff. The result was a fully functioning physical therapy department in this remote jungle station with separate facilities for men and women. At first, the PT department dealt mainly with joint problems, paralysis, and crutch training.

Limb and Brace Shop Established

When Tense and I arrived in Bangladesh in 1974 and began language studies, Larry began to set up a Limb and Brace Shop in addition to the existing PT Department. The Limb and Brace Shop consisted of a workshop that manufactured braces and artificial limbs to meet the needs of orthopedic patients. Larry knew that the PT Department and the Limb and Brace Shop were vital to the functioning of the orthopedic work I would be doing because of the huge volume of post-war amputees that were coming to the hospital for treatment and artificial limbs. Often, a person who lost an arm or a leg could no longer continue in their occupation and would become a beggar. If he had a family, this would also mean economic disaster for them. Those disabled from birth were destined to live a life of begging. The Limb and Brace Shop gave new limbs and new hope to many who were disabled. Some who had never been able to walk learned to walk with the aid of braces. Our Limb and Brace Shop was the only facility of its kind for several million people in this part of Bangladesh.

Larry traveled all over Bangladesh and other countries to obtain the necessary supplies to build the prosthetic arms and legs. The challenge was to produce the prosthetics with locally available materials, and that required a lot of improvising. Larry then trained workers to build the prosthetics. At first, relatively simple leg and arm braces were constructed. I worked with the Limb and Brace Shop to tell them what was needed and to give advice on the construction of these devices.

Larry located a trained PT technician from Dhaka willing to come to MCH to supervise the Limb and Brace Shop. He also hired additional helpers for the PT Department. Larry trained them to do physical therapy and to help patients learn to use their braces and artificial limbs. Finding capable workers willing to come to live and work in our remote location was difficult.

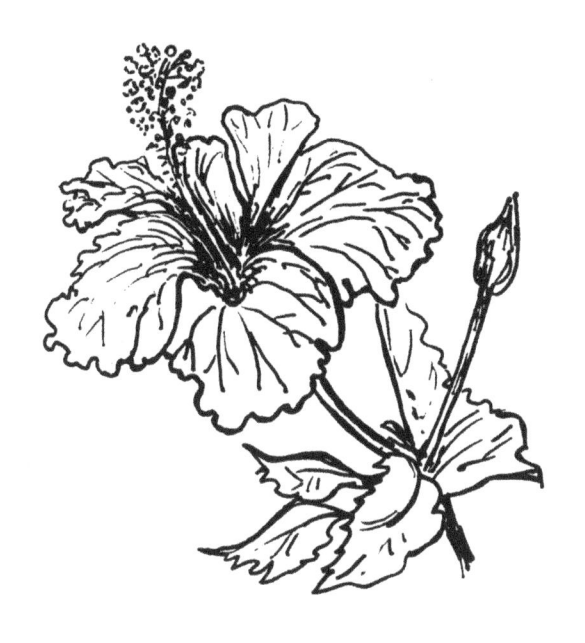

CHAPTER 18

Unexpected Changes

Dr. Peter dies

At 6:30 a.m. on August 30th, there was a knock on our door. When I opened it, Dr. Olsen was standing there. "I have some very bad news for you," he said. "Dr. Peter had a massive heart attack early this morning and died. There was no chance to save him." This was a big blow to the medical work and a shock to everyone. Dr. Peter was only 34 years old. He was deeply loved and respected, and he had a powerful testimony among the nationals at the hospital. We had the privilege of working with him for only one month. The gospel was preached at his funeral and graveside service, and many hospital employees heard the message of salvation through faith in Jesus, as taught in the Holy Bible. At the funeral, Dr. Peter's older brother decided to believe in Jesus for salvation.

Mother dies

On the day following Dr. Peter's death, we received a telegram from the assisted living retirement home in California where my mother was staying. The telegram stated that she had died suddenly on August 28, with no advance warning. Five days later, we received Mother's final letter to us, the fifth one she had written. In her letter, she said she wanted to be baptized and join the church she had been attending and was working through the details with the pastor. We were gratefully assured that she was in heaven waiting for us. I wanted to return to the US to handle her final affairs. However, this was impossible because of the acute doctor shortage resulting from Dr. Peter's death. I was seeing over 200 patients each day and already had 25 orthopedic patients in the hospital.

My mother's final affairs were attended to by my cousin, Roy Chattin, as I had previously arranged with him, and we greatly appreciated his help. We just needed to let our family know. There was no telephone at the hospital. The government was not willing to run a telephone line all the way down to the hospital site, through the forest, and across waterways. We would have had to drive three hours to Chittagong to make a phone call to notify our family of my mother's death. But because we had arranged for Roy to handle her final affairs, he was able to notify the family for us, and we also wrote letters to our family.

Anytime we wanted to make a phone call, we had to travel to the ABWE office in Chittagong. Then, we had to speak with an operator who would assist us in connecting the call. The operator would instruct us to hang up but stay close to the phone. Several hours later, the phone would ring, and the operator would say she could finally place our call. Sometimes, we waited up to four hours in the office for a call to be placed. This was particularly challenging as the time difference between the US and Chittagong was twelve hours. Our call had to be placed at night in

Bangladesh to reach the US in the daytime. The cost at that time was about US $3.00 per minute. Eventually, the ABWE office in Chittagong obtained direct dial service, eliminating the need for lengthy waits to place calls. However, our calls still had to be made at night because of the time difference between Bangladesh and the US. We did not make many calls to the US because of these difficulties.

Communication Challenges

Communication with the outside world continued to be a challenge. The postal service was slow. We wrote hundreds of letters on blue aerograms to our family, our supporting churches, and supporting individuals. An airmail letter mailed from Bangladesh would arrive in the US at least ten days later, and a letter from the US took at least two weeks to reach us in Bangladesh. We typically had to wait at least three weeks before receiving an answer to a letter. National and religious holidays also slowed mail delivery.

Our incoming mail was subject to censorship for many years, considerably slowing down its delivery. Each of us was assigned a censor by the government who opened our mail and read it before passing it on to us. The censor had to get to know our entire family to understand our letters. When a new person arrived at the station, it would be weeks before they started receiving mail from home. We could always tell when our mail had been opened and read by the censor because it would be glued shut with brown glue.

We felt isolated and disconnected from the rest of the world. We could get news via radio broadcasts from the Voice of America and the British Broadcasting Company. Since we did not speak Bengali, we were grateful that we had a weekly church service for English speakers.

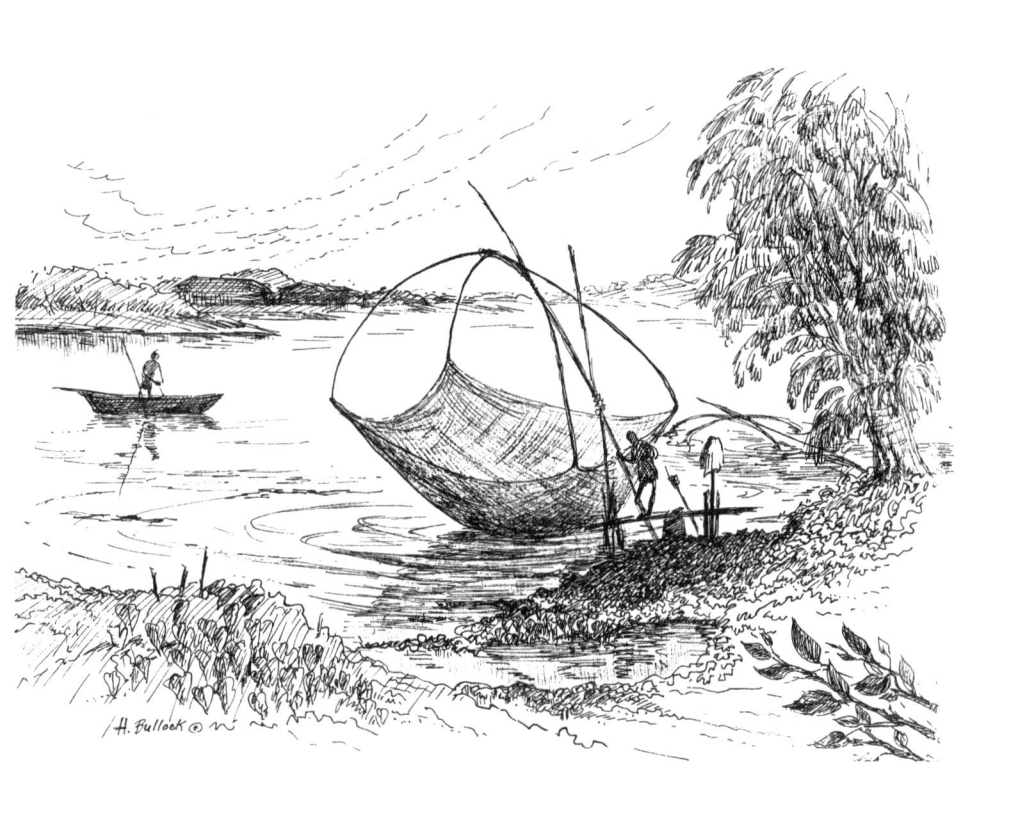

CHAPTER 19

His Perfect Salvation to Tell

Personal Work at the Hospital

At the time of our arrival in 1974, patients waiting to be seen in the OPD would have the opportunity to hear a Bible story in the waiting room. If patients were admitted to the hospital, they would have the opportunity to speak with a national personal worker who visited in the wards and spoke their language. Personal workers shared the message of God's love and salvation as taught in the Holy Bible. Often, the expatriate doctors and nurses would have opportunities to teach biblical truths to their patients. Our national staff of nurses, technicians, and workshop personnel were from multiple religious backgrounds. We wanted them also to have an opportunity to learn about God's plan for man as taught in the Holy Bible. The doctors and other expatriate staff held regular Bible classes with the national staff to share biblical truths.

However, many patients who came to our hospital could not read or write, so printed literature was useless. Patients were given the opportunity to listen to Bible messages and Christian music on individual cassette players in the patient wards if they desired. Most patients were eager to have a personal cassette player at their bedside and played it loudly for all to hear. These tape players were also taken into the villages, and groups gathered to listen to the messages.

Card Talks

Before going to Bangladesh, we visited the Gospel Recordings office in Los Angeles, which produced Bible-teaching materials in many languages for distribution worldwide. At that time, they were producing messages on eight-inch phonograph records. The records could be played on any phonograph. For use in places without electricity, the records could be played on cardboard phonographs called "Card Talks." These were made of flat cardboard panels creased and folded into a triangle. The record was placed on a spindle, and one of the panels contained a phonograph needle, which was set down on the record. A hole was drilled in the record's center so a pencil or pen point could be used to turn it. When the record was turned, the needle produced a sound amplified by the cardboard panel. This acted like a phonograph record player.

The cost for each of these units was five cents. We brought a supply of Card Talks and records to Bangladesh. These were used by the personal workers in the hospital to share gospel messages in the patient wards. These Card Talks were also used in villages. When the record was played, it quickly drew a crowd. Children were especially fascinated by these cardboard phonographs that talked in their language.

Bullock Cart

Making rounds in the hospital wards offered some challenges. I needed to have diagnostic instruments, tools to care for casts, and traction apparatus readily available as I checked on each patient. The solution was to have the workshop construct a rolling cart with drawers in which I could place diagnostic instruments and necessary tools to manage casts and traction. I also carried a selection of books that I might need regarding the care needs of patients.

Then, I stocked the cart with coloring books, crayons, toy cars, dolls, stuffed animals for the children, perfume, lipstick samples, and flowers for women patients. Not many patients could read, but I had some gospel tracts for those who could. This cart could be pushed from bed to bed as I made my rounds to check on my patients. It was called the "Bullock cart" and was extremely helpful and efficient. All the children loved the crayons and toys. This cart opened the door to my visiting with the patients or their relatives, and they looked forward to my coming.

Struck by Lightning and the Other Guy

The hospital had been running at nearly full occupancy with urgent and critical cases, and we were operating with few nurses. One day, a man struck by lightning was brought to the hospital. I told him through the interpreter that sometimes God has to do something extreme to get our attention, and that he would be hearing a very important message while in our hospital. I urged him to give his full attention to this message, which was the good news from the Holy Bible about God's plan of salvation.

Throughout his treatment at the hospital, the man heard the message of salvation as taught in the Holy Bible. I never discovered whether this man responded to the message and received the gift of salvation. However, an amputee patient on the opposite side of the ward had been listening when the personal worker shared the good news of salvation with the patient struck by lightning. The amputee patient did receive that gift of salvation during his hospital stay. I was thrilled to see the new light in his eyes and the joy on his face as he grew in his spiritual understanding each day.

Crank Cassette Players

The Card Talks cardboard record players worked well but didn't last long with repeated playing. Gospel Recordings had also developed a small cassette player/recorder called a "crank cassette player" that could be used to teach Bible lessons. These looked like a cassette player/recorder but did not require electricity or batteries. Instead, the crank cassette player was activated by turning a hand crank. The sound was much louder than the Card Talk record players and could be used multiple times before wearing out. We took some of these to Bangladesh when we returned after furlough. The Audiovisual Department (AV) ordered 25 more crank cassette players from Gospel Recordings in the US to be used in our hospital personal work.

Upon the arrival of the crank cassette players at the port of Chittagong, our shipment clearance agent informed us that the Customs Office had refused to allow us to bring them in. The Customs officials suspected that we intended to sell the players. Selling them would have been a violation of our agreement with the government. The agent said that someone from the hospital would need to go to Chittagong to talk to the Customs Agent in person regarding the matter. I was elected to do that and arranged to travel the next day.

The Customs Agent was a stern-looking man with a beard and a white cap seated behind a desk in the crowded hall. The noisy room was filled with people dealing with customs issues. I showed him the crank cassette player I had brought and explained that we would not sell the units but would use them to play health teaching programs.

Tense had worked with our AV Department to produce health teaching lessons in the Chittagonian language. These were recorded onto cassette tapes. I had one of these cassettes and offered to play it for the Customs Agent. He agreed. When I turned the crank handle and the voice began speaking in Chittagonian, a sudden hush came over the entire hall. People stopped talking and searched for the source of the equipment speaking their language.

The agent then instructed me to talk with the head of the Customs Department. I was taken into that official's private office and again demonstrated the unit. Then I explained to him that we did not intend to sell the units and were planning to use them for public health teaching.

"Do they have batteries?" the official asked.

"No," I replied. "They are activated by turning a hand crank. Would you like to see inside it?"

"Yes," he said, nodding his head. I took a small screwdriver out of my pocket and opened the unit to show him the inside of the cassette player.

"No batteries!" exclaimed the official.

"No batteries," I agreed. The official signed the release documents allowing us to take the 25 crank cassette players. We used these crank cassette players at the hospital for several years until Gospel Recordings produced newer and more efficient equipment.

AWANA

Two of our NGO nurses started an international Awana club for Bangladeshi children at Malumghat. Awana, which stands for "Approved Workman Are Not Ashamed" (2 Timothy 2:15), is a Bible teaching and discipleship program developed in the United States for children two to eighteen. Tense used her art skills to modify the workbook illustrations to make them culturally appropriate with villages, ponds, and South Asian scenery and plants. The Awana program was so helpful in teaching children the Bible that many Bangladeshi churches later started their own clubs. Eventually, thousands of Awana clubs were started in Bangladesh and neighboring countries.

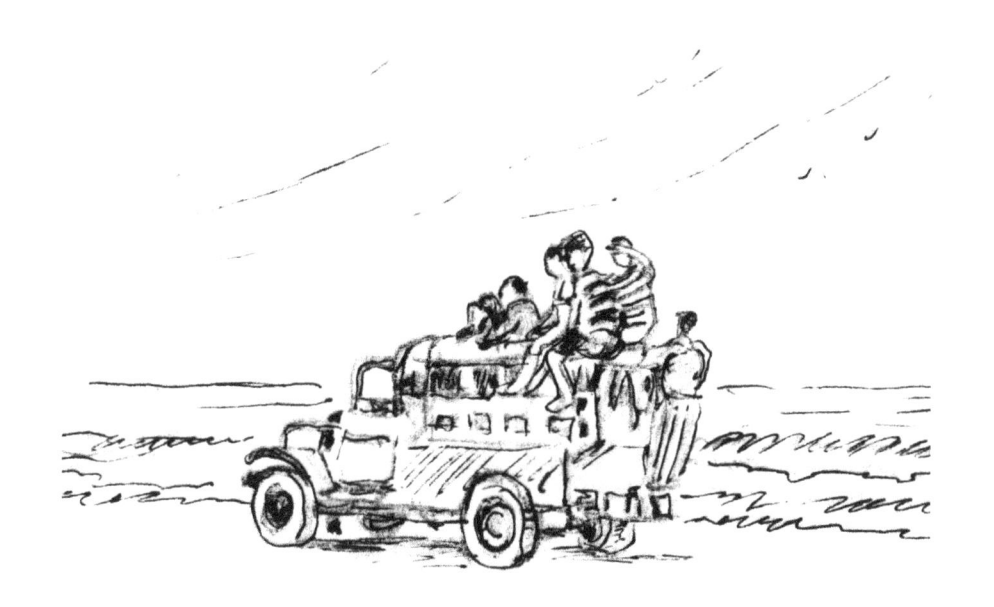

CHAPTER 20

Working with an Interpreter

By November 1974, I had performed over 75 surgeries and had seen hundreds of patients in the OPD. Trying to communicate with patients through an interpreter during those first few months was confusing, but it was a great incentive for me to learn Bengali. I had no idea what the interpreter was telling the patient. He usually would speak to the patients in Chittagonian, which I could not understand. When children came in and were being examined or treated, they squirmed and wiggled. I observed the medics say something to them that sounded like "No loreech," and then the children would stop wiggling. I decided to try to mimic their sounds to get a head start on learning Bengali.

"No Loreech—Don't Move"

One day, a distinguished elderly Muslim man wearing horn-rimmed glasses, a white cap, and a white Punjabi suit entered the OPD. He was carrying a briefcase under one arm and an umbrella under the other. He positioned himself on the examination table, ready for me to examine him. As I approached the table, he began to move around on the table. I decided it was time to try this new language. I looked him in the eye and said, "No loreech!" His eyes widened, and his jaw dropped open. I immediately knew I had said something inappropriate when the medics laughed so hard they could barely stand up.

The man understood my command and sat very still while I examined him. After he left, I asked the medics why they had laughed. They began to laugh again but managed to tell me that the language I had used with this distinguished gentleman was the style of language called the "tui" form that is used with a little child. However, my patient obeyed my command, so it seemed it worked with him.

Another time, I heard the medics telling a patient to "sit there," pointing to a chair or stool. They said something like "Aye kaju boyu," and the patient sat down. I heard this used with adults, so I assumed it must not be the child's language form and decided to try it at the next opportunity.

"Aye kaju boyu," I told my next patient, and the patient just looked at me. Then, the staff told him the same thing, and he sat down. After the patient left, I asked the medic why he had not understood my command.

"I told him exactly what you told him," I said. "He ignored me but obeyed you. What did I do wrong?" He smiled and said that my tone of voice made the difference. I was speaking too politely. Rather, I should speak gruffly for the patient to understand my command. I gave up trying to learn the language that way—at least for a while.

Frustration with Communication

My national translators were not fluent in English and sometimes had trouble understanding what I asked them to communicate to the patients or other staff. This led to some amusing and some not-so-amusing incidents. As I encountered these differences, I became extremely frustrated. Finally, one day, my frustration reached its peak.

A female patient had been admitted with a huge abscess on her thigh. My interpreter was absent, so I had to speak English to the national nurses. I wanted to aspirate some of the abscess fluid for culture. I asked the Bangladeshi nurse to bring me a large syringe and a large bore needle. After a short delay, she brought a tiny syringe and needle. I told her those things were not what I needed and explained again that I needed a very large syringe and a very large bore needle. When she returned the second time, she brought only a slightly larger syringe and a slightly larger bore needle—not large enough to aspirate what I thought would be thick pus. I became more frustrated. I thought the national nurses on the ward would understand English.

I recalled an instance during my orthopedic residency in the US when an orthopedic surgeon in a large American hospital was having maximum difficulty attempting to do a surgical procedure because of the Christmas celebration that was going on in the hospital. There were Christmas bells, decorations, and joviality. He became so frustrated that he stepped to the operating room door and yelled "HELP!" The staff rushed to find out what his problem was. He said, "Turn off those bells and get some people here to help me!" The staff turned their attention to his needs, and the procedure was accomplished.

"Maybe that is what I need to do," I thought. In desperation, I shouted "HELP!" as loudly as possible. NGO nurses and senior Bangladeshi nurses came running from all directions to discover the problem. I explained to them what size of syringe I needed. They finally brought me the large syringe and large bore needle, and the aspiration was easily completed. It took many minutes to perform this relatively simple task, and I was experiencing a high level of frustration. This situation taught me the importance of learning Bengali as quickly as possible so that I could communicate.

That day, I remembered a time in medical school when my psychiatry professor told the class how to respond to possible environmental stresses.

"You have three choices," he said. "1. Change the environment; 2. Adapt to the environment; or 3. Go crazy!" With that, he threw back his head and laughed loudly!

When I went home from the hospital for lunch, I told my wife that it seemed as though a huge mistake had been made. Either I was unsuitable for the work before me, or God had chosen the wrong person. I did not think I was going to be able to stay. Then I remembered an elderly widow back home in the US who had said she would pray for us daily and was giving $5.00 per month toward our support out of her meager Social Security income.

"How can I fail both her and God?" I asked myself.

Remembering the advice of the psychiatrist, I decided that I was probably not going to be able to change the environment very much or very soon. I was going to find it difficult to adapt to the environment without attempting to make changes, and I certainly did not want to go crazy. The only solution for me was to try a combination of choices—I would do my best to make changes in the environment, and at the same time, I would do my best to adapt to the environment.

As I thought about these things, a feeling of peace came over me. I realized that God makes no mistakes. He chose me for this job and sent me here. He was also fully aware of the difficulties I would encounter. He knew that I would have to reach the point where I admitted that I could not do things with my own strength but would have to call upon Him for strength and guidance. I recalled the Bible verse, Philippians 4:13: "I can do all things through Christ who strengthens me."

I have never forgotten this lesson. In the years ahead, I often prayed, "Lord, I don't know what to do in this situation. You called me here, and you know the situation. So, please tell me what to do." Then, a solution to the problem would become evident—sometimes not instantly, but always eventually. After all, it was not my battle but God's.

He certainly did help me during the succeeding years. Conditions at the hospital continued to improve, making it much more like what I had been used to. To my amazement, my expectations also changed drastically over the years. I adapted to the environment and found I could function quite well in extremely difficult situations. It had happened!

Khana at Cox's Bazar

Shortly after I began working at the hospital with the aid of an interpreter, an official with the fisheries department of Cox's Bazar came to the hospital with chest pain after a rickshaw accident. X-rays revealed a fractured rib, but there was no indication of any damage to his lungs. He requested to be admitted to the hospital and specifically asked for a private room. Fortunately, we had a private room available where he could rest in bed and receive pain medication as required. His wife remained with him during his stay.

As part of his government duties, the patient was often required to meet with people from Cox's Bazar. However, his private room was not spacious enough to accommodate groups of more than a dozen people. To address this, he was wheeled out of his room and taken to the front of the hospital, where he held meetings under a shade tree. We suspected he had requested to remain at our hospital because he could not accommodate such a crowd of petitioners at his home in Cox's Bazar.

After a few weeks, his chest pain had subsided enough that he could safely be discharged, but he asked to stay a few more days. Finally, he agreed to go home for further recuperation. Upon leaving, he insisted that I bring my family to his home in Cox's Bazar so he could entertain us. When I told him I could not be absent from the hospital for a long time and had no transportation, he said he would send his car and driver to pick us up. We were excited about experiencing our first khana in Bangladesh as invited guests.

We informed our Guest House hostess that we would not be eating lunch at the Guest House because we had been invited to this man's house for a khana. She suggested we eat lunch before going because it was Ramadan. She thought they probably wouldn't feed us until after sunset, as Muslims fast from sunrise to sunset during Ramadan.

After lunch at the Guest House, the driver arrived to take us to Cox's Bazar. When we arrived at the patient's house, we were taken into the front room and seated at a table. The room was stark, with bare walls made of boards, and the windows were open with no glass. The room's back wall was also made of boards, but there were many knotholes. Each knothole had an eye peeking through, and the door to the room behind the wall was covered with a curtain. We knew people behind that wall were watching us, but we could not see them.

Our host had assured us that an English speaker would be present, but our server spoke only a few words of English. He placed bowls and a water pitcher on the table and then stood silently as if waiting for us to do something.

"I think he wants us to wash our hands with this water," I whispered to David and Tense. I poured water from the pitcher over my hands into the bowl. I could tell from the server's expression that I had done the right thing, and he handed me a towel. David and Tense did the same. Then, to our amazement, he picked up the bowls, threw the water out the open window, and put the bowls back on the table in front of us to use with the meal.

Next, he brought out a big bowl of rice and many other bowls of different foods. We were already full from eating lunch at the Guest House but felt we must eat something from each bowl. We were expected to eat with our fingers and help ourselves to the food in the serving bowls with our hands since there were no utensils, following the Bengali custom. We heard giggles from the back room behind the curtained door as we did this. Finally, when we had eaten as much as we could put into our already full stomachs, our host came into the room and sat at the table with us. We were served cups of Bengali tea with milk and sugar, and it was delicious. Our host drank some with us, as it seemed he was not keeping the Ramadan fast.

After tea, Tense was invited to go behind the curtain into the back room to visit with the women and children who had been watching us through the knotholes. Tense had brought a hand puppet to show them, and she sang "Jesus Loves Me" to them in English. Eventually, we were taken back to Malumghat. We were entertained royally but also learned important cultural customs.

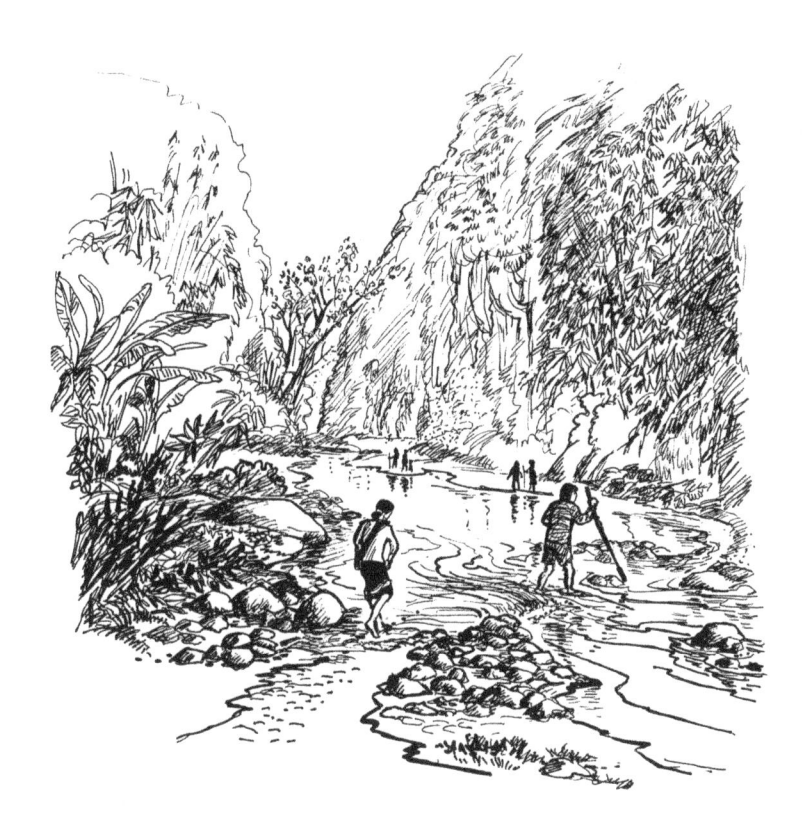

CHAPTER 21

A New Medical World

Orthopedics in the OPD

The hospital had only fifty beds available, ten for each male and female ward and ten designated for obstetrics. I could easily have filled all of those beds with orthopedic patients, but other doctors also needed to use some of those beds for their patients. Once, when I was the only doctor at the hospital, there were 96 patients admitted. We had to accommodate some in beds, some on cots, some on gurneys, and some on the floor.

There was no separate orthopedic department. Orthopedic cases were seen along with the general non-orthopedic cases in the Outpatient Department's examination rooms. Patients would line up in the alley leading to two sets of waiting and examination rooms: one for men and another for women and children. Each examination room was about twenty feet square, with a small, curtained cubicle measuring about six by eight feet on one side of the room. In the center of the room was a small table, about three feet square, where the patient was seated beside an interpreter because we frequently dealt with languages other than Bengali. The doctor who examined the patient sat on the other side of the table or took the patient into the curtained cubicle for a more detailed private examination, if necessary. Surrounding the table stood a dozen or so patients intent on watching the show. Soon, it would be their turn to sit at the table and be the "star of the show."

This was a shock to me. It was like working in a train station! Any casts that needed to be applied were done in the middle of the room or in the private cubicle. If anesthesia was necessary, the patient would be taken to the operating room.

Before I went to Bangladesh, I assumed the facilities and equipment at the hospital would be primitive in contrast to what I was used to in the hospitals in the US. I imagined I would see orthopedic problems I had never encountered while practicing in the US. When I first began seeing patients at the hospital, I soon became aware that I had entered a new medical world. The types of medical problems I encountered and my ability to care for these unusual problems using the available equipment and medications challenged me in ways I had never experienced. The difficulties in communication with patients because of the language barrier and their lack of understanding only added to the challenge. I could only hope and pray that God would give me the guidance and insight I needed to treat my patients despite these difficult challenges.

No Understanding of Anatomy or Physiology

I discovered that the Bangladeshis had little knowledge of the anatomy or physiology of their bodies. Much of what they had learned was based on superstition and custom. Many times, it was difficult to explain the treatment they needed and what we hoped to accomplish for them because they did not understand. We could only say, "An operation will be necessary." Sometimes, the patients would assume that we wanted to do surgery because we wanted their money. The majority of people in Bangladesh were living in poverty and had limited resources. As a result, they were suspicious of everyone's motives.

Improper Treatment from the Village "Healer"

It was unusual to see wounds and fractures soon after they had happened. It was a common practice in Bangladesh to go to a local village "healer" who treated injured joints in a disgusting manner. These healers (called "hammer doctors") would apply heavy pressure or massage on the affected area while using a type of lubricant. Then, they would tightly bandage the area. After a few months or years, the patient would arrive at our hospital with complaints of constant pain and swelling in that joint, along with a significant decrease in mobility.

If the affected joint was in the right arm, it was especially bad. In Bangladeshi culture, losing the ability to use the right hand or arm was particularly devastating. Bangladeshis traditionally eat using their right hand to pick up food and bring it to their mouth. The right hand was not only important for eating but also for cooking or feeding another person or a child.

The left hand was designated for toilet cleansing. At that time, Bangladeshis didn't use toilet paper, only a small pot of water and their left hand. Consequently, the left hand was always considered unclean and was never used for eating, no matter how much it had been washed. If someone lost his right hand or arm, he would be forced to use his toilet hand to eat with his fingers, and he would be treated as an outcast. It was also considered impolite to hand something to someone with your left hand. The recipient would recoil as if you were attempting to hand that person a snake.

I could almost always improve the motion in the damaged elbow by performing a "fascial arthroplasty." That procedure involved removing all the soft tissue in the elbow joint right down to the bone. Then, the bare bones were lined with heavy fascial tissue taken from the side of either thigh. This provided a gliding surface that would allow motion of the joint. After the fascia had been attached, a steel rod was inserted through the proximal part of the ulna, across the joint, and into the marrow cavity of the humerus. After several weeks, the rod was removed to allow movement in the joint. It typically took six weeks of exercise and use by the patient to regain near-normal elbow motion, which enabled a person to eat with their hand. Patients were grateful to have the use of their right hand restored.

Damage from Village Healers

The treatment by village "healers" often caused further damage or infection. I saw some bizarre types of attempted treatment. One patient who came to the OPD had a plug inserted into his skin just below the knee. The plug was fashioned out of bamboo and covered with wax. The object was pointed, and tight bandaging caused skin erosion beneath the plug until it was embedded in an infected crater. When I questioned the patient about the plug, he said it was for control of pain in the lower part of the leg. On examination, it was evident that the plug was located near the saphenous nerve just below the knee joint but was not close to the nerve. Damage to the saphenous nerve could cause sensation loss in parts of the lower leg.

The patient objected when I told him I wanted to remove the plug. He had spent a lot of money and had gone through a lot of pain to get it where it was. He did not want to lose whatever benefit he thought it might produce. Sometimes, we were able to convince patients to have surgery to remove a herniated intervertebral disc, which was the most common cause of lower leg pain. Explaining the situation to the patient took a lot of effort, and the interpreters struggled to convey my message accurately.

We could not ask for lab work or x-rays and then expect the patient to return after several days for an explanation of the results and the treatment plan because they often had traveled a long distance and had nowhere to stay. The patients could stay in a boarding house across the road for a few days if necessary, but it was too expensive for some. Later, we developed a special national guest house on our hospital property for temporary patient lodging.

Delays in Treatment Due to Extreme Circumstances

Often, patients waited days, months, or even years after an injury before seeking treatment at the hospital. Any treatment usually had to be done on the day of their arrival or soon thereafter. Some conditions could have been easily handled if the patient had come soon after his or her injury. Seeing a "fresh" open fracture that had not been "treated" with traditional procedures by the village healer was, in a strange way, refreshing.

On one occasion, a Tribal man arrived at the hospital on an upturned wooden table that was being used as a stretcher. He was suffering from an intertrochanteric fracture of his femur. The injury had happened three weeks earlier, miles up the river in the Hill Tracts. I asked the patient why he had waited so long to come to the hospital. He explained that he had to wait until the flood waters subsided enough for him to be carried on the dirt trail along the river. Then, it took several days for his friends to bring him to the hospital. Patients often traveled long distances, sometimes under extreme circumstances such as road closures due to floods or strikes. Usually, it was expensive for them to come.

We might have been able to operate on his fracture by introducing a stainless-steel nail and plate. Then, the patient could be moved about much more easily, but still, he would not be allowed to bear weight for several weeks until the fracture had healed sufficiently. The problem with this patient was that his hemoglobin was very low. He needed to have blood available to have surgery. No one was willing to donate blood for this patient, and he did not have sufficient money to purchase blood from the blood bank, so surgery was not possible. The only other option was to apply traction to the leg until the fracture had healed enough to allow mobilization, but still not with full weight bearing. With surgery, he could have gone home in two weeks, but the traction treatment required a much longer stay at the hospital.

Several weeks later, while I was making my rounds, I noticed that he was crying. When I asked him why, he explained that he had just learned that his wife had died. She had stayed in the village and starved to death because no one would feed her in his absence. Women did not go to the market, and she had no one to go for her to buy food. She had to resort to begging. Ultimately, after several weeks, she died of starvation. We were devastated when we heard what had happened. Situations like this taught us to carefully consider all aspects of the care we recommended and its impact on both the patient and their family. If we had known that his wife was in such a situation, we likely would have performed surgery so he could have returned home sooner.

Lack of Proper Post-operative Care

Another problem we often encountered was the patient's or family's inability or refusal to carry out discharge instructions or to make suitable dressing changes. They had to be instructed how to prepare relatively clean cloth bandages by sterilizing the cloth with a hot iron if they had one. The iron that was commonly used was made of cast iron with a wood handle. It had a chamber into which hot coals could be inserted to heat the iron. It was heavy, cumbersome, and dangerous.

Rabies

I soon learned to respect what the national nurses knew about the patients coming to the hospital. On one occasion, an elderly woman was brought to the OPD in a comatose condition and was placed on a gurney. The other doctor and I began checking her pupils and other signs associated with comas. Suddenly, one of the national nurses picked up a chart and waved it in front of the woman's face. The patient winced as the air struck her face, and the national nurse shouted, "Rabies!"

We immediately stopped all contact with the patient for our protection and placed her in an isolated location. She died a few hours later because there is no treatment for rabies. It is prevalent in Bangladesh, and the hospital staff are given rabies vaccines regularly.

Tetanus

When we arrived in the 1970s, the hospital wards commonly contained several tetanus patients. I had never encountered tetanus cases in my practice in the United States. Tetanus was one of the major causes of death in Bangladesh and occurred mostly in infants whose umbilical cord had been cut by the village midwife using a non-sterile sharpened bamboo knife. Older children would get infected by cuts and wounds. Boys about age twelve who had undergone ritual circumcision using non-sterile equipment would often become infected with tetanus. In Bangladesh, many people walk barefoot. Stepping on sharp objects with bare feet can result in penetrating wounds to the foot, which may potentially lead to tetanus.

The disease was marked by severe spasms with backward arching. We had no cure for the disease. All we could do was heavily sedate the patient to try to control or reduce the spasms. If possible, we tried to clean up the wound. On one occasion, I was introducing some newly arrived short-term doctors around the hospital, and we saw a twelve-year-old boy patient with tetanus. His back was sharply arched backward, and he was gasping for breath. After showing the patient to them, I moved on to the next patient.

"Wait a minute! We have never seen this before. Don't go too fast," one of the visiting doctors exclaimed.

Another patient who had severe tetanus was a little boy of about four years of age. It seemed unlikely that he would survive. When I arrived at the hospital the next morning and went into the ward where he had been, I was sad to see the bed empty. In my mind, it could only mean that he had died. But then I heard a strange sound behind me. Looking around, I was surprised to see that little boy standing stark naked, holding onto an oxygen cylinder hand truck with both hands and making motor noises with his lips, pretending that he was driving a truck! Boys will be boys in any culture! He recovered and was able to go home a few days later.

Improper Wound Care

Often, a patient would arrive with an open fracture (where bone fragments had penetrated the skin) to which a "dressing" had been applied. These dressings typically consisted of cow manure covered with banana leaves and bound with a vine. It was impossible to provide definitive care for such a wound on the day the patient arrived at the hospital. The soft tissue damage needed to be treated before addressing the skeletal damage. The fracture was often severely infected, along with collateral damage, such as serious skin issues, that could have been avoided.

Gentian Violet and Magnesium Sulfate

When I was in general practice in the US, many antibiotics had not yet been discovered. Some other things were commonly used to help prevent or treat infections. One of these things was gentian violet, a bright purple solution. It was commonly used to treat mouth ulcers and had several notable features:

- It was bacteriostatic, meaning it inhibited the growth of certain bacteria;
- It had fungicidal properties, effectively combating some fungal infections;
- It promoted the regeneration and multiplication of epithelial cells; and
- It had an attractive appearance.

When I got to the hospital in Bangladesh, I had no idea what sort of bacterial and fungal problems I was going to encounter. We didn't have a large supply of antibiotic ointments, so I decided to use gentian violet on wounds and incisions. I also used a tincture of Merthiolate (now withdrawn because of the mercury content). It was red in color and was a powerful bactericide. The NGO nurses told me that the patients liked these colorful medications because they made them feel that something had been applied to their problem.

The word got out about the purple solution, and people began using gentian violet in the villages, too. One day, a man came to the hospital with his arm wrapped in a cloth from fingertips to the shoulder. I asked him about his problem, and he unwrapped the cloth. As he uncovered his shoulder, I could see it was completely purple, covered with gentian violet. As the rest of the wrapper was removed, we could see that the entire arm and hand were covered with gentian violet. Finally, we saw his basic problem—a small cut on one of his fingers. He probably thought, "if a little bit does a lot of good, a whole lot should do a whole lot better."

When this Osmopak was applied to a wound, it would draw the fluids out and any purulent matter like pus. This type of poultice paste was not available at the hospital site. But magnesium salts were available. I had our Central Supply staff make a saturated magnesium sulfate solution—as much as will dissolve in sterile normal saline—and used that as moist packs for dressings. The patients did not like it because it stung, like applying salt to an open wound, but it was effective. Such dressings were changed several times a day if there was an infection.

I had been taught that honey applied to an open wound would stimulate granulation tissue to form and provide a base for epithelial cells to grow out onto. In Bangladesh, honey was in short supply, so I used granulated sugar instead. It was plentiful and worked just as well as the honey. The ants didn't seem to like it, so it did not cause any problems. Measures like this helped prevent infection. In fact, the infection rate among my orthopedic patients was lower than what I was used to in the US. The Bengali people have so much exposure to bacteria growing up that they develop a strong level of immunity in their systems. The infections we did see were mainly in non-native individuals like us. Unfortunately, as new doctors came in, many stopped using these methods, leading to an increase in the infection rate.

Conditions I'd Never Seen

Often, patients would come to the hospital with conditions that I had never seen or read about in my US training or practice. I was required to do procedures for which I had no formal training or experience. Sometimes, I was the only doctor at the hospital for weeks or months, and I had no one I could consult about the treatment. In situations like this, I felt out of my comfort zone.

I had to make a choice. Should I do my best to perform the procedure, or should I send the patient to another hospital? Sometimes, it would be too hazardous for the patient to be sent to another hospital. After consulting the old medical books in the hospital library, I would try my best to perform the procedure. Later, I would teach what I learned to other doctors at MCH.

My "Secret Weapon"

When I came to a point in a surgical procedure where I didn't know what to do next, I would stop and pray, asking God to guide my hands and show me what to do. Often, as I prayed, an idea would pop into my head. I would try the new idea, and it would work. I saw patients get well when I didn't expect them to. However, some patients died despite the best care we could give them. It was all in God's hands. I learned to pray for guidance and trust in God while caring for a diabetic patient at the clinic in San Luis Obispo.

While finishing my last few months at the San Luis Medical Clinic before going to Bangladesh, I wondered if I had enough experience and expertise to handle all the unusual cases or rare conditions I would encounter. Medical practice in the US does not usually involve unusual or rare entities. One gains experience handling these kinds of cases through many years of practice. But I did not have many years of practice.

It was at that time that an elderly man in our church who was diabetic came in with dark areas high up in his forefoot. It was evident that the arterial supply of blood to his leg was steadily decreasing because of diabetes. I had to advise him that a very high amputation would be necessary to get into an area that still had a good blood supply. There were two options: below the knee or above the knee. Below the knee would save the knee function and allow him to walk with an artificial leg and foot, but the circulation at that level would not be as sure as above the knee. An amputation above the knee would mean loss of knee function and would require a much higher artificial leg. He might not be able to develop expertise in walking with an above-the-knee prosthesis at his age unless he also used crutches.

I explained these options to the patient and asked him for his preference. If we operated below the knee, he might still require an above-the-knee amputation if the circulation at the below-knee level proved inadequate.

That, of course, would be another amputation. He said that he would prefer the below-knee amputation because he still wanted to be able to walk easily so that he could visit people and share the gospel with them. I agreed to this plan, and we prayed together. We asked the Lord to guide my hands and prayed for healing. Then we trusted Him for the outcome.

I performed the amputation below the knee. On the second post-op day, I changed the dressing and was alarmed when I could see an area about the size of a fifty-cent coin turning dark. The next day, it was darker still, and I knew it was dying. In desperation, I called a plastic surgeon to get his opinion on whether it might be possible to construct a skin flap of good skin to cover the developing defect. He advised sending the patient home with a dry dressing and checking it again in one week. That would give time for the full development of the dying skin area, and then we would know the size of the flap that would be necessary. We followed this advice. And we prayed again.

I saw the patient in my office one week later and removed the dressing, expecting to see a black area with blisters. To my astonishment, I saw instead an area of baby-pink skin where the dark area had been developing. Healing continued without difficulty, and the patient could walk with full knee function easily with a below-the-knee prosthesis. God had shown me that I need not worry about the sufficiency of my operative skills. I needed to pray and ask God to guide my hands with the knowledge I had learned, and He would do the rest. It felt as if I had a "secret weapon" of prayer. This was encouraging as I considered what new medical situations I might face in Bangladesh.

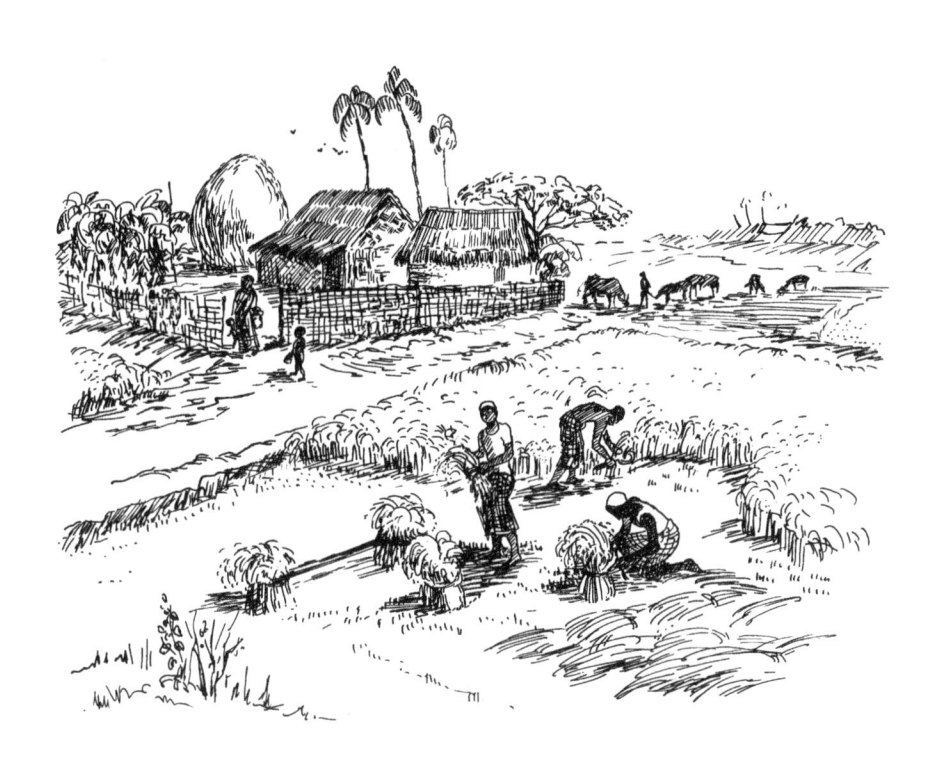

CHAPTER 22

Unexpected Responses to Medical Care

Amputation Refused

I was still new at the hospital and had much to learn about the culture of the Bangladeshi people. I did not understand their behavior and was shocked at some of the unexplainable responses of patients to medical care. One young man in his early twenties came to the hospital with his arm wrapped up in a dirty cloth. When the cloth was removed, the arm was mostly bones from above the elbow to the tips of his fingers. A few shreds of tissue clung to the bones, and the stench of his gangrenous arm was powerful! He had suffered a snake bite three weeks earlier, and his arm swelled enormously, shutting off the circulation. He was very anemic and had a high fever.

When we told him the arm had to be removed, he drew back and said, "Oh no! I promised my mother that I would not let my arm be cut off!"

"How would you be able to work with just one arm?" she had asked him. Unfortunately, he left without treatment, going home to a certain death.

Fear, Ignorance, and Cultural Taboos

Though we did not know why, patients would sometimes feign unconsciousness upon arrival at the OPD. To determine if a woman was truly unconscious, a technician would pretend to lift the bottom of her saree, prompting the patient to reach down quickly and stop him. The same thing happened in the case of men wearing a lungi. They, too, would resist any move to lift the lungi. These protective movements revealed that the patients were not comatose.

One lady scheduled for abdominal surgery insisted that she be taken directly to the operating room on a gurney without changing into a hospital gown. In the operating room, the technicians tried to prepare her abdomen for the incision. However, she refused to allow her saree to be lifted enough to expose her abdominal skin. There was no choice other than to cancel the surgery and return her to her bed.

One of the female hospital staff members had a pronounced limp due to a shortening and weakness of her leg. It may have been the result of polio. Every day, she had a laborious and painful walk to the hospital from her home across the main road. I asked her if she wanted a leg brace that would allow her to have a more normal gait. She said she would like that, so I sent her to the brace and limb shop to be measured for the brace. Very soon after that, the Limb and Brace Shop employees said she refused to allow them to measure her thigh. I asked the female physiotherapist to measure her, but the lady refused. She never got any help for her limp.

The Doctor Fixed It

On one occasion, a man came to the orthopedic clinic complaining of shoulder pain. I examined his shoulder, manually putting it through the range of motion. Arriving at a probable diagnosis of early frozen shoulder syndrome, I sent him to the PT Department to learn shoulder exercises to regain mobility of his shoulder without pain. When he got to PT, the technicians asked him what his problem was, and he responded, "None." They told him the chart noted he had complained of shoulder pain.

"The doctor fixed it," he said and left the clinic. Patients often left the clinic after receiving an X-ray procedure without waiting for the ordering doctor to review the image, mistakenly believing that the X-ray itself was the treatment.

Very Sick Little Girl

Not long after I began working at the hospital, we still saw patients in the old outpatient clinic. A woman clothed in a black burka had brought a little girl about four or five years old to be seen. In Bangladesh, it is not customary to keep track of ages. It was obvious that the child was very ill. She was listless and had pneumonia and severe anemia. She might have also had a urinary tract infection because she had a high fever. It was evident that she was very ill and needed emergency care to save her life. I told the Bangladeshi nurses to have her admitted immediately to the female ward, and I wrote orders to be carried out as soon as possible—laboratory studies, antibiotics, and cultures.

After seeing the rest of the female outpatients, I went to the female ward to check on the little girl. To my amazement, she was lying on the bed, still fully clothed, and absolutely nothing had been done. I learned that the woman who had brought her to the clinic was not her mother. She was the second wife of the girl's father. She had told our nurses not to do anything at all, as she was going to take the child home to let her die. The father had said that it would be less costly to let her die and then have another child with his second wife instead of spending a lot of money on this child, who might die despite treatment. And then they left! I never knew what happened to the child, but I am certain she did not live long. This kind of behavior horrified me, but I saw many more things just like that. It was a culture shock for me, coming from a society and personal background where life is valued and every life is considered precious.

He Touched My Foot

An elderly man was brought in with a large sore on his foot. The national staff instructed him to sit on the examination table and introduced me to him. I didn't want to kneel to inspect the sore, so I reached down and grasped his foot to lift it to where I could examine it. To my amazement, the patient jumped down from the table, got down on his knees, grasped my ankles with both hands and began to press his forehead down onto the top of my feet with huge sobs and tears!

I asked my interpreter what I had done wrong to have him respond like that. The interpreter explained that, in Bangladeshi culture, the feet are considered the filthiest part of the body and should not touch anyone else. No Bangladeshi doctor would have touched a patient's foot in that manner. The fact that I had done so was a complete surprise to the patient, who was overwhelmed by my humility and compassion.

We got him back on the table and treated his infected foot. Our hospital was unique in that culture because we treated our patients as human beings in need and extended our hands of comfort to them. We hoped that during our language study classes, we would learn all the appropriate things to do and not to do in that new culture to avoid offending the Bangladeshi people. We did not want anything to hinder our sharing with them the good news of salvation from the Holy Bible.

Fear

A village lady of uncertain age with work-scarred hands and well-worn clothing was first seen sitting trembling on the examination table with her right hand clutched to her breast and covered with the folds of her black bourka. She had swelling at the base of her index finger for six days, which had steadily been getting bigger and more painful. She had been running a fever. Although she lived close to the hospital, she had put off coming out of fear.

Examination revealed evidence of a deep-seated abscess in the base of her finger, extending into the palm. It was necessary to advise incision and drainage. Although this sort of operation could easily be accomplished under local anesthesia with a cooperative patient, it would be difficult to perform that on a patient as fearful and uncooperative as this lady. For that reason, I had advised admitting her to the hospital. Her eyes had grown wide at the suggestion of an operation, and I quickly explained that we would not cut off her hand (which many Bangladeshi patients fear will happen in such a situation) but were only going to make a small cut to drain the pus in her painful hand.

As I wrote the instructions for her admission, I directed the nurses to prepare her immediately for the surgery. Checking at the nurse's station a short time later to see if the patient had received her pre-anesthetic medications, I was told, "She isn't here. She came back here but left to wait outside for someone to come to give her permission to have the operation." It was common for women to refuse to have an operation until their husbands arrived to sign the consent.

We found her sitting on a bench in front of the hospital and persuaded her to return to the nurses' station. Eventually, her husband gave his consent, and one of the Bangladeshi nurses led her by the hand to prepare her for surgery.

I imagined what sort of things might have been going through her mind when she was transferred to the operating room. There she was, lying on the operating table with all sorts of handles and levers, underneath a light bigger than any light she had ever seen, surrounded by all kinds of shiny and impressive-looking equipment. How different it was from anything she had encountered in her village. Moreover, she was alone in a room with four strange men without her husband. No wonder she did not want to become unconscious. She had been fearing that place for six days and had barely mustered enough courage to enter. It took great courage for her to submit to what must be done despite her fear.

"How many children do you have?" I asked.

"I don't know—maybe six or eight," she replied, not wanting to shift her attention to answer my question, which she perceived was designed to distract her. One of the operating room technicians moved to the head of the table and asked her in Chittagonian, her native dialect, how many boys she had.

"Eight," she answered.

"How many girls?" the technician asked.

"Three," she answered. That totaled eleven children! She had left a nursing baby with the people waiting for her.

She asked if I would just put her arm to sleep and not her entire body. She was afraid to become unconscious in the strange and frightening surroundings. Although we were only going to operate on her hand, it seemed best to administer a drug called ketamine, which produces dissociative anesthesia. The patient is not really anesthetized or asleep, but they do not care what happens, and for all practical purposes, they are anesthetized. We administered the injection into the muscles of her arm, waited for three or four minutes for it to take effect, and as she slipped off into dreamland, we began to prepare her hand for the surgery.

The surgery was uneventful. After she slipped off to sleep, the hand was quickly scrubbed and draped, and the tourniquet inflated to provide a bloodless field. A small incision in just the right spot provided access to the pus pocket, which extended deep into the finger and palm and surrounded the important structures of the hand. After the pressure had been relieved, the cavity was irrigated with an iodine solution, and a gauze wick was inserted. The skin was closed, and the hand dressed. This took about 15 minutes. Orders were written to the effect that she could return home as soon as she was fully awake and should come back to the hospital in a few days for a dressing change.

When she woke up, the lady was relieved to find the pain in her hand gone. She was still alive and in familiar surroundings. It was a frightening experience for her, but perhaps her fear had been placated, and she realized that the people at the hospital would not harm her. Perhaps she would not hesitate to come sooner next time and would encourage others to come, putting aside their fears.

This scenario happened daily, often many times in a day. Patients came despite their fears and were met with compassion, tenderness, and mercy. They discovered that the MCH doctors, nurses, and staff were friendly and cared about them. That opened their hearts and minds to receive the message of salvation as taught in the Holy Bible—not from the mouths of strangers, but from the mouths of friends.

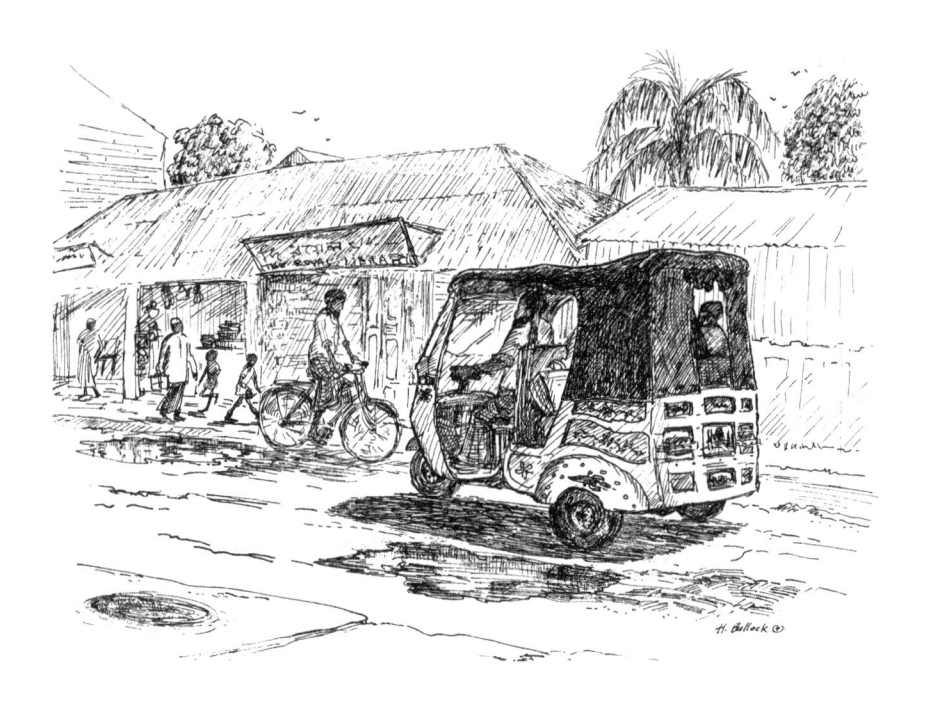

CHAPTER 23

No Blood, No Admission

When a patient was brought to the hospital with an injury or condition requiring a blood transfusion, we would tell the family our policy was that the patient would need to have at least one unit of blood donated before we started the surgery. Many types of operations could not be done safely without having blood for transfusion. Without the required unit of blood, he could not be treated and cared for at our hospital. Our hospital had a small amount of blood in the blood bank that patients could purchase, but we would not give it for free.

We did not keep much blood on hand, so we had to rely on a willing donor to give some of his blood to the patient.

Obtaining blood for transfusions was a major problem. The Bangladeshis believed that taking blood from a person would leave him weak and unable to work, exposed to sickness, or he might die. We were told that during the war, when West Pakistan invaded East Pakistan, the soldiers were killing anyone who was not a Muslim, and they were using their victims as a source of blood for their injured troops in need of blood transfusions. As much of the blood of the victim would be drawn as possible, and the victim would die in the process.

It was common for a patient's relatives and friends to run away upon learning that blood would be needed to treat a patient. Sometimes, men would refuse to give blood for a wife, thinking it was easier to get a new wife than risk giving blood.

If the patient's family could not give blood or buy it, we would tell them they must take the patient to Chittagong to another hospital. We kept the patient in the OPD and gave him the necessary emergency care while the relatives and friends made that difficult decision—to give blood or not to give it and instead, run away or abandon the patient.

We found it difficult to convince the fearful family. To remedy this, Tense and I helped our AV department produce a video to show fearful donors as they waited in the OPD. The video showed that it was safe to give blood in our hospital. The video explained that an average adult has about 10.5 pints of blood and that the body continually produces a new pint of blood every two weeks. When blood is drawn for contribution, only one pint or unit is drawn. Then, the body replaces all the blood that has been withdrawn. It would have been taken out of circulation by the body in any case and replaced with a pint of new blood. Thus, one pint could safely be drawn without harm to the donor. In the video, we explained that we would not take their blood if it were not of high enough quality. Our laboratory was fully capable of typing and crossmatching blood from donors and matching it to the recipient's blood type.

The Bangladeshis often accepted this information and consented to give blood for transfusion, but not always. Many times, we had to postpone or even cancel surgeries for lack of blood on hand for transfusion, if needed. When a patient needed a transfusion, we learned from bitter experience not to admit him to the hospital until the blood was available. To admit him without the blood could leave us with a deserted patient who could not be properly cared for and would die as we stood by helplessly watching. It was heartbreaking. Sometimes, this put irresistible pressure on us to provide free blood from our limited blood bank, which the family hoped we would do.

One morning, while making rounds at the hospital, I got a note asking me to come immediately to the OPD to see three critical patients. When I arrived at the OPD, the first patient I saw was a man who had been in a machete fight. He had deep cuts on both of his legs and had a gaping head wound. Fragments of the skull were visible along the bloody edge, and some brain tissue was oozing out. He was bleeding profusely and in shock but was still conscious. This man needed immediate attention and blood. This was definitely one of those "out-of-my-comfort zone" situations.

I was the only surgeon at the hospital that day and would perform the surgery. Although my orthopedic specialty typically did not cover cranial or brain surgery, I had general surgical knowledge and skills from my one-year general surgical residency before my orthopedic training.

Ideally, the patient should have been sent to the Chittagong Medical College Hospital, which was the nearest government hospital. However, if the patient arrived at night, he might not be seen until the next day. It was nearly impossible for local patients to travel to Chittagong for treatment. It was expensive to travel, and once there, they would not know how to get around in a large city. The trip involved traveling on a crowded bus over a narrow, dangerous road for at least three to four hours. Buses would not take a person who had to be lying down on a stretcher. Patients usually could not afford to have a sangi go with them to prepare their food and assist in their care in the hospital. Additional trips to Chittagong would be required for follow-up care. For most patients, it was our hospital or no treatment at all. Without treatment, they would have to go home and suffer the consequences of non-treatment. Considering all of this, I felt it was better to treat his wound at our hospital rather than send him to the hospital in Chittagong.

The second patient was a young man who had been gored in the groin by a cow the day before. A doctor had treated him on an offshore island where the incident had happened. The doctor had sewn up the wound, but the man was still bleeding profusely. It was apparent that he had lost a lot of blood, and there was no evidence of circulation in the injured leg. He needed immediate attention and blood.

The third patient was a child who had been gored in the cheek by a cow one week earlier. A village doctor had sewed up his wound, but when the sutures were removed, he suddenly began to bleed profusely. A quick test on his blood revealed that he had a coagulation defect. He was a hemophiliac. He needed fresh blood to provide the missing clotting factors.

We started emergency treatment on all three patients, giving them some intravenous fluids, antibiotics, anti-tetanus medication, pain medicine, and dressings, but told their relatives and friends that we could not admit the patients to our hospital unless they donated the required amount of blood because it was needed for their treatment. The patient with the head wound did not have enough money to purchase blood from our supply, and the men who had brought the patient were reluctant to give blood. We told them they must decide quickly whether they would either donate or buy blood or take the patient on to the hospital in Chittagong.

Assured we had done everything possible for the patients except start blood transfusions, I returned to my rounds, leaving the medics and the cashier to argue and bargain with them. Hearing nothing more about the three patients, I assumed they had been taken to Chittagong, which was a poor choice but the only choice if no blood was given.

Late that afternoon, after seeing many orthopedic patients in my department, I went out to OPD and discovered, to my amazement, that all three patients were still there. Finally, after much encouragement, the friends who brought the man with the head injury agreed to donate one unit of blood so we could begin the surgery. The family members of the other two patients had also found someone willing to give blood. At last, the laboratory technician could draw the blood needed for each patient.

This arrangement had taken many hours, but the important thing was that the blood for each patient was now available. We quickly took the patients into the hospital, prioritizing the treatment order of all three patients. We could care for only one at a time.

The little boy with the bleeding abnormality (hemophilia) could be cared for by a simple compression dressing and starting that precious fresh blood flowing into his veins to offset the coagulation abnormality. We started the transfusion immediately.

The man with the head injury was in the greatest need of emergency surgery, so we took him to the operating room first. When my scrubbing was complete, I prayed, stepped into the operating room, and accepted the sterile gown and gloves to be worn for the surgery. The head injury surgery took many hours, but I was able to clean up and close the wound. The surgery went well, and he survived the procedure.

Next, we took the young man with the injured leg to the operating room and started his blood transfusion. Exploration of the patient's wound revealed that the femoral artery had been torn halfway through. More than thirty hours had passed since his injury. It did not seem possible that restoring the circulation could prevent his losing the leg, but we would not know if we did not try. So, we carefully repaired the tear in the artery. An anti-coagulant was given into the artery, and a releasing operation was done in the lower leg to counteract the tremendous swelling that had already started. Then, the patient was taken back to his bed. We planned for the gangrene to declare itself and demarcate itself so we would know where to amputate his leg.

What was the result? The man with the head injury made an uneventful recovery with no sign of infection or other significant problems. He had a weak right hand, but he was alive.

The hemophiliac boy quit bleeding after two units of fresh blood, and it looked like his immediate problem was over. This bleeding problem would plague him for the rest of his life, however, as every small cut would bleed profusely. He would require many transfusions. We did not have prepared factor fractions to treat hemophiliacs, as they were available only in the US. We had only fresh blood.

The young man with the injured leg now had a warm leg, except for his toes. We thought he probably would lose his toes, but it was possible that he would not require a major amputation of his leg. Based on my experience and judgment, I did my best for each patient with the equipment and facilities available.

The central common factor in these cases was the need for blood. Without blood, patients could not be effectively treated, and there was no point in admitting them to the hospital. As I thought about the unusual day, it occurred to me that a similar scene would be enacted in the case of each one of us. A time will come when each one of us will be asked about some blood. I will be asked if the blood of Jesus Christ has paid for my sins. No other form of payment will be accepted—no money, medicine, influence, or good deeds—nothing else. The Bible clearly states in Hebrews 7:27 that Jesus shed his blood "once for all" when he offered up himself on the cross as payment for our sins. A person can refuse to believe in Him and refuse to accept that payment for the penalty of sin. In that case, he will have to pay the penalty himself—the penalty of spiritual death and eternal separation from God. At the time of judgment, God will say, "No blood, no admission."

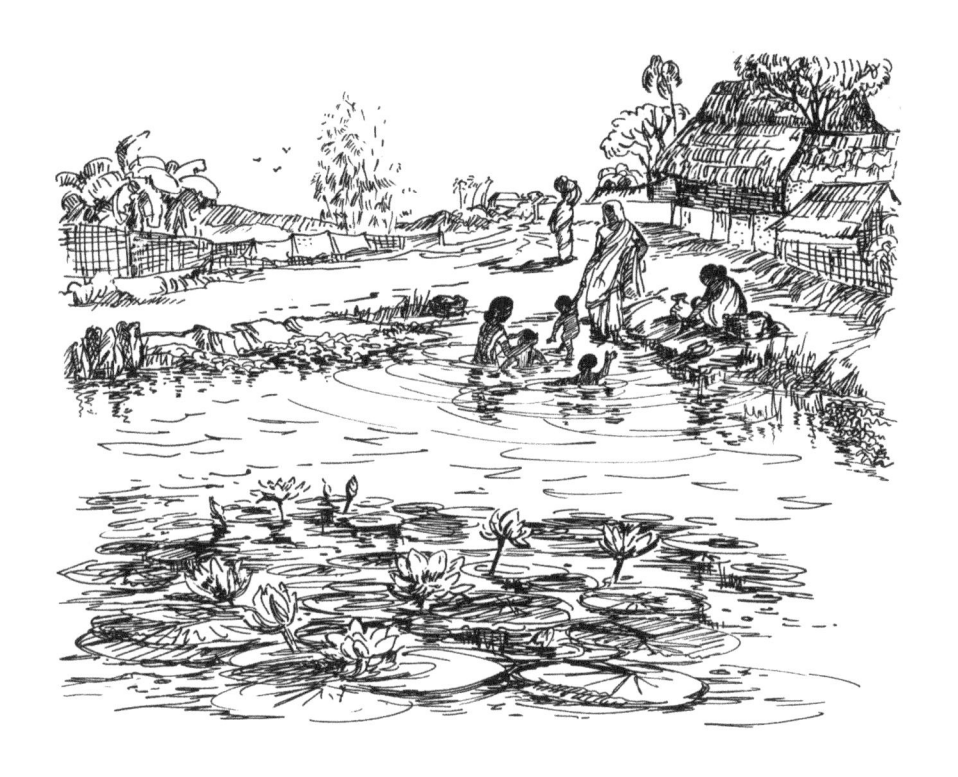

CHAPTER 24

Learning Bengali

I was grateful that I could spend whole days helping at the hospital during the critical time of the doctor shortage. Some would walk who would not have walked, some would return to work instead of existing as beggars, and some would live who would have died.

Finally, the language committee located an instructor, and we started language study in December. I had to stop doing full-time medical work for a while, although I continued to see some patients when they had orthopedic cases or emergencies of various types.

One of our nurses, Lyn S., who was skilled in linguistics, wrote a Bengali language textbook that we found extremely helpful. Joan Olsen, who was proficient in several languages, agreed to be the supervisor of our class. She spent many hours assisting our instructor and writing drills for us to practice.

Learning to speak, read, and understand the Bengali language, also known as Bangla, was one of the most challenging things I have ever had to do. Language school occupied our entire day. We attended school for three hours each morning, and each afternoon was dedicated to private study or tutoring. In total, we committed at least thirty hours each week. It would be a while before we could speed-read this language, but it was a real joy to begin communicating with our national coworkers.

Bengali is a difficult language to learn. The Bengali alphabet is written in a script completely different from what I was used to, with sounds that are not used in English and a word order that differs from English. It has an informal style, which is the common, everyday language, and an honorific or formal style, which is the literary style. There is also a style called "tui" that is used only with children. When William Carey translated the Bible into Bengali, he used the formal style for spiritual texts. Unfortunately, the high-level, formal style is mainly used by educated Bangladeshi people and is not commonly used. The newspaper is written at this high level.

To make it even more challenging for us to learn the language, there are four main dialects of Bengali. In our region, the Chittagong District, the most commonly used dialect was Chittagonian. The village people spoke mainly Chittagonian, but Bengali was their trade language. At our hospital site, most of the national staff conversed in Chittagonian. We were not expected to learn Chittagonian but were required to become fluent in Bengali. We needed to know Bengali to do our personal business in the city, speak with government officials concerning hospital matters, and deal with customs officials.

Answered Prayer

One evening, our language teacher visited me in our home. He had many questions about spiritual matters, and we talked for over an hour. I shared with him the verses from the book of Romans that had helped me understand my spiritual condition and need for salvation. We read the verses in both English and Bengali and discussed them. A few days later, our teacher decided to trust Christ for salvation. Later that day, he met with Jess E., our hospital administrator, who talked and prayed with him. Jess brought the teacher to our house to share his decision to trust Christ. He was radiant with joy! After his salvation, we arranged to meet weekly to read and study the scriptures and work through a new believer's course.

Swimming Pool Project

God is kind. He knew we would need something to do that we understood instead of studying Bengali full-time, so He arranged a therapeutic project for me to do. I discovered some termite-ridden crates on the ground near one of the houses and beside them, a cement-lined tank, half full of water and brimming with frogs. I was told it was supposed to be a swimming pool. Everything needed to construct the pool was in those crates, including a pump and a plastic liner. Since it was similar to the above-ground pool we had in our backyard in the US, I was familiar with the setup.

I asked the Language Committee for permission to supervise the workmen as they finished the installation. I assured them that the project would not detract from my language learning but would give me a healthy diversion to preserve my sanity. It would also be a great father-son project that I could do with David. This pool became a refreshing retreat for our teammate families at Malumghat, where the MKs could learn to swim.

Tense Teaches Art

Tense also needed projects to preserve her sanity while studying language. She was asked to make a series of Bible story illustrations on large flashcards for the tribal Bible teachers to use in winter Bible school. She also drew pen-and-ink illustrations of scenes of Bangladesh and the Bengali people for the Scripture calendar published by our Literature Center.

Our teammates on the field welcomed Tense for her artistic talents and ability to teach children and adults. She enjoyed teaching art to the MKs at the Malumghat school. Later, she taught adult art classes for some of her teammates at Malumghat. Inspired by the class, they started an Art Club to paint together regularly. This was an excellent outlet from their duties at the compound and a good teaching base for those who often functioned as their children's teachers in the MK school.

Tense was asked to fill in as a substitute teacher at the MK school. Once, she taught kindergarten for a month.

Among her other duties, Tense also became the resident Grandma for many of the MKs, helping new mothers with their newborns and caring for their other children when their grandmothers could not be with them.

David the MK

David was 15 when we arrived in Bangladesh and quickly made friends with Jim, another MK who was the same age. While Tense and I studied Bengali all day, David and Jim homeschooled together with the help of short-term teachers. Jim's family invited David to join them on the first of many trips to Cox's Bazaar, a coastal town thirty miles from the hospital site. It was a popular tourist destination known for its long beach, which stretches over ninety miles. David was also included in many other exciting MK adventures, such as motorcycle trips into the jungle, game nights, soccer games, bike riding, and hunting trips. Sometimes, David accompanied me to the hospital and observed surgery when I was on call. David told us he thought Bangladesh was a great place to live.

Do It Yourself Photo Lab

Tense was our photographer on the field, taking pictures of events, celebrations, and travels. She also recorded videos of our activities to take home with us on furlough to report to our family and supporting churches. Sometimes, she joined me in the operating room and recorded surgeries. Tense shared photos and videos with other team members for them to use in reporting to their supporters and families.

During our first few years in Bangladesh, we could not purchase or process color film. We set up a black-and-white processing lab in a dark closet in our house to process the photos we took with a 35 mm camera. David produced prints for us with a donated enlarger. Eventually, color film processing became available at Cox's Bazar, and our postmaster set up a business of taking our films to Cox's to be made into slides and prints.

Village Bible Class

One day, Tense was invited to go with Becky, one of our nurses, to a women's Bible class in the village near the hospital. They crossed a small bamboo bridge and walked between the rice paddies on levees, then continued down a dirt lane to reach the village. Tense and Becky removed their shoes as they entered the mud-floored thatched house and sat on a jute mat on the floor. Tense looked around at the group of women dressed in colorful saris. These were wives of male hospital nurses, operating room technicians, and x-ray technicians who worked at MCH. She was thrilled to finally be there with these Bangladeshi women for whom she had prayed for several years.

Becky asked Tense to share how God led her to Bangladesh. As Becky translated into Bengali, Tense told the women that she had gone to church every Sunday as a child, but it wasn't until she was a young teen and heard the gospel again while at a Christian camp that she understood that Christ died for her sins. She prayed and trusted Christ as her savior that day. She told the ladies about how we met in high school and got married a few years after graduation. They enjoyed hearing about our four children and our new baby granddaughter.

Then, Tense told how God had impressed upon her heart as an adult that she should "get ready to go," though she did not know that meant going to Bangladesh. She shared how God used her surgery to show her that she needed to dedicate her life to do things that matter for eternity. She told God she was willing to go wherever He sent her.

As Tense finished speaking, Becky prayed for each of the women and their husbands and that Memorial Christian Hospital would be a light to help bring the gospel message of salvation to the Bangladeshi people.

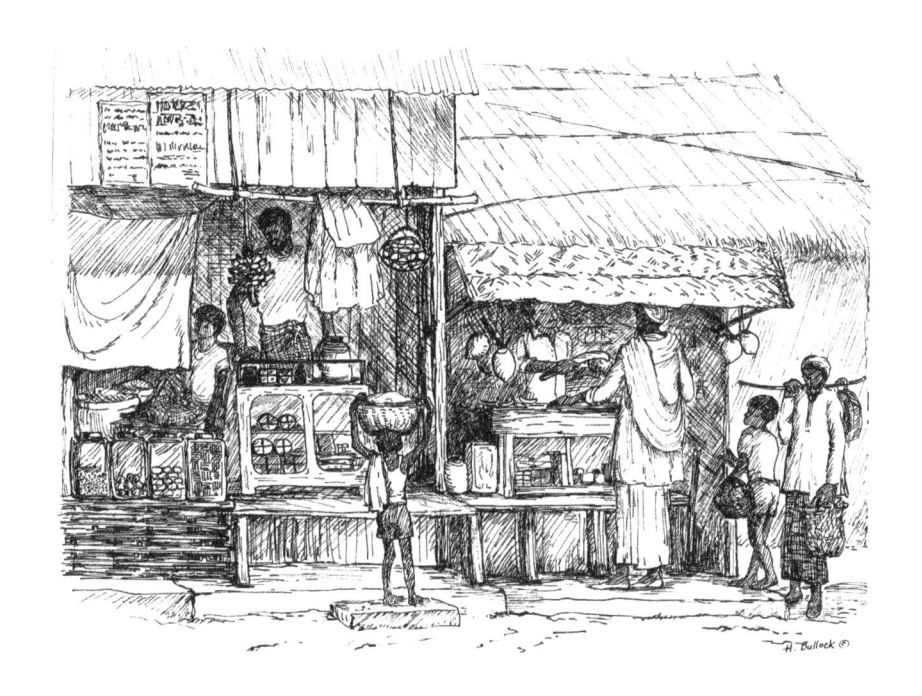

CHAPTER 25

A New and Strange Culture

Learning about this new culture was part of our preparation for serving in Bangladesh. Growing up and living in smaller towns in the US, we were used to orderliness, trustworthiness, safety, good roads, police protection, and modern communication. We had to develop wariness in our new culture. Stealing was common. We had to learn to be constantly on guard to protect our belongings and ourselves. Things left outside, like hoses and water bowls for pets, were subject to being stolen.

We had a few personal experiences with this sort of thing. Once, we were asked to purchase a ceiling fan for one of our colleagues. We purchased one at a small dokan. When the clerk was writing the receipt for the money I had given him, he looked up and asked how much he should write down for the price of the fan. He assumed we would ask our friend to reimburse us for an inflated price.

While shopping in the city market, Tense saw some shopping bags she liked and wanted to purchase four as gifts. The clerk placed the four bags on the counter, slightly out of our sight. He rolled up the bags, tied them with a string, and gave the package to us. When we got home and untied the package, there were only three bags. We learned to take our own shopping bags with us and place our purchases in the bags ourselves.

We saw thin plastic bags that had been mended to repair tears in them so they could be used again. I once asked a store clerk for a scrap of paper to write a note. The clerk carefully removed one sheet of typing paper, then tore off a small rectangular piece from one corner and gave it to me for the note. The clerk would not give me the entire piece of paper.

We were advised that if we mailed a letter at a post office other than the one at the hospital site, we should hand it to the postal employee and wait until we saw his hand stamp the postage we had affixed to the letter. Otherwise, he might remove the stamp to sell it to someone else if we left before that happened.

We realized that we would face complex challenges while working in that new environment.

Shipment Arrived

During our pre-field ministry travels, we received many donated drums to ship our items to the field for the first time. We had to create a detailed inventory of the contents of each drum for customs purposes. Three weeks before Christmas, the shipment with our personal belongings and household goods arrived in Chittagong, cleared customs, and was delivered to the hospital site. That seemed like Christmas to us as we unpacked the many wonderful gifts of food and the supplies we had received on our travels in the US and packed in the drums. We had to bring everything we would need for a four-year term since not much was available for purchase in the local shops or stores, especially in a nation recovering from a recent war. In a land of scarcity and extremely high prices, these items spilled out before our eyes like jewels. We unpacked the crates and drums and stored some of the contents in additional drums on the veranda of the Guest House. Some things had to be stored in a central godown.

We discovered early that the humid climate was not friendly to things that must be stored. Mold developed rapidly, and vermin got into things. Open shelves were not suitable for storing perishable items. Clothing and bedding had to be stored in an airtight container, including at least one Humisorb package to control moisture. The best containers for this type of storage were fifty-gallon steel drums that we could get from the hospital since many items coming from the US were shipped in them.

Whenever a family left to go home on furlough, they were required to pack their household items in drums and other containers. These were stored in a central storeroom so another family could use their house while they were gone. An inventory had to be prepared as if the drums and containers would be shipped. That way, if the owners could not get back to Bangladesh at the end of their furlough and the items had to be shipped back to the US or Canada, they were ready to process for shipping and customs. Packing and unpacking became a very familiar activity.

Snake

We brought with us a twelve-gauge shotgun from the US to use for hunting and protection from rabid dogs and wild animals. It was packed into one of our drums. Our drums had arrived but were not unpacked, as there was no room to put everything contained in those drums. However, I had taken the shotgun out of one of the drums and brought it into our room so I would know where it was in case of need.

Next door was the single girls' residence, where our NGO nurses and teachers lived. One day, the darwan suddenly burst into our room and excitedly told me a poisonous snake was right by the single girls' residence. He knew I had a shotgun and could kill the snake—he hoped. I grabbed the gun, slammed a cartridge into it, and hurried across the driveway to the SGR residence. The doorkeeper pointed to the snake at the edge of a flower bed beside the door, where someone might have accidentally stepped on it while leaving, unaware of the snake's presence.

I was about fifteen feet away from the snake. I raised the gun, took aim, and fired it. The head of the snake was blown off. When we looked closely at the snake, we could see it was a banded krait, a very poisonous and aggressive snake.

When I ejected the spent cartridge from the gun, I was astonished to see that the cartridge had been loaded with a single slug instead of a packet of shot. It would have been easy to miss the tiny target of the snake's head at that distance with a slug. My mind went back to the time my dad taught me to shoot a gun and told me that bullets were not cheap and that I had to make sure each shot counted.

The lady who had discovered the snake and called the darwan looked at its body and asked, "Is it dead?" When I assured her that it was dead, she reached down, picked it up, and draped it around her neck. "Take my picture," she said courageously. We were all feeling relieved and praising God for His obvious protection of us once again.

Christmas 1974

Our first Christmas in Bangladesh was quite different from anything we had ever experienced. There was none of the commercialism we were used to. For the Bangladeshi Christians, Christmas was a day of rejoicing and celebration. On Christmas Eve, a group of national Christians went caroling until 3:30 a.m. Christmas morning began with a special church service, followed by visitation. The NGO workers visited the nationals in their homes in the morning and were served tea and sweets called "mishti." Then, in the afternoon, the nationals visited the NGO workers in their homes. In the Guest House, we had about fifty visitors. Those in the regular houses had hundreds of visitors. Of course, we served them tea and mishti also. Gift exchanges were minimal, but the Christmas spirit was warmly felt. We were very thankful for our family and supporters back home who sent lovely cards and letters to us. This made it seem more like the Christmases we were accustomed to and made everyone seem much closer than 12,000 miles away. Some of the Christmas cards arrived as late as April because they had not been mailed with an airmail stamp.

Political Upheaval

We continued studying the Bengali language and were having a progressive examination in our language study class when we heard on August 15, 1975, that President Mujibur Rahman, the first president of Bangladesh, had been assassinated. He had been friendly toward our work at MCH, and now the future was uncertain. The army overthrew the government, resulting in the declaration of martial law. Travel became more complicated for us in the southern part of the country.

Peter W.

On the evening of August 31, 1975, a lone Dutch man on a bicycle rode into the compound, looking for a place to stay for the night. He had long hair and a long beard, was dressed in a lungi and a tee shirt, and wore an old floppy hat. Bob N., the Guest House manager, invited the young man to have dinner with them. He also arranged for him to stay in the Guest House overnight. Bob learned that the young man's name was Peter and that he had spent four years in a monastery but had run away before becoming a priest. Peter had been bicycling from Holland throughout Asia in search of spiritual truth in Eastern religions. He worked occasionally along the way to pay for his food and lodging. After the meal, Bob invited Peter to attend our English evening church service at the nurses' living quarters. He hesitated and said he'd been to too many services and had seen too many rituals.

"I don't think you'll find much ritual here," Bob told him. Peter agreed to go and seemed to enjoy the meeting. Later, he told us that as he looked around at all the shiny-eyed people, he felt comfortable there. He said that they seemed genuine. After the meeting, we had refreshments to welcome the new teachers for the MKs and a nurse who had returned from furlough. Peter talked and visited with each of the teammates.

Bob gave Peter a copy of Dr. Olsen's book, Daktar, Diplomat in Bangladesh,[25] and said that he would probably enjoy reading it since it was written by one of the people at the meeting. Though he was very tired from bicycling all day, Peter poured over the book most of the night and kept shaking himself awake when he got sleepy. "I was searching for truth," he later told us, "and the doctor who wrote the book seemed to be in the same situation."

The next morning, Tense went down to the dining room alone for breakfast, as I was convalescing in our room with infectious hepatitis and jaundice. This was our last day to have meals in the Guest House because we were moving into our new home that day. We had been living at the Guest House for one year since our arrival.

As Peter packed his gear and got ready to take off on his bicycle, he noticed Tense sitting alone in the Guest House dining room, having breakfast. He felt it wasn't right for her to eat by herself, so he walked into the dining room and sat down to keep her company. As they talked, Peter began to tell her that he had stayed up most of the night reading Dr. Olsen's book. He said he had finally discovered the truth for which he had been searching and decided he wanted to follow it.

Tense told him she was happy to hear that wonderful news. Then she picked up a banana, and as she offered it to Peter, she said, "It will only be yours if you reach out and take it. Similarly, Peter," she explained, "it is important for you to receive Christ as your own Savior and Lord. If Christ is knocking at your heart's door, you should open the door and let him come in. Why don't we kneel together right now, and you can tell God about your new faith and invite the Lord Jesus into your life? Then I will pray and thank Him for all He's done for you."

"Ok, let it happen!" Peter cried. Together, they knelt in the dining room, and Peter prayed a simple prayer telling God that he believed that Jesus was the truth for which he had been searching. Then Tense prayed with him and thanked God for Peter's newfound faith.

"Let's go to the front office," Tense said as they stood up, "and I'll get you a Bible."

Together, they rode their bicycles to the office at the front of the compound. Tense shared the exciting story about Peter's new faith with Jess E., the hospital administrator. Jess gave Peter a Bible and information about the ABWE guest house in Chittagong since he planned to head that way.

When Peter reached Chittagong, he stayed three days in the home of one of our teammates, who encouraged and discipled him from the Holy Bible. Before leaving Chittagong, Peter met with other people in Chittagong from the Netherlands and shared his testimony with them. After Peter returned home to Holland, he sent us a letter telling us how he was sharing his new faith with his family.

God's Protection

At long last, seventeen months after we arrived in Bangladesh, our Volkswagen Super Beetle arrived at the Chittagong port. We traveled to Chittagong on a Bangladesh bus to get the car cleared out of customs and have it licensed. Having a car at the hospital site would be helpful in many ways, particularly during the rainy season. We frequently used it to travel to Cox's Bazaar or Chittagong for shopping and business trips.

On one of these trips to Chittagong we left late in the day, which meant we would arrive after dark. At first, the absence of heavy traffic on the road after dark was a blessing. Most bazaars were closed, so going through villages did not slow us down. We were able to speed along, making good time.

Our situation changed dramatically as we approached the road leading to Chittagong on the city's outskirts. There was no pedestrian traffic on the road and no animals. It was getting dark, and there were no streetlights. The road ahead looked clear, but suddenly, it seemed darker than usual. I could see a fork in the road up ahead, and I knew one of the roads led to Chittagong. However, I was unsure of where the other road led.

I stopped the car and got out to determine which road I should take to get to Chittagong. When I walked to the front of the car, I suddenly gasped! Just a few feet ahead of where we had stopped, there was a pit about eight or ten feet deep in the center of the road. There was no warning sign at all—nothing to warn oncoming drivers. I got back in the car and carefully drove around the pit. I took the fork in the road I hoped led toward Chittagong but drove very slowly the rest of the way with my headlights on the high beam. This was one of the many times we were again reminded of God's protection over us while we lived and served in Bangladesh.

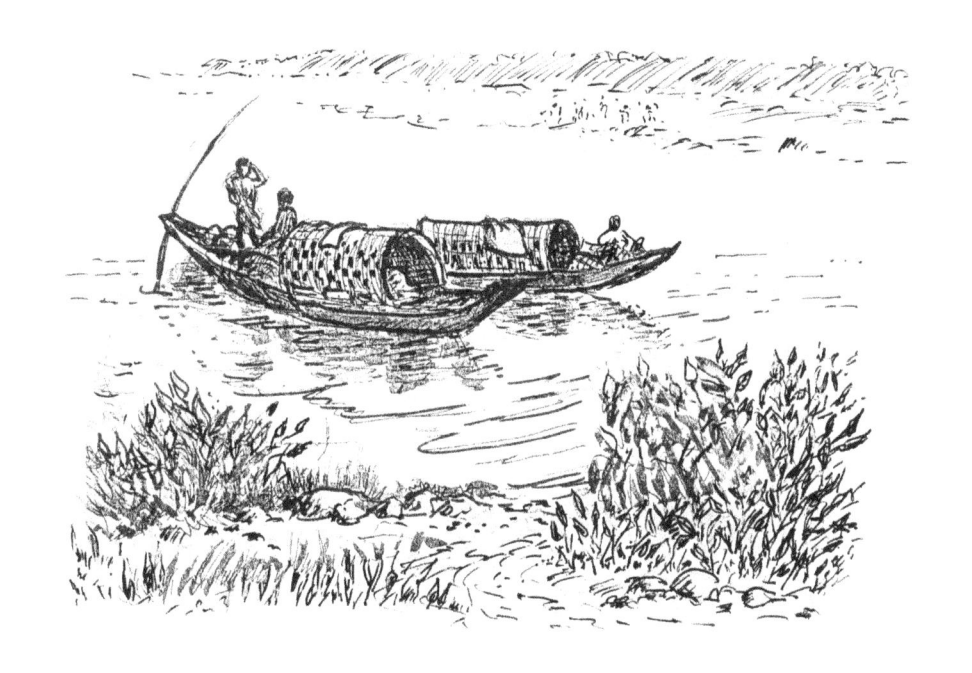

CHAPTER 26

Family Reunion

End of First-Year Language Study

It was a huge relief to finally complete our first year of Bengali language study with written and oral exams in December 1975. Soon after that, our college-aged children, Peter and Karen, came to Bangladesh for a visit. We drove our Volkswagen to Chittagong and flew to Bangkok to meet them. We had a wonderful Christmas celebration together in Bangkok and enjoyed a much-needed vacation as we recovered from our complicated first year of language study and adjusting to our new life at Malumghat.

Upon arriving in Dhaka, Karen and Peter immediately experienced the same culture shock as we had felt upon exiting the airport into the streets crowded with people, rickshaws, baby taxis, trucks, buses, and cars. Beggars surrounded us, asking for "baksheesh." We avoided handing out coins and later learned that it was better to give the beggars a piece of bread or a cookie they could immediately eat. After a few days, we flew to Chittagong and stayed in the ABWE guest house. We toured the city and introduced Karen and Peter to some of our teammates.

Finally, we loaded our Volkswagen with our luggage and drove three hours south on the one-lane Arakan Road to the MCH compound. Centuries ago, warrior elephants moved up and down this road to the Arakan district of Burma. Along the way, we passed by lush green rice paddies and villages with crowded bazaars where men in lungis shopped for food and household goods in the open-air dokans. Occasionally, we had to wait on the shoulder of the road for a colorful Bangladesh bus to pass.

We arrived at Malumghat just in time for the Spiritual Life Conference, a semi-annual three-day meeting of all the ABWE teammates in Bangladesh, including those from Chittagong and Hebron. Peter and Karen were eager to meet our teammates and help with the conference. They made a large banner that read, "Follow Me, and I Will Make You Fishers of Men," and Karen taught a Bible class to the younger children each day.

Hebron Trip

After the conference, Peter, Karen, and Tense traveled by boat with two of our teammate families, who were returning to our jungle station, Hebron, in the Chittagong Hill Tracts. I was feeling unwell and didn't want to risk getting sick on the boat. David had to stay home to prepare for school.

They climbed into the narrow canoe-like sampan boats with the other teammates and their young children. Strong men using long poles propelled the boats 16 miles up the peaceful Matamuhuri River. The boats were 25 feet long and only four feet wide in the middle, with a thatched canopy for shade in the boat's center. The three-hour boat ride in the low-riding canoes was terrifying as the water lapped just inches below the boat's sides. Monkeys jumped from tree to tree in the lush jungle on each side of the river, and brightly colored birds flew in and out of the tree branches.

The men docked the boats at the muddy boat landing, and the group climbed up the bank to the crowded Lama Bazaar. Curious tribal and Bangladeshi faces greeted them as they walked through the crowded bazaar and continued on a narrow path through the jungle to Hebron, the most primitive of our stations in Bangladesh. Tense, Karen, and Peter spent two days in Hebron with our ABWE teammate families living there. They visited a tribal church, a small building with woven bamboo walls and a thatched roof, called "the Jesus House," and learned about the outreach efforts to the tribal community.

Every year, a Tribal Bible School was held at Hebron for the tribal church leaders in the Hill Tracts. Our medical staff would give health lectures and instruction to the people who came to the Bible school. One year, Tense and I were asked to present a series of health lectures on hygiene and sanitation to the tribal people. We took a projector and a screen with us, and using a generator, we showed them pictures of the microscopic world around them. Tense brought health teaching booklets she had designed to illustrate these important lessons. The tribal audience sat listening with rapt attention. They were amazed to realize that germs were everywhere, especially on their hands. This was an entirely new concept for many of them. The tribal nationals had no knowledge that anything like germs existed. Bangladeshis do not use forks or spoons for eating. Instead, they grasp the food with the fingers of their right hand and put it into their mouths. If they did wash their hands before eating, it was only with plain water poured over them. We taught them the importance of using soap to clean their hands before eating.

Poor hygiene and lack of sanitation caused much illness and death. We tried to help our tribal believers learn and understand good health measures and preventive medicine.

Second-Year Bengali Language Study

After Tense, Karen, and Peter returned from Hebron, we began our second year of Bengali language study. Our two classmates were nurses who were greatly needed at the hospital. We accelerated our language program to begin work at the hospital as soon as possible. While we resumed language school, Peter worked on projects all over the compound using his carpentry skills, and Karen assisted Tense and other teammates with secretarial work.

During our second year of language study, we were introduced to more complex concepts, such as idioms and practical speech patterns. Although learning Bengali was challenging, we were beginning to communicate on a new level with the Bangladeshis and relate to them personally.

PART THREE

Developing The Orthopedic Department

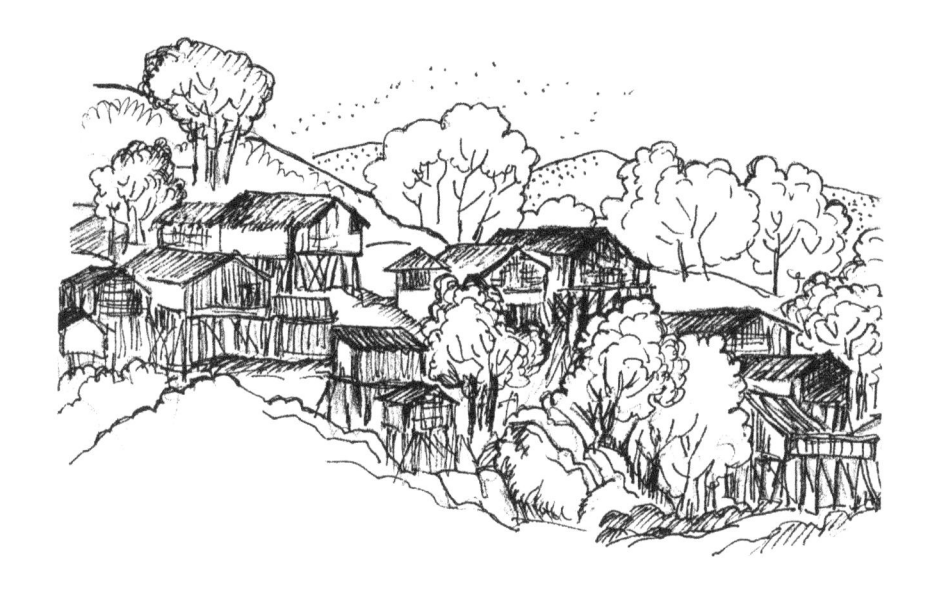

CHAPTER 27

Working Full-time in the Hospital

Language Difficulties

By November, I had completed my second year of Bengali language study and was finally permitted to begin working full-time at the hospital. I did not need a translator this time, or so I thought. I tried speaking in Bengali but found that the nationals had difficulty understanding me. It seemed that most of them spoke Chittagonian. I had progressed from speaking English to my interpreter and having him translate it into Chittagonian to speaking Bengali to my interpreter and having him translate into Chittagonian. I was never sure if the interpreter was conveying the message I intended.

One day, a well-dressed man from Dhaka brought his daughter to the hospital for treatment. I asked him if he spoke Bengali. "Of course," he replied in Bengali. It was refreshing to speak with him in Bengali and hear Bengali from him.

Tribal Languages

In our location, at least four tribal languages were spoken, which complicated things. Patients from the Hill Tracts area spoke one or more of these languages and often had difficulty understanding Bengali. Fortunately, we had local staff fluent in those languages and could assist with translation. On one occasion, a man from one of the tribal villages arrived at the hospital very close to closing time. He was brought to the orthopedic cast room for examination. I wanted to give him some instructions, but he didn't understand Bengali. I asked to have one of the tribal-speaking nationals come to translate for me but was told that they had all gone home. A sweeper cleaning the orthopedic cast room observed my predicament and volunteered to interpret for me. I wondered whether he knew this man's language. When I told him what I wanted to say, he began an animated conversation with the patient with much grunting and nodding of heads. After receiving my instructions, the patient left with a smile.

"How many languages do you know?" I asked the sweeper.

"Five," he answered with a smile.

Room 13—A Separate Space for Orthopedics

When I began working full-time in the hospital, I realized I would need a separate room to examine and treat orthopedic patients. A ten-by-twelve-foot room with a sink was available and was ideally suited. The wide doors to this room opened to the exterior corridor on one side and directly onto the surgical corridor on the other. It was originally intended to be an anesthesia prep and post-op recovery room and held wooden shelves and cabinets where patient X-rays were stored. Labeled "Room 13," it was also used as a temporary morgue where corpses were placed until the families came to take them away.

After receiving permission from the medical committee, I began seeing orthopedic patients in that tiny room, but it had to continue to be used as a morgue until other arrangements could be made. Things were going well until one morning when I took a patient into Room 13 to apply a long-leg cast, only to find a gurney with a sheet-covered form on it already occupying the room. We moved the live patient's gurney into the room and stationed it alongside the other gurney. As I proceeded to apply the cast, the patient kept looking nervously at the other gurney, knowing full well what was under the sheet. The Bangladeshi people are very superstitious, believe in ghosts, and try to avoid dead bodies.

Eventually, the medical committee arranged to have a small temporary shed constructed under a tree behind the OPD to use as a temporary morgue. Corpses were placed in this shed until the family could take them home for burial.

We Learn to Conserve Medical Supplies

When we started our work at MCH, we faced the serious challenge of dealing with the scarcity of essential items in Bangladesh after the war. Some supplies were donated, but everything was in very limited supply. One such item was surgical gloves. Instead of discarding them after use, we had to come up with creative ways to reuse them. We didn't have access to gas sterilization in the beginning years of MCH, so we had to autoclave and carefully package the gloves for reuse. We were aware that the used gloves might have pinholes, but they still provided a significant amount of protection to both the physician and the patient.

Crutches were not available from outside sources. Patients needing crutch-type support would simply use a stick held in both hands. I found it amazing how well patients could ambulate with such a device, which was always obtainable. If crutches were needed in our hospital, we could supply the patient with aluminum crutches that had arrived in the hospital shipments. Or we could make wooden ones in our carpenter shop.

Adhesive tape and ordinary adhesive bandages were scarce. Even string and rope were hard to find. Hardly anything was disposable. Scalpel blades had to be resharpened, along with dermatome blades. Hypodermic needles for injection were washed and sterilized, then stored in test tubes with a ball of cotton at the base. Glass injection syringes were used, as they could be sterilized and autoclaved. Surgical drapes and towels were made from cloth and could be washed in the hospital laundry and sterilized for use again.

Hospital Laundry

The hospital laundry was in a shed outside near the workshop. Soiled linens were laid on a concrete pad, and boiling water was poured over them. Then, they were scrubbed by hand with a stiff brush. Next, the linens were put into concrete washtubs about four feet square and 18 inches deep, and a laundry worker would step into the tub and agitate the contents with his bare feet. Finally, the linens were rinsed again, then wrung out by hand as much as possible and put on a clothesline to dry in the sunshine. They did not use clothes pins. Instead, there were two ropes twisted together. A gentle twist could separate the ropes, and then a corner of the cloth was inserted into the space between the twisted ropes, which held the cloth securely. When the cloth items were dry, some were taken to the ironing room. A heavy cast iron filled with hot charcoal was used to press the cloths. Finally, if necessary, the cloth items were autoclaved to sterilize them.

Women's Mite

To help with this problem of non-existent or extremely scarce medical supplies, Dr. Joe DeCook started a program where individuals and church groups could help gather supplies for the hospital. He called the program "Women's Mite."

Dr. DeCook contacted women's ministry groups in churches all over the US and asked them to collect surplus materials from nearby hospitals and clinics. These were items such as dressing supplies and sutures that had been opened but were not used by the hospital and would usually be discarded. The items were then sent to a central packing location at Good News Baptist Church in Grand Rapids, Michigan. When large amounts of these supplies began to arrive, the church constructed a special building on their property where the items were sorted and packed into drums or boxes and then packed into a steel shipping container. These containers were then shipped to the hospital on a freighter. The women's groups also collected funds to pay for the shipping.

Sometimes, old eyeglasses were donated to the Women's Mite shipments. One day, a middle-aged woman came to the hospital with a fractured hip. It was unusual for a woman of her age in Bangladesh to have a fracture like that, but she had fallen from a great height. She was a genteel woman and quite mild in speech and manner. Her fracture was reasonably straightforward, but she was running a low-grade fever. I did diagnostic studies on her for eight days to be sure she didn't have a hidden infection or other condition that would complicate her surgery. During those days, I learned she could read quite well and was interested in reading the Bible literature we offered her. But she lacked one thing. She had left her glasses at her home far away.

The day after her surgery, I remembered that we had received some used eyeglasses in a Women's Mite shipment. I looked through them and found some that seemed to be mostly magnifying lenses. She put one of the pairs on and found she could read quite well with them. She began avidly reading the common language Bengali New Testament. This might have been the first time she had ever read this book. During the remainder of her hospital stay, she had time to read, ponder, ask questions, and learn what the Holy Bible teaches about God's plan for her salvation.

Once the Women's Mite shipments were cleared through customs in Chittagong, they were sent to the hospital, where the containers were opened, and the items were sorted and stored in the hospital godown. Each shipment was like Christmas for our hospital. These hospital-related items shipped to the hospital were allowed to come into the country duty-free because of Dr. Olsen's negotiations in Dhaka with government officials. He also persuaded them to give duty-free status to the medical workers at our hospital. This agreement saved thousands of dollars for the hospital and our NGO workers.

Rolled Bandages

Rolled bandages were an essential part of our dressing supplies and were prepared by women's groups from our supporting churches in the US. They made the bandages by tearing old sheets into strips of varying widths and rolling them into bandage rolls. One women's group couldn't find used sheets, so they purchased new ones to tear into strips. They were eager to help us in any way they could.

When we opened the drums from the hospital shipment in the godown, these rolled bandages were a welcome sight. We used the rolled bandages for wound dressings, emergency diapers, restraints, arm slings, traction and suspension ropes for suspending arms or legs from overhead frames, and for fastening objects together. We also sterilized them for use in the operating room as post-operative dressings.

One day, I received an urgent note from a nurse informing me that I was needed at the hospital immediately. It was written on a piece of a rolled bandage. The women's groups who collected, sorted, and prepared medical supplies for our hospital were a vital part of the MCH team.

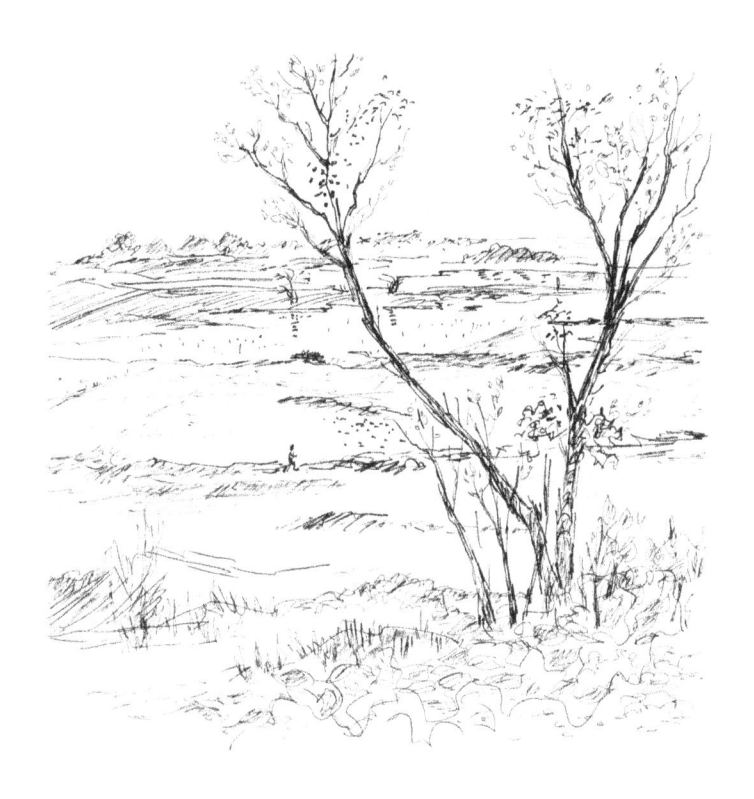

CHAPTER 28

Training Helpers

Training National Orthopedic Technicians

When I started working at the hospital seeing orthopedic patients, I quickly realized that the job would be too big for me to accomplish alone. I discovered a small booklet in the hospital library written by the World Health Organization, which provided guidance for healthcare professionals working with individuals of diverse languages and skills. The book suggested that the nationals should be taught simple skills they could do safely, such as putting on and removing casts, setting up traction, and changing dressings, which did not require diagnostic judgment. I needed to train an orthopedic staff of technicians to assist me while I concentrated on the diagnosis and treatment of serious orthopedic cases.

One problem I encountered was that most men applying to be orthopedic assistants were unfamiliar with using hammers, drills, and screwdrivers. They did not understand physics principles such as levers, fulcrums, and vector forces. They did not grasp the concept of traction principles, such as the resultant force of two forces pulling in different directions. They also had no experience handling electrical equipment, such as plaster cutters. I would have to teach them all those things. Also, their English language skills were limited, and they quickly became lost when they encountered medical terminology.

I devised a test to determine if they could use simple tools to perform simple tasks. I asked the workshop to give me two boards with holes drilled through each of them, a bolt that was long enough to pass through both boards, and a nut that could be screwed onto the bolt. I would hand all these things to the applicant, along with some pliers and a screwdriver for tools, and then ask them to fasten the two boards together. Then, I observed them as they figured out how to accomplish it.

The first man who passed the test spoke Bengali, Chittagonian, and English. That was going to make my first training course much easier. I immediately put him to work with me to prepare the orthopedic department room. It had been a storage room for used X-ray films and other materials. I started my new trainee clearing out this room and taking down shelves. While he worked on preparing the room, I made a quick trip to Chittagong to get our drums out of customs. When I returned, I found, to my dismay, that my trainee had decided he did not want to become an orthopedic technician after all. So, he quit. That meant I had to test more applicants.

I finally found one man with the skills needed. This man was working at the hospital as a sweeper, but he was interested in becoming an orthopedic technician. He became my first trainee, and I worked with him for many months. I started with one technician and then added others as needed. First, my trainees had to enroll in classes taught to medics who worked in the outpatient clinic. In these classes, they gained skills for treating various conditions and received Licensed Medical Fellow (LMF) certificates. Then, I used the orthopedic textbooks and journals I brought from the US to train the technicians in simple orthopedic procedures. This took a lot of time, but eventually produced a team that could handle many of the procedures by themselves, significantly saving my time and energy. I also had weekly Bible studies with these men.

The World Health book also suggested medical helpers could be taught basic surgical skills. As I considered the best way to teach these skills, I found that men related well to 3-D models, such as a skeleton.

Fortunately, I had a skeleton that I obtained during my freshman year in my medical school anatomy class by salvaging the bones from a spoiling cadaver. Another medical student helped me during our school vacation, and we scraped all the flesh off the bones, cooked them in a pressure cooker, wire-brushed them, and soaked them in bleach. We each took half of the skeleton. When the bones were clean and dry, I drew the origin and insertion point of all the muscles on my set and labeled them. Over the years, those bones were incredibly useful for teaching and training orthopedic technicians and physical therapy personnel.

Several years later, I trained a new orthopedic technician. He was fluent in English, which made it easy for me to train him. This technician became quite adept at doing simple surgical skills by himself with minimal supervision. I assisted him when he needed me.

Since we could not pay salaries equal to those outside the hospital, we allowed the technicians to work at other jobs outside. Some decided they could do procedures in their villages or homes and make extra money. This eventually backfired, and they got into trouble, which reflected badly on the hospital. Eventually, the ruling was made that they could not work inside and outside the hospital simultaneously. They had to choose, which resulted in the loss of significant staff. One morning, when I came to the orthopedic room, I found one of my two technician's keys lying on the table with a note that said he had decided to go to the Middle East to work for more money. That left just one technician until we could get more men trained.

X-ray Department and Equipment

Upon arriving at the hospital in Bangladesh, I discovered the hospital had a 100-milliampere portable X-ray machine and a smaller 15-milliampere portable X-ray machine. The X-ray images from those machines were of poor quality, particularly when taken of thicker body areas, such as a lateral view of the spine. Neither machine had a moving "Bucky grid," which would have improved the quality of images by blurring the grid lines so they would be invisible. Quality X-ray images were important for my orthopedic evaluations.

I wondered if there might be a Bucky grid in the hospital storage godown. Praying as I explored the godown, which seemed like a "treasure room" to me, I discovered traction devices, instruments, and hardware that could be useful for orthopedic surgery. I was elated to find a vertical chest X-ray table that was designed to stand against a wall to hold the X-ray film cassette. This unit contained the Potter-Bucky spring-loaded diaphragm needed for our X-ray machines. Since this unit was made to function upright for chest X-rays, it was unsuitable for skeletal X-rays that required a horizontal table. I had the hospital workshop welders help me design and build a pipe table to hold the X-ray table in a horizontal position. Finally, we had a working, spring-loaded Bucky device for our X-ray machine.

When we took the first lateral lumbar spine X-ray with the Bucky grid attached to the unit, the technician asked me what those white boxes were. I explained to him that they were vertebral bodies. He had never seen them with that clarity. This was a real boost to my morale, and I was thankful that I would have good X-ray images for my orthopedic work.

Training X-ray Technicians

Since the orthopedic patient load was increasing, the hospital hired more men to serve as X-ray technicians. I began training them on the techniques they needed to take X-rays suitable for my orthopedic practice. One of the previous short-term doctors had brought an X-ray technician training manual, which proved to be extremely valuable to the X-ray department staff. Eventually, we had four X-ray technicians in the department.

Tense Teaches English

One of Tense's duties involved teaching English to the orthopedic and X-ray technicians I was training. They met with her every morning for lessons, reviewed vocabulary, and had English conversations. Tense also taught English to Bangladeshi nurses and adult schoolteachers who were teaching English to Bangladeshi children.

Tense Teaches in Bengali

Tense finished her second-year Bengali Language Study class in April. One of her final assignments was to prepare and teach a Sunday School lesson from the book of Acts to third and fourth-grade children of the national hospital staff. She enjoyed preparing for the lesson about Paul's escape from Damascus in a basket. She enjoyed it so much that she requested permission to teach it again to some of the women patients at the hospital, and her teacher interpreted it for her into Chittagonian, which most of the patients spoke. She also taught Sunday School to MKs and taught a tribal girl how to teach Sunday School lessons in Tribal Sunday School on our station. After all the effort Tense put into learning the language, being able to communicate was extremely satisfying for her.

Another assignment for Tense's language study was to write and produce a puppet show, which she called "A Bride for Isaac." She trained two Bengali women Bible teachers to be her assistants in the puppet ministry program. They performed the show for the hospital employees in the chapel. Puppet shows and other drama programs were popular and enjoyed by all ages.

Making puppets and marionettes was a favorite activity for Tense, and she made the puppets for the Bible story puppet shows. The puppet outreach team performed in the hospital wards, at girls' camps, and school assemblies. Later, the puppet shows were put into video format and were shown to patients in the waiting room at the OPD.

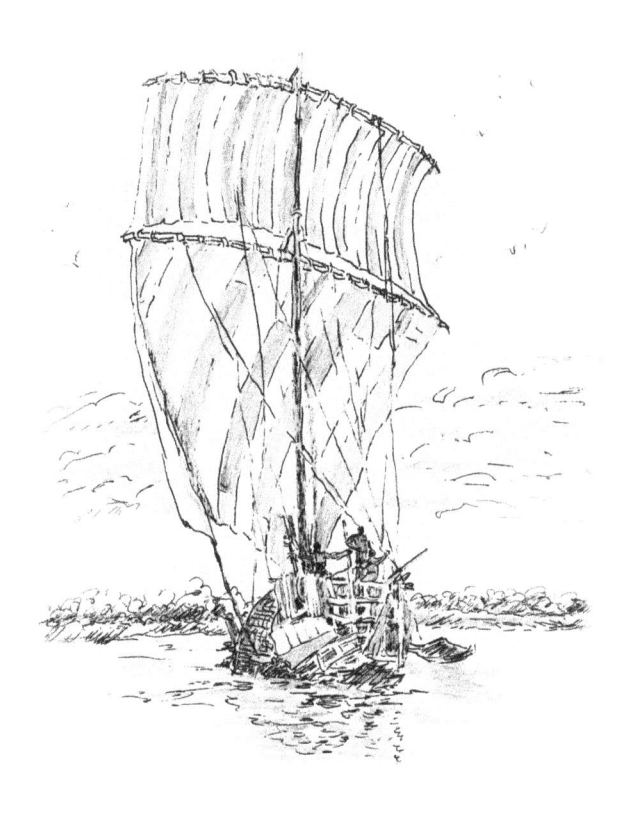

CHAPTER 29

Indian Rope Trick

In July 1976, Tense and I attended a meeting of the Indian Orthopedic Association in Calcutta at the Great Eastern Hotel. As we waited to be seated in the large banquet room, we were entertained by a band playing on the stage. One of the musicians was a man with very long black hair. I told Tense I did not like seeing men with long hair, not realizing that the man behind me heard my comment.

"We invented it," he said. Embarrassed, I turned to look at a man wearing a maroon turban standing behind me. He was an Indian Army

Colonel from a Sikh background. Not appearing to be offended, he smiled and introduced himself. His name was Colonel Chahal, and he was the doctor who developed the Spinal Cord Injury Centre for the Armed Forces at the Military Hospital in Pune, India. As we talked, he asked me if I knew about the "Indian Rope Trick." I knew of the rope trick for its reputation in stage shows but did not know of any medical applications. He said that if I visited his hospital, he would show me the "trick." Little did I know the importance of that "trick" and how it would change our treatment of spinal cord injuries.

Return trip to Spinal Cord Center

In 1977, I arranged a visit to the Spinal Cord Injuries Centre and took Larry Golin with me. Colonel Chahal, whom I had met at the orthopedic meeting in 1976, took us on a tour of the wards. He showed us one patient with braces on his lower legs, walking with crutches. He was an officer who had been in a vehicle accident. He was thrown out of the vehicle into a ditch that was partly filled with ice-cold water. When he was found, he had been in the water for several hours, and his legs were paralyzed.

An X-ray of his spine revealed very severe fractures of his spinal column, with actual dislocation of the vertebra. He was immediately sent to the Spinal Cord Injury Center. The doctors assumed that his spinal cord had probably been severed and that the damage was permanent. To make his recovery more manageable and transfer him out of bed easier, it was decided that he should have surgery to correct the dislocation and stabilize it in a correct alignment position. He was scheduled for surgery, but before that could be done, he developed pneumonia from being in the ditch filled with cold water for a long time before being rescued. Surgery would have to be postponed.

To make him more comfortable while he waited for surgery, the doctors decided to apply strong traction to his pelvis, hoping to pull the vertebra into better alignment. A leather belt was tightly bound around his pelvis, and a forty-pound weight was attached with ropes. The foot of the bed was elevated about two feet to keep him from being pulled out of bed. The belt had to be removed every couple of hours to massage his skin to protect it from becoming ulcerated with pressure sores. His legs were still completely paralyzed and without sensation. Weeks passed as he lay in bed in this contraption, and his surgery was delayed, even though his pneumonia had cleared with treatment.

One day, during the doctors' rounds, the patient exclaimed, "Look at my toe!" The doctors were amazed as he moved his big toe on one foot. He also said he could feel their touch. This was clear evidence that the spinal cord had not been completely severed. The doctors decided to continue the traction, which they named the "Indian rope trick," to see what would happen. Surgery could always be done in the future if necessary. Eventually, he recovered to the point where he only had to wear a posterior splint, as he had a "foot drop" and couldn't pull his feet up to the normal position. With this splint, he could walk. While there, we saw many other patients who benefitted from the Indian Rope Trick. I was very impressed and resolved to try this procedure on my next spinal cord injury patient.

MCH Patient with Spine Injury

Soon after returning to our hospital, a patient came in with a severe fracture of his spine and paralysis. The injury was already more than a few days old, but we decided to attempt the "Indian Rope Trick" anyway. To avoid skin pressure problems, we used thick stainless-steel rods, called Steinmann pins, in both femurs and applied traction to these rods. The foot of the bed was elevated high enough to prevent his being pulled out of bed by the fifty pounds of traction applied.

We were utterly amazed when the paralysis gradually disappeared and the patient regained motion in his legs. We had already told him that he would most likely never walk again, but he became able to walk with braces and crutches and was sent home. Encouraged by this result, we decided to treat every case like this with the Indian Rope Trick regardless of how old the injury was, and we were constantly amazed by the results.

Several years later, Tense and I were visiting Cox's Bazar and decided to get some ice cream from a newly opened ice cream parlor. As we stood on the sidewalk in front of the store, I heard someone calling, "Doctor! Doctor! Doctor!" The voice came from a man high up on the bamboo scaffolding of a four-story construction site across the street. As he shouted, he scrambled down the scaffolding like a monkey swinging from branch to branch. When he got down to ground level, he ran over to us. I discovered that he was the spinal injury patient I had predicted would never walk again! He had come to thank me for his spectacular result. The best part was that while in the hospital, he heard the gospel message of salvation as taught in the Holy Bible.

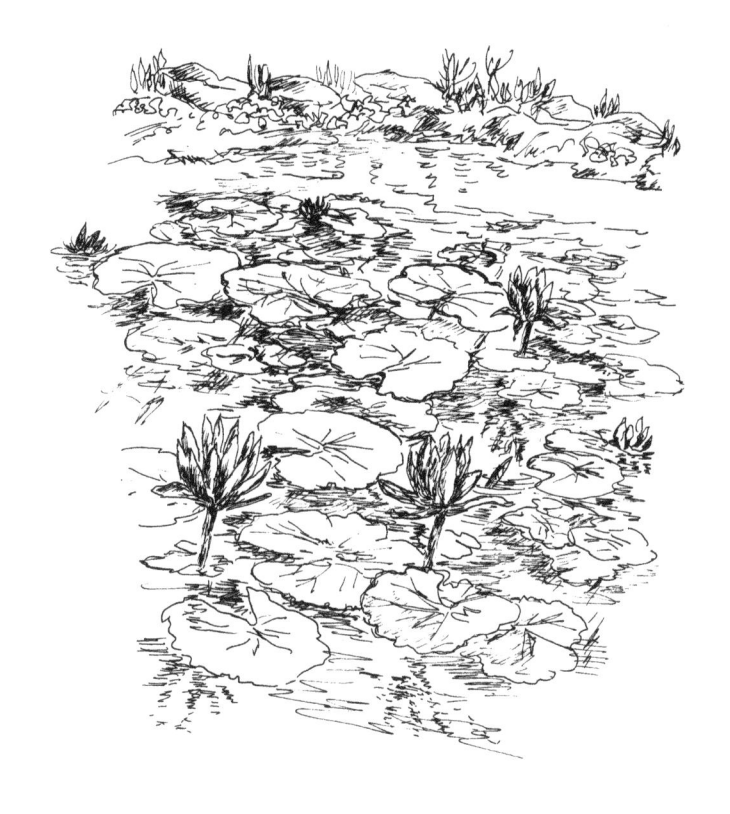

CHAPTER 30

Provision And Protection

Noah's Sterilizer

During the construction of MCH, a surgical resident in the US who planned to work at MCH after his residency just happened to see an old sterilizer unit sitting on the hospital's loading dock as he was leaving work. He asked what would happen to it and was told it was to be thrown away. When he asked if he could have it, he was allowed to take it and had it shipped to MCH in Bangladesh.

The sterilizer consisted of a cylinder about thirty inches long and fifteen inches wide mounted on a four-foot-tall frame. Two heater rods in separate cylindrical containers were mounted inside the large cylinder. It was very simple to operate: add water and turn on the heaters, which generated steam and sterilized the contents. We joked that the unit was so old it must have been with Noah on the ark, so we called it "the Noah unit."

Years later, upon our return from a furlough, we found out that the hospital had acquired two new, larger sterilizers known as "autoclaves." One was a medium size, and the other was much larger. The medium-sized one had been installed and was working, but our maintenance supervisor was still installing the larger one. Soon after we started using the larger autoclave, we noticed a small leak coming from somewhere inside it. Our maintenance supervisor could not locate the leak, which got bigger until it was finally identified as coming from a small metal bellow, part of a device called a "safety release valve." The bellows were part of a thermostatic mechanism, and there was no way to plug the leak. Water coming from the bellows was leaking onto the electric wiring, making it unsafe to operate the machine. We searched the storeroom but couldn't find the required part to repair it. Nothing like that was available in Bangladesh, so we had to order a replacement part and arrange for someone to bring it with them upon returning from the US. That would take several weeks, at least. Providentially, a short-term doctor was planning to come to Bangladesh in the near future and could bring the needed part for the leaking autoclave.

Meanwhile, we had only the medium sterilizer, except for the ancient "Noah unit" that had been patched and repaired many times but then put into storage when the new autoclaves arrived. We brought the Noah unit from storage until the larger autoclave could be repaired and found that one of the two heating elements had overheated and burned out. It could only heat at twice the time that had previously been required. We thought the burned-out element could be bypassed, and the remaining element could generate enough heat to be functional. It worked, except that it was very slow. Together, the Noah unit and the medium-sized autoclave could barely keep up with the steady demands for sterile equipment but were the only recourse we had until the part arrived for the larger autoclave. This caused a significant upheaval in patient care.

Operations had to be canceled or reduced to procedures that required only a bare minimum of sterile equipment. We even put pressure cookers into service as mini sterilizers, which helped a little.

We still needed to find a replacement for the burned-out element of the Noah unit. Of course, nothing like that was available in Bangladesh. I collected all the model information from the sterilizer and contacted the REAP headquarters in Los Angeles, which supplied equipment for missionary hospitals. We received a reply from REAP that the sterilizer was old and no longer in production. However, it just so happened that one of these "Noah" units had been donated to REAP from the City of Hope Hospital in Los Angeles and was sitting on their dock. Even more amazing was that there were two new elements for the unit with it on the dock still in their unopened boxes. The man at REAP said he would send the new elements to us in California when we were home for a family visit but to take good care of them because they were no longer being manufactured. When we received the two elements, we guarded them carefully and took them with us when we returned to MCH. By the time we returned, the new autoclave had been repaired and was functioning. We had prayed that it would function correctly after installation and would not have to be set by a qualified engineer because it contained a small adjustment screw that had been preset at the factory as part of the safety mechanism. To our relief, when the new part was installed, it worked perfectly. The Noah unit was then used to sterilize surgical gloves for reuse.

Anything can go wrong with the equipment at a hospital in a remote station. How thankful we were to have an excellent maintenance supervisor on staff with the training and experience to keep the equipment operating and who could improvise and utilize whatever supplies were on hand. God continued to demonstrate His power by providing the means for us to work in the place to which we had been called.

God's Protection—Saved from a Centipede

God also demonstrated His power through His protection of us. When we returned to Bangladesh for our second term in the fall of

1978, we had a better idea of what to expect at MCH than when we arrived for our first term. We knew working in a remote jungle setting like Bangladesh could be dangerous for many reasons. However, we also had confidence that God always guided and protected us with His unseen hand. Often, that divine hand of protection was unmistakably evident.

Tense's art skills were called upon immediately after we returned, and she was asked to design the program cover for the MK High School graduation. As Tense sat working on the program cover at the dining room table, she hummed a verse of the hymn "Day by Day"[26] while meditating on the words.

> Every day, the Lord himself is near me,
> With a special mercy for each hour;
> All my cares he gladly bears and cheers me,
> He whose name is Counselor and Pow'r.
> The protection of his child and treasure
> Is a charge that on himself he laid:
> "As your days, your strength shall be in measure"
> This the pledge to me he made.
>
> ~ Carolina Sandell Berg

A fly began bothering her as it buzzed around the table, so Tense got up from where she was working, picked up a chair beside her to clear the path to the flyswatter, and set it down hard next to where she had been sitting. After she got the fly swatter and killed the fly, she noticed some movement on the floor and looked down to see the wriggling body of a huge tropical centipede about eight inches long with its head crushed under the chair leg! If she had not gotten up to get the fly swatter, it could have delivered a dangerous bite and much pain to her sandaled foot. She immediately thanked God for protecting "His child and treasure," as the words of the hymn were still fresh in her mind.

Near Electrocution

While taking a shower at our home in House #12, I reached up to adjust the shower head, which was metal. Suddenly, a bolt of electricity shot through my body. The convulsive shock was so strong that it tore my hand loose from the grip on the shower head and threw me out of the shower onto the bare floor.

"Don't touch anything metal!" I shouted.

Tense came dashing in to check on me. The cook switched off all the electricity in the kitchen. We sent a message to the workshop to send a crew to investigate. They found that the compressor on the refrigerator had shorted out. Somehow, the short 220-volt current was directed to the water pipes. They also discovered that the ground wire for the system had been twisted loosely onto the wire that went into the ground and, over time, had developed a high resistance joint due to deposits at the junction between the two wires. At least the defective ground had siphoned off enough of the 220 volts that I was not electrocuted. After that incident, I covered all bare metal fittings with electrician tape to prevent further shocks until the grounding system could be overhauled. Once again, we rejoiced in God's protection.

Yellow Tape

We went home to the US for our furlough in August and traveled through Israel and Europe as a graduation trip for David before he started college. We flew from Dhaka to Delhi, India, and were scheduled to fly from there to Israel with a layover in Tehran to change airlines. All of our suitcases had hasps and padlocks, and I applied yellow tape around the red suitcases to make them more easily identifiable. We thought we had checked our luggage all through to Tel Aviv in Israel, but as we sat in the arrival lounge in Tehran, I noticed that other passengers had claimed their luggage. When I inquired, I was told we were changing airlines and had to recheck our bags.

I hurriedly found all but one of our suitcases on the luggage carousel, and then the carousel quit running. I sought out the attendant.

"I'm missing one of my suitcases," I told him.

He replied, "Everything has been unloaded. Perhaps one of your bags missed the flight."

"Do you have a lost and found department?" I asked.

He scowled and looked at me intently. "Yes, but it would not be possible for your luggage to be in there."

I insisted I be allowed to look, so he showed me a doorway behind him, indicating that it was the door to the lost and found department. When I said I wanted to look inside, he said, "There's no way your luggage could be in there."

I continued to insist.

Finally, he opened the door. The room was about twenty feet wide and thirty feet long. At the back of the room was a staircase to an upper level. Instantly, I recognized our missing red suitcase with the yellow tape sitting under the lowest level of the staircase.

"That one there, the red one with the yellow tape," I said, pointing.

"It could not possibly be yours!" he insisted.

But he finally agreed to look at the nametag. He acted astonished to discover that it was indeed our suitcase. I thanked him, took the suitcase, and left. Evidently, the padlock suggested that there might be something of value in the suitcase, and it had been secreted away for later inspection. I was thankful for this reminder of God's constant protection.

Meetings for Reporting and Recruiting

We had a demanding schedule during our furlough to visit our supporting churches and individuals, speaking in over 75 churches. Before we left the field, we had let people know about our need for better X-ray equipment. As we traveled, supporters donated funds to help us buy, refurbish, and ship the needed machine. We also sought to challenge the people we met in the churches to dedicate their lives to serving God. As a result, several individuals and couples decided to do so, and some even went to Bangladesh.

Donated X-ray Machine

When our travels led us through Milwaukie, Oregon, I stopped to see my former partner, who had contacted me about our need for X-ray equipment.

"Why don't you take the machine we used to own together?" I was surprised to hear him say. "I no longer need it and am willing to donate it to the hospital."

I gladly accepted his offer. We were still reporting to our supporting churches and had to stay on our schedule, but I began trying to figure out how to get the X-ray machine from Oregon to Los Angeles, where it would be prepared for shipment to Bangladesh. The next day after our meeting in Sacramento, California, I went to the U-Haul store near the church to inquire about renting a truck to move the equipment. I explained my need to the man behind the counter and was surprised at his reply.

"Dr. Bullock," he greeted me. "I was sorry I missed your report at church, but I had to work. I have a truck that must get back to Los Angeles somehow. If you pay the fuel cost, I can let you use that truck to deliver the X-ray equipment to Los Angeles." I was elated to hear this good news. He understood that I would have to drive the truck up to Milwaukie, Oregon, to pick up the machine and then drive it to the agency in Los Angeles that would arrange the overseas shipment. The man supervising the shipping would be gone in just a few days, which narrowed the time I had to get it to him.

I decided to drive Tense up to Medford, Oregon, and leave her there with her mother for a visit while I worked on the X-ray machine transfer. We had arranged for the X-ray repair company to disassemble it immediately and help me load it into the truck. When I arrived with the U-Haul truck, the X-ray machine had already been taken apart, and we loaded it quickly. Next, I had to get to Los Angeles as soon as possible. I was driving alone and stopped to rest occasionally along the way, staying within the speed limit while concentrating on the highway signs and avoiding cars that sped by me on both sides. Driving along in the truck shortly after midnight on California freeways, it struck me that my mind was alert and clear and that I could easily negotiate this most difficult part of my trip. I had been driving almost continuously for 18 hours, with only one half-hour nap at a rest stop earlier in the afternoon of the preceding day.

Everything was going well, and I made good time. I had just begun the last lap of the trip from Bakersfield up the Grapevine grade to Upland when the temperature gauge on the truck shot up into the red. I stopped the truck, got out, and opened the hood. No steam was coming out, and I couldn't see any leaks. The belts looked okay. I knew better than to open the radiator cap. I had to wait while the engine cooled off, wasting precious time. I thought I might have to call U-Haul and ask them to send a replacement truck, but I wondered how we would get that heavy equipment into the new truck.

I prayed and told God that this was His machine for use in His hospital, and I needed His help getting it to Upland. After waiting about ten minutes, I remembered that there was a service station a few miles further up the road where I could stop and get some help. I had not yet come to the steepest part of the grade, so I got back into the truck and started the engine, thinking I could limp along slowly until I got to the service station. To my surprise, the temperature gauge read normal!

I got back on the road and gingerly started up the grade, carefully watching the gauge. The gauge never budged for the rest of the climb, as steep as it was. I had a very heavy load and would have expected the engine to heat up a little bit, but it did not. I passed several cars on the side of the road with their hoods up that were stopped because of overheating. The temperature gauge remained normal for the rest of the trip, and I made it to Upland just under the deadline. We got the machine unloaded without problems. It was shipped to Bangladesh on a freighter and arrived safely about a year later. That X-ray machine served us at MCH for many years. God's provision for us at MCH came in unexpected ways.

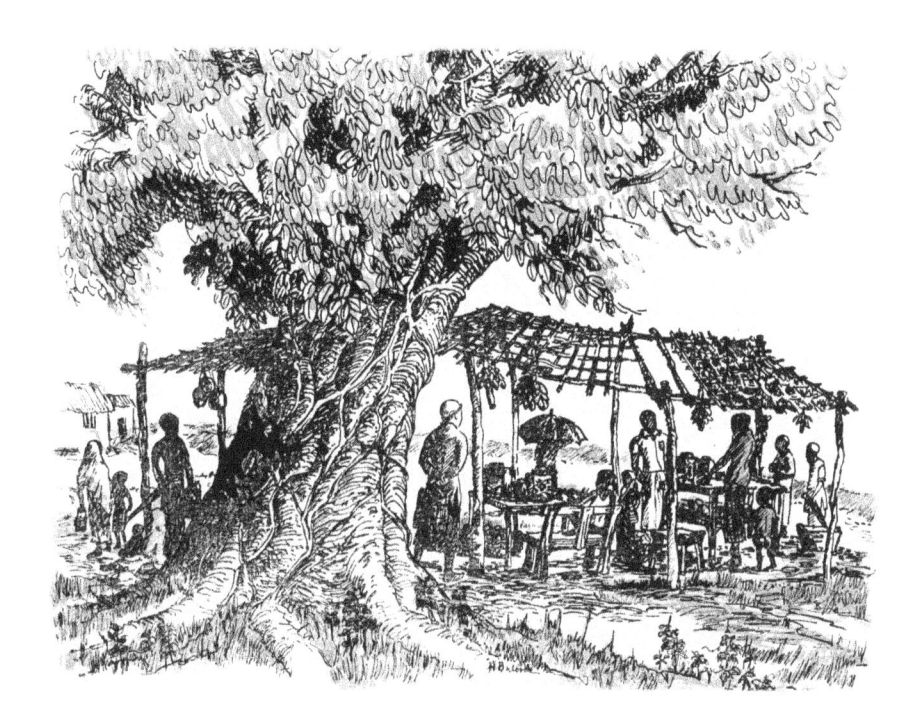

CHAPTER 31

Return To Bangladesh

Return To Bangladesh

Upon our arrival in Dhaka in October 1978, we were greeted by the monsoon season in Bangladesh, characterized by umbrellas, flooded fields, lush green rice paddies, and hot, humid weather. It felt good to be home again, and our national friends and teammates greeted us warmly. We went immediately to Malumghat, where I began working at the hospital full-time because of the doctor shortage. Again, I was assisted by an interpreter. Tense stayed busy working on an art project involving

Sunday School materials. While we helped at Malumghat, Dr. Olsen began working on our visa paperwork, made embassy visits for us, and was successful in getting our one-year visas extended.

Dr. Joe DeCook was happy to see me return to the hospital because he had been the only doctor for several months and was desperate for help. He needed to take his wife to the US for medical treatment, as she was having severe complications from a disease we called "Chittagong Hepatitis," a form of perihepatitis peculiar to that region of Bangladesh. His return to MCH was uncertain because her condition was so severe.

Many of our teammates were getting this mysterious viral disease that acted like hepatitis but without jaundice. They suffered from a variety of symptoms, including severe fatigue and weakness, low-grade fever, liver, kidney, spleen, and back muscle pain, severe headaches, insomnia, and loss of appetite. At first, we thought this syndrome was limited to our expatriate personnel, but we later learned that a disease called "non-icteric hepatitis" was commonly diagnosed in the national population.

The only treatment we found for this condition was bed rest. Recovery usually lasted three or four weeks, but it was not unusual for the patients to have relapses associated with stress or minor common illnesses such as colds. Some patients had liver biopsies, which revealed only capsular inflammation. Thus, the name was changed to "perihepatitis."

In the spring of 1983, MCH closed for two months because of an epidemic of perihepatitis among the staff and NGO families. Two epidemiologists from the Centers for Disease Control in Atlanta and Yale University came to Malumghat for several weeks to collect data for a study that could identify the cause of this disease.

Language Study Review Course in Dhaka

After a few weeks, we returned to Dhaka for a short-term language review and shared a rented house with two of our MK school teachers who were also studying Bengali. We had language class in the mornings and tutor time in the afternoon. The year of furlough with little Bengali practice made it seem like we were starting over again in language school. However, we quickly began picking up fluency, as Bengali is spoken clearly in Dhaka, unlike Chittagong, where most people speak the Chittagonian dialect. Each of us engaged in extra activities to have opportunities to practice our Bengali.

Tense attended a drawing class at the Dhaka Art College near our house every afternoon. This allowed her to make friends with the art students and practice her Bengali. One afternoon, we had a fascinating visit to a Bengali artist's home. Tense met her at the Dhaka American Women's Club, where she displayed her oil paintings. The artist's home was on concrete pilings by the flooded Ganges River. We had to walk out on a long wooden walkway to reach her home, where we saw her work and discussed art. After we visited her home, the artist invited us to attend a poetry meeting at the home of a famous Bengali poet, and we were asked to sign the guest book. All of this was a good cultural and language experience for us.

I spent time with Dr. Garst at the Rehabilitation Institute Hospital of Dhaka (RHID), where I assisted him in some of his surgeries and lectured his students. This time was valuable for me. I learned much from him about orthopedic surgery in that part of the world and had an effective language review.

Krukenberg Procedure at MCH

The loss of both hands was a huge problem in the Bangladeshi culture. Hooks are not usually sufficient to enable the person to have functional independence and employment. While I worked with Dr. Garst in Dhaka, he told me about an operation called a "Krukenberg" procedure developed during World War I by a German orthopedist named Herman Krukenberg. In this procedure, the radial and ulnar portions of the arm are separated to provide a sort of "lobster claw" or pincher that could be opened and closed by the remaining muscles in the arm. The arm also retained sensation, so the patient could feel what he or she was grasping. Understandably, acceptance of this procedure was even more limited than acceptance of a hook or claw. The individual had to be desperate to regain some degree of function to agree to this procedure.

Dr. Garst had performed this procedure on both arms of one of his patients, and the patient was now working in his hospital in the X-ray department. I decided to go see this patient while I was in Dhaka. Upon arriving at the hospital, I went to the X-ray department, where I saw a man sorting and filing X-rays at the desk. I asked him if he would direct me to the patient with the Kruckenberg arms. He looked at me strangely and then showed me his arms. He was that patient! I was astonished. He was writing on the files with a pen, using his arms, and then filing the films. At first glance, it seemed that he had two very functional arms. I was very interested in trying this procedure when I had the opportunity.

One day, when we were back at Malumghat, the power company was erecting a power line across the hospital property, putting up metal towers, and stringing the power lines. The Bangladeshi children who lived at Malumghat had learned that it was great fun to hang onto the power cable as large pulleys were stretched into place. It would lift them into the air until they let go and dropped back to the ground. One boy, about fifteen years old, had grasped such a cable and was lifted off the ground. He was close to one of the metal power poles and decided to go hand over hand on the cable to the pole instead of dropping to the ground.

He did not know that the power had been turned on to the cable this time, and it was "live." When his feet touched the metal pole, a jolt of electricity passed through his body. His body weight caused him to drop to the ground instead of being electrocuted. However, the boy sustained severe burns to both arms and legs. One leg required amputation below the knee, and one arm had to be amputated just above the wrist.

We were able to save the hand on the other arm, but it was deformed and nearly useless. What sort of future could this young man look forward to? I was able to talk him into letting me perform a Krukenberg procedure on the amputated arm, and we made a below-knee artificial leg for the amputated leg. He was very cooperative in learning to use the "Krukenberg" arm and eventually became a rickshaw driver.

The only other Krukenberg procedure I performed was on a middle-aged woman. The procedure went well, but she was so embarrassed by the "pincher" arm that she kept it covered. She may have used it at home when no one was watching.

Patients needing treatment from the Limb and Brace shop and the PT department required multiple visits. This gave the hospital personal workers and staff repeated opportunities to share with patients the good news of salvation.

Hand Tumor Case—"EMERGENCY!"

As I entered the orthopedic cast room one morning, I recognized a man and wife who had come several weeks earlier seeking treatment for a tumor the size of a large hen's egg on the husband's left hand. It occupied the entire shaft of the ring finger metacarpal bone. The patient was a typist who sat under a tree in front of the courthouse, preparing documents for customers. The tumor had grown so large that it prevented the use of his left hand.

X-rays showed the tumor was like a giant cyst with very narrow walls. It could have been benign or malignant. Reconstruction was not possible. I had explained to them that the only way to care for the problem properly was to completely remove the ring finger and the metacarpal bone that housed the tumor. That would leave him with a four-fingered hand, and he should be able to type with his three remaining fingers and thumb. They seemed to understand and quickly agreed to his having the surgery.

Unfortunately, all the beds in the hospital were occupied with critical patients. The hospital had declared an "Emergencies Only" status, so this patient could not be admitted. I gave them the names of two doctors, one in Chittagong and the other in Dhaka, whom I felt could do the surgery. Disappointed, they left.

They returned and told me they had visited the two doctors I had named. The doctors both demanded more money for the surgery than this couple could possibly afford. This couple returned to plead with me to do the surgery in our hospital. Again, I had to tell them that our hospital was still closed to all admissions except emergencies.

Suddenly, the wife stepped behind me and threw her arms around me, locking her hands and wrists together in an iron grip. This was totally unexpected. In that culture, a woman would never put her arms around a man who was not her husband. Such a thing would be totally prohibited.

"I will not let you go until you agree to operate on my husband's hand!" she shouted. As I could not pry her grip loose, I had no choice. I hobbled to the telephone with her still clinging to me and phoned the male nursing station.

"This is Dr. Bullock speaking," I said. "I have an emergency patient who must be admitted for surgery. Put him anywhere--in a bed, on a gurney, or the floor, but he must be admitted NOW!" The man was admitted, and the surgery was accomplished the next day with an excellent result. He and his wife were very grateful.

Challenging Surgical Cases—Machetes

We saw many patients who had lost limbs or parts of limbs. If a patient lost their hand, we would try to get them to accept an upper extremity prosthesis with a standard hook as a substitute for a hand. This option was poorly accepted by adults, and most people refused.

One day, a patient arrived with a massive wound to his right hand from a machete fight. The opponent's machete had struck the base of the little finger and then extended obliquely through all the bones to the wrist at the base of the thumb. All tendons, nerves, and blood vessels had been severed, with the single exemption of the radial artery. The artery was still embedded in the narrow soft tissue hinge on the wrist's thumb side. That very slender strap of soft tissue, with the embedded radial artery and some of the thumb extensor tendons, was all that held the hand onto the arm.

A partial amputation most likely would have been completed immediately if he had gone to one of the national hospitals in Chittagong. Considering that this was his right hand, I decided to try my best to salvage it. After thoroughly cleansing the cut surfaces, I inserted a thin stainless steel metal rod through the central canal and into the base of the metacarpal bone to which the finger belonged. This brought everything into good alignment, but the nerves and tendons were still cut. I decided to wait 24 hours to see if the radial artery could supply enough circulation to the cut fingers to survive.

The next day, when the dressings were changed, the color of the patient's fingers remained good. At that point, I decided to reconnect the tendons and the nerves to see if they would heal. Later, after all the incisions had healed and the metal rods were removed, the patient was very pleased to see that he could move his fingers a little, which looked like they were not dead. It would take much longer for the nerves to connect and tendons to unite firmly, so the dressings were continued.

We fully expected the sensation to return, and the result was amazing. Eventually, the patient achieved about a 95% restoration of his right hand and could touch the tip of each finger to his thumb and move all the joints. Meanwhile, another special treatment was taking place. While he was in the hospital, the patient learned about the plan of salvation from the Holy Bible, and we prayed for both his spiritual and physical healing.

"Ambulance" at MCH—Change of Plans

One morning, I woke up feeling rested because I had not been called to the hospital in the middle of the night after I had gone to bed. When I arrived at the hospital to make rounds in the wards that morning, I noticed that the men's and women's wards were unusually empty. It seemed we would have a peaceful day at the hospital, which was rare. I finished my rounds in record time, and since I did not have any critical cases on my service that day, I was looking forward to an opportunity to visit a little with the patients.

My first patient was a little girl about seven years old who had been brought to the hospital three days previous with a dislocated hip. Her hip had been dislocated for three weeks before her parents brought her to see us. We took her to the X-ray department to examine her hips while she was under anesthesia. Attempted closed reduction of the dislocation by manipulation had not been successful, so she was put into skeletal traction using a metal pin through the tibial bone, and weights were applied to gain traction. That day, I was going to check the reduction by X-ray while she was under anesthesia before putting her into a cast. We had already given her the anesthetic (ketamine) and had taken the first X-ray of the needed films.

Suddenly, the day ceased to be quiet and peaceful. A large truck had just pulled up in front of the hospital. This makeshift ambulance was full of survivors from a truck accident that had happened down the road from the hospital.

I quickly turned the plaster cast work on the little girl over to my senior orthopedic technician and went outside to triage the injured men. Three of the survivors had already been brought into the hospital, but three others were lying very quietly in the back of the truck. I climbed up into the truck and discovered that two of them were in shock with bleeding and obvious fractures from multiple injuries. I was very glad there were four doctors at the hospital that day. Three of them took care of the lesser-injured patients.

As the hospital nursing staff moved quickly into action, I was impressed with their ability to handle difficult emergency cases like this. They functioned smoothly and efficiently as a team, absorbing the added workload without a word of complaint. The rest of the day was spent taking care of the three severely injured men and working on multiple patients who came in through the OPD. I was grateful for my orthopedic assistant, a young Bangladeshi man who had learned his job well and performed with enthusiasm and expertise. Without his help, the day would have been a disaster. Two of these injured men stayed several months in the hospital for treatment of multiple injuries. During their recovery time at MCH, they heard the truth about what the Holy Bible teaches about God's plan for man's salvation.

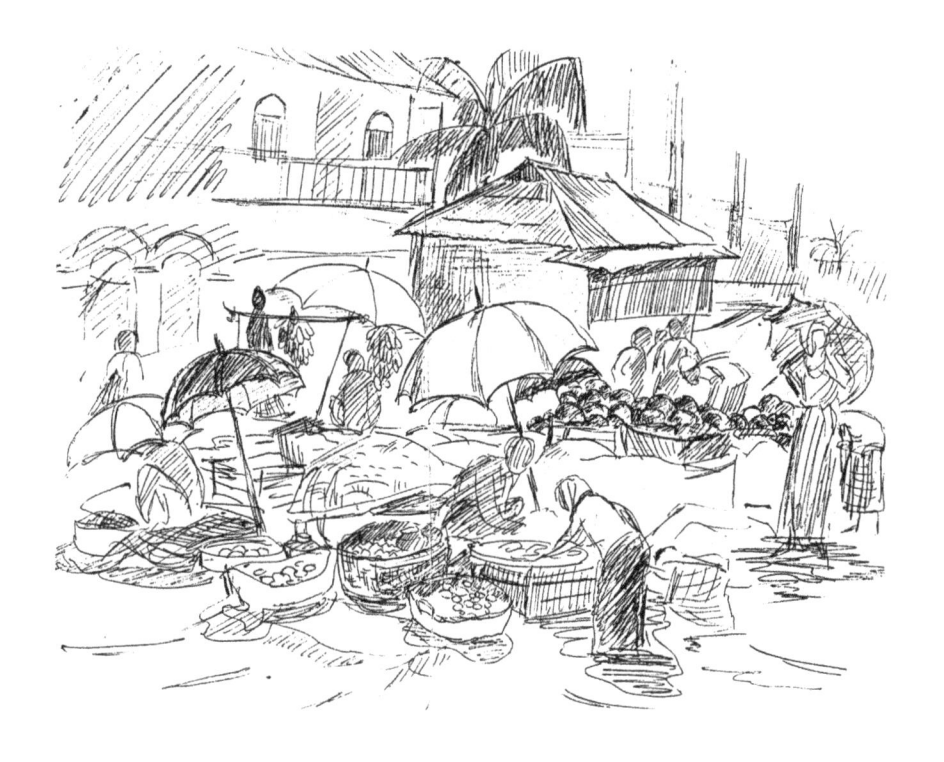

CHAPTER 32

Hope for the Hopeless

I was the first full-time orthopedic surgeon to practice at Memorial Christian Hospital. When word got out that orthopedic care was available at MCH, patients with many challenging orthopedic problems started coming. Some came with problems that had not been treated correctly by national doctors or had remained untreated for years. These patients were often resigned to living the rest of their lives as devalued cripples, dependent on begging for their livelihood. They were overjoyed to learn that we might be able to restore them to a place of health in which they could support their families and live a much more productive life.

Birth Defects and Clubfeet

Babies were often brought to our hospital for clubfoot treatment. In my training years in medical school, many children with clubfeet were treated by surgical methods or by brute force, with terrible results. I learned about a better way developed in the 1950s by Dr. Ignacio Ponseti of the University of Iowa Hospital and Clinics. This method used gentle manipulation and stretching of the baby's foot, and then a cast was put on to hold the foot in the new position until the next cast was applied. A new cast would be put on each week until the foot moved to the final, desired position. At that time, the baby would be fitted with a brace and boots to keep the feet from reverting to where they were before the casting. This procedure was non-surgical except for a possible tenotomy of the Achilles tendon before the last cast was applied.

I taught the orthopedic technicians the Ponseti method. The Clubfeet clinic developed to the point where we saw about a dozen children every week. The orthopedic technicians became so proficient with this treatment that they required minimal supervision and achieved excellent results. We even applied the principle to older children, which was usually successful. It was rewarding to be able to help the children with their disabilities so they could have normal lives.

Rickets

Rickets is a disabling disease caused by a lack of Vitamin D or calcium which affects developing children. It was a prevalent condition in our area of Bangladesh. The body can produce vitamin D through exposure to sunlight. Since children in Bangladesh typically wear minimal clothing and spend ample time in the sun, lack of sun exposure was unlikely the cause in our area. However, calcium intake was often inadequate and may have contributed to the condition.

A team of US epidemiologists investigated the cause of the rickets cases we treated at MCH and concluded that it was caused by what they termed a "coastal effect," seen only along coastal areas. It may have been related to the relatively high amount of aluminum in the water at the coast, which could affect the body's ability to absorb and utilize calcium.

Deformities occur when the growth centers at the ends of the bone cease to develop normally, resulting in marked curvatures of the affected bones. I had little exposure to rickets in the United States. However, in Bangladesh at that time, we treated many children with skeletal deformities caused by rickets.

Our prevention treatment consisted of vitamin D, if we could get it, and calcium, which was also in short supply. The deformities could only be treated by surgery. That involved cutting the affected bone, putting it into the correct alignment, and then holding it with a plaster cast until it healed. We saw some remarkable improvements, both in children and adults, but especially in the children. They became able to walk and function normally.

It was common to see adults or children with one or both legs bowlegged or knock-kneed. Sometimes, the angle of the bend was forward or backward rather than sideways. Often, children with rickets would not be brought to the hospital until their deformities were far advanced. One young girl came whose right leg was bent at a right angle below the knee from rickets, and she could not walk. I performed surgery on her right leg, and the result was satisfactory. She came back several times over the next few years for further surgery on her other leg and follow-up procedures.

An older teenage girl came with severely deformed legs that were so bowed that her knees were more than eighteen inches apart when her ankles were touching. She was brought for treatment so that she would be marriageable. A man would not marry a woman with such a deformity, as it was thought that her children would also have that deformity. I operated on her legs and succeeded in getting them straight enough that the knees could touch. She and her parents were delighted.

Burn Contractures

In Bangladesh, cooking in the village was usually done over an open fire at ground level. As a result, burns were common in both adults and children. When a woman squatted in front of the fire to tend to the cooking, her clothing could easily catch fire, and she might try to beat the fire out with her hands. Depending on the fabric, sometimes all of her clothing would catch fire quickly, enveloping the woman in flames and causing burns to her entire body. These patients often succumbed to their injuries despite our efforts to treat them.

Mothers often held their infants while cooking. If the mother's clothing caught fire, the infant could get severe burns. It was also possible for children to accidentally tip a pot of boiling liquid onto themselves. Without proper care, these types of burns could result in severe scarring, contractures, and deformities of the extremities, especially the hands or feet.

Before our hospital was established, no good burn care was available in the southern area of Bangladesh. When the hospital opened, patients with scarring from burns they had sustained years earlier would come for treatment. Overcoming these contractures and trying to give them a functioning hand, foot, or other part of their body was quite a challenge. Infants and young children were brought with severe contractures and deformities from burns. In one particular case, the child's hand was bent backward so much that the back of the hand was stuck to the back of the wrist. The fingers were drawn into a tightly clenched fist, and the hand was useless.

Treatment for such contractures involved surgical removal of the scar tissue sufficiently to allow the extremity to be moved into the normal position as much as possible. Then, dressings were applied until enough granulation tissue was formed to allow the application of split-thickness skin grafts. These grafts were obtained from an unscarred part of the body by an instrument called a "dermatome," a vibrating knife that lifted a very thin slice of normal skin for the graft. The graft was then applied over the granulation tissue and held in place until it became attached. This could not be done in one procedure but would require multiple procedures and a strong measure of cooperation by the patient's family.

A woman came to the hospital to get treatment for scarring on her right hand, which had severely contracted in the opposite direction. Her wrist was acutely flexed, and her fingers were useless. This deformity had been present for many years, and she was forced to use her left hand for everything, including cooking and eating, which caused her much shame and disgrace. Our goal was function rather than appearance.

For a hand, the functions desirable are pinch (fingertip to thumb tip), grasp (gripping an object such as a ball or a stick), and hook (using the flexed finger or fingers to hook something and draw it toward the body). The hand may not be pretty, but it can be very useful if it can perform these three functions. Even if only one or two of these functions could be obtained, it was more valuable than a useless extremity. Patients were usually grateful to have any use of their hands again.

Treatment of burn contractures often involved prolonged or frequent hospitalization. While the patient was being treated, the personal worker had the opportunity to carefully explain God's plan of salvation from the Holy Bible. As a result of witnessing and compassionate care, many patients received the truth about salvation as taught in the Holy Bible.

HOPE Fund Established

I soon became painfully aware of the fact that many patients who came to the hospital with orthopedic problems were extremely poor. Some had traveled many miles seeking our help and could barely afford to come to the hospital. We were deeply troubled by the many people, particularly children, who came to the hospital needing treatment for conditions such as congenital deformities, cancers, paralysis from cerebral palsy or poliomyelitis, birth defects, club feet, burns, spinal curvatures and fractures of all sorts. Treatment of these patients was often time-consuming and relatively expensive since it involved repeated plaster casts, special bracing, and multiple operations. Treatment of most orthopedic problems involved long hospital stays or repeated hospital visits.

Although we had the facility, the team, and the expertise to handle most of these problems, many families could not afford to pay for the needed treatment and repeated trips to the hospital for follow-up care. The hospital had funds for relief available to emergency patients who could not pay. However, these relief funds would soon have been exhausted if they were used to treat non-life-threatening cases. Since the relief funds could not always be used, we had no choice but to turn these patients away. It was heartbreaking and extremely frustrating to see patients who had come with treatable conditions be turned away because they were unable to afford the necessary care. They had to return to their homes for whatever sort of care might be available to them there or none at all. They might be doomed to life as beggars. This was especially traumatic in the case of children who were dependent upon their parents to pay for their care.

I felt strongly that when God brought people to our hospital for physical care, He expected us to use the opportunity to tell them of the love of Christ as taught in the Holy Bible and the spiritual healing available to them, as well as provide them with whatever physical care they needed. I always felt sad when we had to send patients away if they couldn't afford the care, were unwilling to accept the necessary treatment, or because there were no beds available in the hospital. That meant they might never hear of God's love for them.

Memorial Christian Hospital was not a free hospital and was not self-supporting. As a non-profit organization, no NGO personnel working there received any salary from the hospital. Funds to operate the hospital came from several sources, including individual donors, donations from charitable organizations, or allotments from work funds taken from the NGO medical staff's monthly support. Additionally, patients were charged nominal fees for doctor visits, labs, x-rays, and surgery. However, the revenue was barely enough to cover the expenses of running the hospital. Several hundred national personnel worked at the hospital. Wages paid to our national employees were less than they could get working elsewhere, but many continued faithfully working at the hospital.

In 1979, we decided to create a special fund that would enable us to provide the needed surgical care for elective cases of patients with disabling orthopedic problems who could not pay for such care. It would also enable us to provide needed braces and artificial limbs for impoverished children and adults and for rehabilitation for paralyzed persons to allow them to have a normal and productive life. This fund would also help us sleep better at night, knowing we did not have to turn away someone needing treatment. We decided to call it the "Hospital

Orthopedic Patient Enablement" (HOPE) Fund. When we told our supporters in the US about the HOPE Fund and asked them to donate if they could, the response was good. With the help of the HOPE Fund, many who had no hope of a better life here on earth were given hope through their contact with Memorial Christian Hospital. But most importantly, they heard the gospel's good news from the Holy Bible.

To avoid abuse of the HOPE Fund, a committee of national hospital employees was set up to interview applicants requesting assistance. The nationals were more effective at determining the applicants' financial status than the medical staff and could easily detect fraudulent claims. The committee then decided what amount the patient or the patient's family should be able to afford, and the HOPE Fund would cover the remainder.

HOPE Fund—Treatment Refused

One day, a man about thirty years old was brought with great difficulty to the hospital by some friends from one of the nearby islands after he had fallen out of a tree. In the cool winter season, there was great demand for firewood. When the fallen branches had all been picked up, the woodcutters climbed the trees to cut the dead branches for firewood, which was a hazardous occupation. We often had patients with injuries from falling out of trees. When this man fell, he broke his back and was instantly paralyzed from the waist down. Living in Bangladesh was hard enough for able-bodied persons, but for a paraplegic, the outlook was hopeless.

When we examined the injured man at the hospital, we were hopeful that he could recover some function in his legs. At that time, MCH was one of the few hospitals in Bangladesh with a paraplegic rehabilitation program. In this program, if the individual was motivated, he could learn to walk with braces and crutches and to transfer himself from bed to a wheelchair. He could learn to care for himself. He could even learn a new trade with which he could support himself and his family if he had one.

The man was quite ill, having suffered chest injuries as well. He was also in spinal shock from the back injury. His mind was not clear, and he required restraints to keep him from throwing himself out of bed. When his general condition improved with treatment and his mind cleared, he realized where he was and what had happened to him. He began to demand to go home, saying that he did not have any money to pay for treatment. We carefully explained to him that going home would mean certain death within a short time from complications of his injuries. He still wanted to go home.

The HOPE Fund Committee investigated and found he could not pay for treatment. Thus, he qualified to receive free treatment under the HOPE Fund. We explained this to him and said that it would involve hospitalization for six to eight weeks, then braces, physical therapy, and occupational training. All he had to do was accept this offer of free medical care as a gift.

The man refused to accept the offer of free treatment. No amount of pleading with him or his friends would change his mind. He refused to eat or drink, and we finally had to let him go home to a certain miserable death.

Another patient, a young boy with severe flexion contractures of his legs due to rheumatoid arthritis, was brought by his father from a location 90 miles north of the hospital. After approval by the HOPE Fund committee, treatment was given that would allow him to stand and walk with braces and crutches. However, because he was growing, he would need several replacement braces and crutches. The father was asked to return with his son in six months for a recheck. However, they did not return until six years later, at which time the deformities had progressed to the point that treatment was going to be far more complicated and require a greater commitment on the part of the boy and his family. They left and did not return.

When these things happened, I thought how similar this is to the response of many people to the offer of the gift of salvation. Man's sinful condition has but one outcome—spiritual death, which is eternal separation from God. There is only one "treatment" for this "disease," and that is to receive Jesus Christ as Savior and claim His sacrificial death on the cross as atonement for sin.

Some patients who spent a long time recuperating in the hospital have accepted this gift of salvation. The HOPE Fund program resulted in even the poorest of patients and their families having the opportunity to receive much more than physical healing—they learned about salvation, spiritual healing, and the joy of eternal life with God, as taught in the Holy Bible.

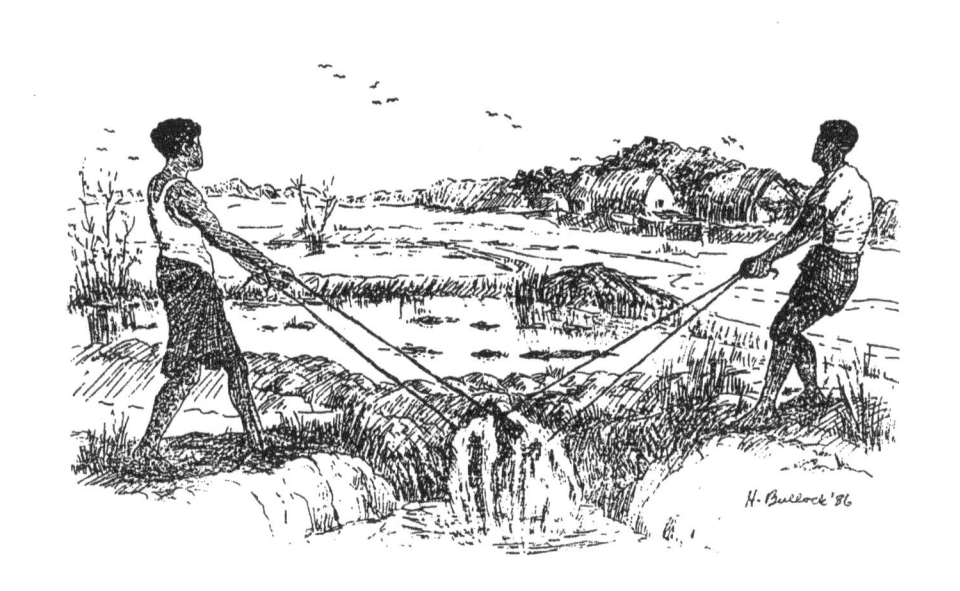

CHAPTER 33

Prosthetic Limbs

Limb and Brace Shop

Bangladeshis were accustomed to seeing people with artificial legs. However, artificial arms were not as commonly used. Losing an arm or hand would greatly diminish a person's ability to function.

When I arrived in Bangladesh, the usual type of artificial hand used was a hook, which could be opened and closed by cables attached to the arm above the amputation. This was crude, but it allowed people to pick up objects and hold things. At first, these artificial-hook arms were poorly received by adults, particularly women. Such prostheses were unusual and peculiar, which made the wearer extremely sensitive to others' reactions. Some felt embarrassed about wearing a prosthesis and concealed the end of the missing limb with a shawl to keep it hidden. However, for some arm amputees, regaining function mattered more than the scorn of onlookers. A manual worker could learn to use tools again with a prosthetic device, and people gradually became more accepting of it.

One of our national nurses had lost her left arm due to very severe X-ray burns before she came to work at MCH. She received the first artificial arm manufactured at our Limb and Brace Shop. The fabrication of this arm was a real test of ingenuity for our technicians in the Limb and Brace Shop. They needed a left-hand hook for her prosthesis, but we had only a few right-hand commercially manufactured hooks that had been donated to our Limb and Brace Shop from the US. They were not available for purchase in Bangladesh. The hook would have to be made in Bangladesh.

Bangladeshi artisans were so skilled at sand casting that they could manufacture key blanks from brass with that method. We arranged to have them make brass hooks for prosthetic arms, and it was a great success. We manufactured artificial arms in our Limb and Brace Shop for injuries above and below the elbow.

Our technician created a mirror-image replica of the sample right-hand hook and took it to a brass work in Chittagong, where they made a sand casting of it in brass. Then, our Limb and Brace Shop technicians used the new left-hand hook to build an artificial arm with parts of donated artificial arms for the hinged elbow and wrist unit. Next, they began the complicated job of teaching the patient how to use the arm. She inspired everyone around her as she progressed in her ability to function with her new arm in her home and as a nurse at MCH.

Soccer Player

A twelve-year-old boy broke his arm. It was a simple fracture of his radius and ulna. He was taken to a local "bone setter," who had learned his skills in a hereditary fashion, and the man applied a primitive splint to the boy's arm. The problem was that he applied it too tightly. When they realized it and came to MCH for help, it was too late to save the arm. The hand and forearm were black and had to be amputated. Ordinarily, that would mean that this boy would have had to live out the rest of his life minus his left arm, which could greatly impact his ability to earn a living. However, because our hospital had the Limb and Brace Shop where our technicians could make an artificial arm, his future held much greater potential. He and his father eagerly accepted our suggestion that he be fitted with an artificial arm as soon as the stump had healed.

Then came the big day. Since there had been some stump revision because of a bony spur, it delayed the fitting of his prosthesis, but finally, it was ready. However, his face clouded with disappointment when the odd-looking device was firmly strapped onto the stump of his arm. He tried to make it do something but could not. It took hours of patient instruction before the boy finally grasped the principle of moving and shrugging his shoulders in just the right way to lock and unlock the elbow, move the new arm through flexion and extension, and open and close the hook. At last, he caught on to just what movements were necessary and seemed encouraged. After three days of practice, we showed the boy a video of a man demonstrating how easily and deftly he could do almost anything with his two artificial arms. After watching the movie, the boy's eyes were shining. His father beamed as he realized that all was not lost regarding his son's future.

This boy quickly learned to use his new arm to open and close an umbrella, throw a ball, use a saw to cut a board, and more, and we were fairly certain he would do well with it. However, no one in his village had ever seen an artificial limb. We sent a note home with them to the child's teacher, asking the teacher to enlist the cooperation of his classmates and friends to encourage him and not make fun of him.

Two years later, the boy and his father returned to the hospital for a new prosthetic arm. When the boy pulled off his shirt to show me the problem, I was amazed at what I saw. That artificial arm was not only well-worn; it was practically demolished! The harness was broken. The only thing holding it onto his arm was the control cable. The prosthesis socket was too small, and the stub of his arm barely fit into it. All this was ample evidence that he was using the arm regularly. He wore it all day long and used it for everything. I found out later that he was the goalie for his soccer team. His prosthetic arm truly was a part of him Seeing the boy's progress was heartwarming for Larry and me.

"Just a few good users like this," I told Larry, "and word will get out far and wide that a person doesn't have to be permanently disabled just because he has lost an arm." With an artificial arm, a person can earn a living, provide for his family, and have a nearly normal life. All this was made possible through the HOPE Fund. The boy's father could only afford to pay half the cost of the artificial arm, and the HOPE Fund paid the balance.

Prosthetic Feet

Prosthetic appliances, especially feet, had to be specially modified to make them suitable for Bangladesh. For example, giving a man an artificial leg that required him to wear a store-bought shoe over a prosthesis created numerous complications. He was not used to wearing shoes, could not afford to keep purchasing them, and needed to be able to walk and work in a wet environment, such as a rice paddy.

Larry Golin learned of a doctor in Jaipur, India, who was making a rubber foot. Larry visited the doctor and studied the foot. He found that patients wearing a prosthesis with this kind of rubber foot could run, jump, and even climb trees. They could wear sandals or go barefoot since the rubber foot looked real and was barely noticeable. It could be made in different colors to match the wearer's natural skin color. The "Jaipur foot" was constructed of several parts and fastened together by rubber straps that functioned as ligaments. Larry tried to bring a supply of these rubber feet back to Bangladesh but found the difficulty of importing them made it almost impossible. After much painstaking research, he was able to have special molds made so these feet could be built at MCH. This was an instant success, and a steady stream of amputees began to come to the hospital to get a foot like this. The new foot offered hope to many amputees.

Foot Camp

Larry recognized that many amputees lived too far from the hospital to learn about the Jaipur foot or to travel to the hospital to get one. The answer seemed to be to take the Jaipur foot to the amputees, so Larry devised a plan to hold foot camps in various locations in the country. Setting up a foot camp involved getting permission from the government to use a public facility such as a school and then printing and distributing brochures to advertise. Then the supplies and equipment from the Limb and Brace Shop were taken to the camp site and set up in the building for production of the prostheses.

At the foot camp, a leg would be built from aluminum sheeting and fitted to the patient's stump. Then, the rubber foot would be attached. All this was accomplished in a day or two at the patient's cost of about US $1.25. That small sum did not cover the cost of materials, but it made the patient feel like he had purchased the prosthesis with his own money. This helped ensure he would use it and take good care of it.

I attended one of the foot camps to examine the amputees to determine whether their stumps were suitable for receiving a prosthesis. Many of the stumps were not suitable, in my opinion. However, the orthotics crew said they could manage. I was greatly impressed by their improvised solutions.

As I attended the camp, I thought about Jesus walking around the countryside of ancient Israel, healing people in the crowds that assembled and then teaching them about the Kingdom. Our purpose in providing physical healing was to develop relationships that enabled us to offer spiritual healing. The fitting of the Jaipur foot and braces and the instruction of its use and care required many visits, allowing us multiple opportunities to share with the patients the message of hope and salvation taught in the Holy Bible.

Unmarriageable

When I returned to MCH from a furlough, I was assigned the care of the patients of one of our doctors who was returning to the US. My orthopedic technician took me to the wards to meet the patients. As we approached bed #2 in the female ward, he said, "Here is a pitiful case. She now looks worlds better than when she came." He went on to explain that a tree had fallen on this young girl's leg, resulting in a fracture of the tibia. She lived in the Hill Tracts and could not get good medical care quickly. The result was a horribly infected wound which developed osteomyelitis. When her family finally brought her to our hospital, she was an emaciated, stinking mess. Dr. Goddard and the orthopedic technician did their best to clean up the infection, but they were finally forced to amputate the leg to control it. The technician had been so moved by this girl's situation and poverty that he had donated blood for her. When I saw her, she had a short, draining stump below the knee, which was not long enough to support a below-knee prosthesis. It needed revision.

Although her condition had significantly improved, she was still a withdrawn, unsmiling little girl in acute discomfort. She and her mother were being fed from the hospital kitchen, where the staff ate because they were too poor to buy food. At least she was getting a nourishing diet, and the results of this were evident. She had regained some weight but still needed to improve her health and strength.

We scheduled her for a through-knee disarticulation surgery. This was a procedure that would allow us to give her a good artificial leg and would allow the leg to grow at the normal rate at both ends. The surgery went well, and she healed promptly. Gradually winning her trust and confidence, I teased her as I made rounds and coaxed some smiles and giggles out of her. From then on, she was cheerful and optimistic. She learned to walk with crutches and was finally able to leave the hospital to continue healing at home.

What could a young girl do in this culture with only one leg? She would be unmarriageable and unable to do much work around her house—not a very bright future. But we assured her mother that we could provide her with an artificial leg with financial assistance from the HOPE Fund.

After a couple of months, once her stump had healed and was ready, she and her mother returned to Malumghat and spent several days visiting the hospital while the Limb and Brace Shop created the artificial leg. The new leg had a Jaipur foot and looked like a real foot with toes. It even matched her skin color. When the big day came, and she could put on her new leg and walk again, the shine in her eyes and the beaming smile on her mother's face were indescribably joyous. While this girl and her mother were in the hospital, they had numerous opportunities from many sources to hear the good news of salvation as taught in the Holy Bible.

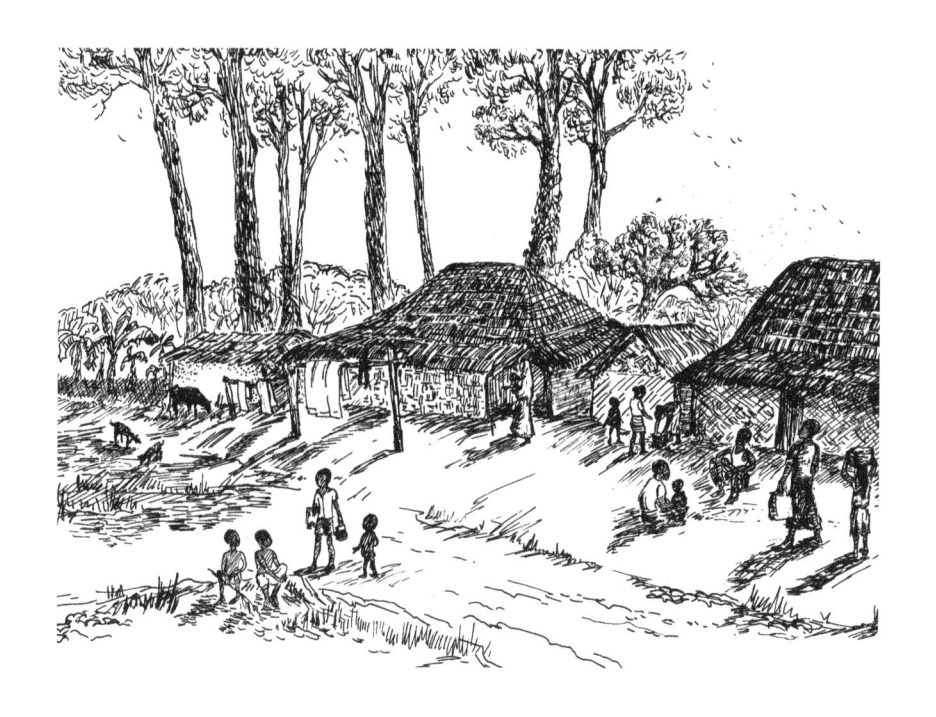

CHAPTER 34

Every Life Matters

Chittagong Hepatitis

In 1980, our medical staff began steadily decreasing for various reasons. Nancie, one of our NGO nurses who was in language school, contracted "Chittagong Hepatitis." Many of our teammates were getting this mysterious viral illness. The only cure seemed to be six weeks of bed rest. Nancie had already lost a lot of weight and did not seem to be making a recovery, so we decided that she must return to the US for an intensive medical workup. One of the other NGO nurses, who had been supervising the OPD, accompanied her to the US. This meant that the responsibility for supervising the OPD had to be shifted to other staff. Nancie later recovered enough to return to Bangladesh and served faithfully at MCH for many years.

"Orthostetrics"

After our general surgeon went home on furlough, Dr. Dick Stagg, a family practitioner, and I were the only full-term doctors left at the hospital until Dr. DeCook returned on June 1 for three months. We would still be without a general surgeon for an uncomfortably long time. Dr. Stagg had had quite a bit of surgical experience and would be able to perform many of the general surgeries, but the more complicated ones would be beyond both of our capabilities.

With all the other doctors gone, Dr. Stagg had to handle all the obstetric cases alone. I was doing all the orthopedic surgery. We prayed that we would not be flooded with serious general surgical cases, but I was thankful to be able to fall back on my general surgery training, realizing anew that God had prepared me for this place.

The caseload for Dr. Stagg was heavy, and I felt he was being overworked. I had good training in obstetrics in medical school and general practice but limited experience with cesarean sections. I offered to take half of the obstetric cases if he would teach me how to do them. He agreed, and I began to take every other case. What I hadn't counted on was that some of the patients that fell into my care were not simply cesarean sections. I also treated a host of other obstetric problems, including destructive delivery of infants who had died, ruptured uterus, and retained placentas. That year, I did over 100 cesarean sections. Dr. Stagg and I were sure that a visiting OB/GYN resident could probably see more obstetrics pathology in a short time at our hospital than he might see in a lifetime in the US.

"I've decided to rename my specialty," I told Dr. Stagg one day. "Instead of orthopedics, I will call it "Orthostetrics."

Dr. Stagg and I tried to find a way to lessen the hospital load during our times of reduced surgical staff. We removed several beds from the male and female wards, which we thought would lighten the load on the national staff. It worked for about one day. Soon after that, five students were brought in who had been injured in a brick-throwing argument between two student groups. That was followed shortly by six men who had been badly chopped up in a machete fight during a land dispute. Then, eight men who were mixing gunpowder and smoking at the same time (an incompatible situation) were brought in, suffering from multiple burns and traumatic injuries. At times like this, we had to put cots down in the center aisles of the wards to handle the additional patients.

Arm Out

I never knew what would happen when I was on obstetrics duty. Often, I would be in bed when a messenger arrived at my door with a note from the medics up at the hospital. The note would briefly describe the problem and ask me to come immediately or soon. This time, the note read, "Twin boy was born three days ago. The second twin's arm came out, but the twin would not come. Baby dead. Please come to do destructive delivery."

I dressed and went to the hospital, expecting to do a destructive delivery because the baby was presumably dead. When I arrived at the hospital, the patient was already on the operating table waiting for the delivery. The obstetrical nurse told me that this tribal woman had delivered one twin three days previous in her village. However, the second twin would not come out. People had been pulling on the baby's arm for three days, and it was very discolored and floppy. If there was no fetal heartbeat, we could assume the baby was no longer alive. The nurse had not heard a heartbeat. Sometimes, a fetal heartbeat was impossible to detect by listening with a stethoscope.

Because of the uncertainty of the situation, I decided to make a small cut on the skin of the baby's protruding arm to determine if the baby was alive or dead. Dead babies don't bleed, but live ones do. I straightened out the fingers of the baby's hand and then turned my head to pick up the scissors with which to cut the skin. When I turned my gaze back to the arm, I was surprised to see the fingers had curled up in the flexed position again. This was not a dead baby!

"Prep for a section," I immediately told the nurses, and they hurriedly did so. We were using ketamine for anesthesia when possible because it was quick. I ordered a dose to be given to the mother by IV. Time was short. I proceeded as soon as possible with the cesarean section and delivered a baby boy, barely alive but responding to resuscitation and bawling. We had rescued him not a moment too soon. He was reunited with his brother, and his mother was delighted to have two live boys.

One Telephone, One Motorcycle, One Life

We had recently moved to House #12, which was closer to the hospital than our previous house, a half-mile away at the back of the compound. There were no telephones at the MCH and no hospital intercom system, but I had installed a wired intercom that connected my house to the hospital for emergency contact. One day, Tense and I were seated in our living room when a call came over the intercom from one of our NGO nurses.

The voice blurted out, "Body out – head won't come out. Hurry!" I realized the call came from the hospital delivery room. My Honda motor scooter was parked in our driveway, ready to go with the front pointed toward the hospital. I rushed to the motor scooter, jumped onto the seat, and kicked the starter lever. The engine roared to life, and I raced up the road toward the hospital.

A minute later, I arrived at the hospital's front door, parked the motor scooter, and rushed down the hallway toward the delivery room. Bursting through the door, I saw the mother lying on the delivery table. The baby's body was out, but the head was not out. There was no time to check for fetal heart sounds, change shoes, put on surgical clothing, or even wash my hands. I had received excellent obstetrical training in medical school and knew how to use forceps, but there was no time to locate them.

Immediately, I shoved my hand under the baby's body and thrust my fingers under its neck. Quickly, I found the baby's mouth and put a finger in it. Then I gently pulled on the chin to bring the head downward while I pushed on the mother's abdomen with my other hand. As I pulled and pushed, the head began to come out. I pulled as hard as I dared, hoping that I was not injuring the baby's neck or brain. Finally, the head was delivered, and the baby girl was born. The elapsed time was less than five minutes from the intercom call.

After the baby was born, I examined her carefully. She seemed to be doing fine. I hoped she had not suffered any harm during the delivery. On the mother's return for her post-delivery appointment, I examined her happy, healthy baby, who showed no sign of injury from her traumatic delivery.

Equal Treatment for Everyone

A patient from the affluent class had returned to the hospital for his follow-up appointment. Individuals in this social class often did not like to wait and preferred to receive immediate care. They expected to be placed at the front of the line. After registering upon his arrival at the hospital, this man anticipated I would see him next. Instead of sitting in the waiting room until his name was called, he entered the hospital and came into the wards where I was making my morning rounds to see my patients.

"I am here," he announced when he saw me, expecting me to drop everything and tend to him. I acknowledged him and told him I would examine him as soon as I finished seeing my patients. I then proceeded to go from bed to bed to check on my patients. He followed me and stood at the foot of each bed. I ignored him and continued to check on my patients—changing dressings, reviewing the orders, and physically examining the patients' blood pressure, pulse, respiration, urine output, and other vitals. Then, when I had finished seeing each bed patient, I moved on to the next bed in line, all the time followed by the man who had returned for his follow-up appointment. At one bedside, I removed the patient's dressing and examined the wound. Then, reassuring the patient that everything was okay, I moved on to the next bed.

"You really do!" my follower exclaimed after watching me examine my patient's wound.

"Really do what?" I asked.

"You really treat everyone, rich or poor, like they were the most important person in the world," he answered.

"That's correct," I said. "Now it is time for me to see you. Let's go to the examining room." He followed me, and I examined him.

Mr. S.C.—A Change of Heart

One day, a middle-aged Bengali businessman traveling to Cox's Bazar in a jeep driven by his chauffeur was injured in an accident about one mile past our hospital. Mr. S.C. had been leisurely sitting in the passenger seat with his right knee leaning a little outside the jeep. As they started to cross a bridge, the driver drove too close to the bridge railing, and Mr. S.C.'s knee struck one of the supports of the railing, resulting in a fracture of his right femur.

The driver immediately turned the jeep around to take Mr. S.C. back to Chittagong. Mr. S.C. was experiencing so much pain in the fractured leg as they approached our hospital that he directed the driver to turn into the driveway. He was taken into the waiting area, where he was seen by one of our medics. Mr. S.C. said he wanted to be admitted to our hospital and asked to be put into a private room. He was told that he could be admitted, but no private rooms were available then, and he would have to agree to be placed in the male ward, which consisted of about twenty beds. He asked if it would be possible to screen his bed from the rest of the ward and was told it would be possible. He was placed in a corner bed, and curtains were pulled to seclude his bed.

When I saw the patient and examined his X-rays, I told him that we could treat his fractured femur, but it would require prolonged hospitalization for traction, followed by casting. At that time, I was not doing open reduction and internal fixation for long bone fractures due to a lack of supplies and equipment. Rather, after spending enough time in traction to allow skeletal healing to become strong enough, a walking cast could be applied, allowing the patient to get out of bed and bear a little weight on the fractured leg.

Mr. S.C. agreed to this approach, and we began his treatment. It was easy to have a conversation with him since his English proficiency was excellent. I offered him a copy of the Bible in Bengali, but he said he did not read Bengali but would accept a Bible written in English. He also accepted the Bible literature I left with him. He told me he had attended a Catholic parochial school for a few years. We developed a friendship over the next few weeks, but he never seemed willing to discuss spiritual things.

One day during his confinement, he asked that the curtains be taken down, and he began to get acquainted with the other patients in the ward. During one of our conversations, he told me he was overwhelmed by their poverty and said that he noticed one man near him had not eaten for several days, as he had no sangi to cook for him. Mr. S.C. arranged for food to be brought in from a restaurant across the street for that patient. "I have lived in Bangladesh for many years among people like these other patients," he told me, "But I have never really seen them."

Eventually, the fracture had healed enough to allow us to place him in a long-leg, weight-bearing cast with a hinged knee and hip. With crutches, he was able to walk reasonably well. When the time came for Mr. S.C.'s discharge, he presented me with an envelope, which he said his father had sent as relief for the poor patients in the hospital. We were not aware that his father had ever visited him. The envelope contained a considerable amount of money. Every year after that, he would send a cake to us at Christmastime to be shared with patients and staff at the hospital.

Over subsequent years, I saw Mr. S.C. from time to time, both as a patient and as a friend. Finally, after returning from furlough, I wrote to him, saying, "During our years of friendship, you never told me anything about your relationship with Jesus Christ." He replied in a letter and said that he was certain his name was written in the Book of Life but that he could not come out openly as a Christian because it would be "business suicide."

Elephant man

One day, a man from a refugee camp was brought in with multiple fractures and the footprint of an elephant on his chest. He had been searching outside the camp for firewood when an elephant threw him against a tree and stomped on his chest. Somehow, he lived.

He did not speak Bengali, and conversing with him through the translators was difficult. We did the best we could for him and treated his many fractures. He refused to talk much, even though some of our staff could speak his language. I never saw him smile when I came through the ward to check on him. He just lay in bed recovering from his wounds.

Finally came the big day when his fractures had healed to the extent that he could be safely discharged from the hospital. He still was not smiling. The scars from the elephant's foot were still plainly visible on his chest. Speaking through an interpreter, I told him that he was probably the only living man with a footprint of an elephant on his chest. He looked down at his scars and then broke into a big grin. He was going to be famous! I never saw him again. I can only hope that while he was recovering at the hospital, the personal workers were able to help him understand the message of God's love and forgiveness as taught in the Holy Bible.

Yellow Jeep

It was the week after Christmas, and I was the only surgeon on duty at the hospital. A small boy about five years old was brought in with a large head wound. His pupils were dilated, indicating pressure on the brain from hemorrhage, so I made a burr hole on the trauma side of his head to relieve the pressure. But he still had pupil dilation. So, I made an exploratory burr hole on the other side of his head and determined that there was a hemorrhage on that side, also. His condition was too critical to send him to Chittagong for care. He would die if not treated immediately. It was up to me to treat his injury with the best care I could provide.

The cleaning had to be done as carefully as possible to avoid further damage to the exposed brain tissue. As I scrubbed before entering the operating room, I sensed the urgency, wondering how much of this little boy's skills were going into the bucket catching the cleansing fluids flowing from his head. After cleaning the wound, I pulled the torn dura mater together with fine silk sutures to cover the brain tissue and close the tear in the dura. I could feel "special help" as the edges slowly came together, leaving only a small open area I could easily cover with a flap of tissue from the dura. Then, I carefully wired the bony fragments together and sutured the tissues together to cover the defect in the skull.

After closing the scalp and applying the dressing, I realized how exhausted I was, feeling completely drained. But the boy was still alive, and he had withstood the procedure well. The next few hours would tell the story. Would he survive the shock, the blood loss, and the possibility of infection, I wondered? Was there significant damage to the brain? All I could do was try my best, and that is what I had done.

Over the next few days, the boy's condition steadily improved, as first one hurdle and then another was passed. When I returned to check on him, his eyes were wide open and followed me as I moved near his bed. His father said he had taken some oral fluids and could tell us his name, but he would not smile. He had been through a traumatic event and had a dazed look, as if he could not figure out what was going on.

"Do you know what this is?" I asked as I held a small toy jeep before him to test whether he could connect his thoughts and respond appropriately. I wondered if there had been too much damage to that little brain.

"It's a yellow jeep," he answered, smiling. What joy I felt when I heard his words! This was a wonderful Christmas present for me.

"Thank you, Lord," I breathed. His answer assured me he would make it, but he still had a long recovery ahead. My next question to him was also a test. "Do you need a yellow Jeep like this one?" He nodded his head and reached out his hand to take it. Happy Day!

The next few days allowed me to become better acquainted with the little boy and his father and to tell them about another wonderful Christmas gift—the gift of eternal life that is still available to everyone who receives the truth of the gospel as taught in the Holy Bible. As we labored in that far-off place, God brought many people to our door to allow us to tell them the truth about Him. That made it all worthwhile.

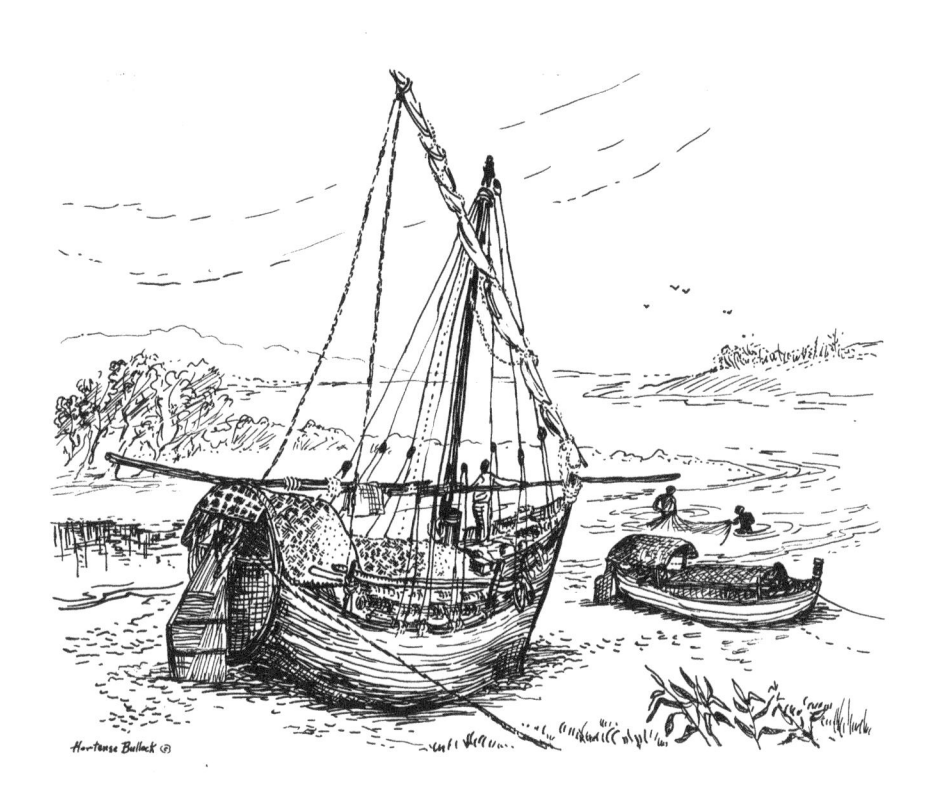

CHAPTER 35

Equipment and Supply Challenges

1981 Doctor Shortage Continued—A Difficult Year

A short-term orthopedic surgeon and a general surgeon came during the fall of 1981 to carry us through the doctor shortage. Our last short-term doctor left at the end of December, which meant Dr. Dick Stagg and I were the only doctors at the hospital again. We took turns being on call every other night. I was in surgery one night when the generator stopped working. The surgery had to be finished with a flashlight and lantern. On examination the next day, we learned that the fault in the generator was because of a leaking oil seal. We had no spares, and none was available in Bangladesh. We sent a telegram to one of our nurses who was home on furlough and asked her to bring spare oil seals with her when she returned to Bangladesh in three weeks.

We let our supporters know that additional short-term doctors were urgently needed as Dr. Stagg was planning to leave for furlough in May. Dr. Stagg's wife was suffering from a serious illness, and it was very likely that they would not be able to return to the field after their furlough. Dr. K had been on medical furlough for a heart problem, and we were unsure of his return. Dr. H., a surgeon, and his family had just arrived and planned to stay for six weeks. However, we did not know if any short-term doctors would be able to come in May or June.

About that time, Dr. Olsen returned from his furlough but had to travel to Dhaka on an important assignment to negotiate with the Bangladesh government concerning mission business. He did not stay at the hospital to do medical work. Thankfully, the difficult matter was successfully solved. We were very much indebted to Dr. Olsen for his negotiation skills on our behalf.

Additional Responsibilities

In addition to my medical work at the hospital, I also helped with other responsibilities at Malumghat, as did all of our teammates. Dr. Joe DeCook had started a cassette ministry in the hospital. When he had to leave Bangladesh to take his wife to the US for medical treatment, he asked me to take over as Director of the cassette ministry for the AV Department. My duties involved maintaining and repairing the audio cassette equipment used in the AV Department. Another responsibility I had was manufacturing and repairing orthopedic surgical equipment. I set up my workshop in our home for this maintenance and repair work, as there was no space at the hospital to do that work at that time. Later, I set up a small workshop in my office at the hospital where I could sharpen and repair the surgical instruments and equipment.

Generator—God's Provision

Two large Onan generators were on duty at the side of the road from the hospital back to the housing area. These were necessary whenever the government power shut down, which was at least several times every day and for unknown periods. At the hospital was another smaller generator that could supply power to the operating rooms in case of a blackout.

One of the generators had been overhauled several times but had ultimately deteriorated to the point that a new one had to be sent to us. It had arrived and was sitting in crates beside the road, waiting to be installed. Our workshop crew had become proficient at keeping the old hospital vehicles running, but when something as complicated as the new generator had to be installed, that presented a difficult challenge. The instructions were complex. It had to be done with the utmost precision.

The workshop crew studied the instructions and prepared the mounting base as carefully as possible. They were about to attempt the installation when two American men arrived at the hospital site and said they had come from Dhaka to see the hospital. They had heard a lot about MCH and wanted to stay in our Guest House for several days to make this a "vacation" for them. We asked them what their occupation was in the US. To our surprise, they said they were Onan engineers and had come to Bangladesh to do an installation in Dhaka. Praise the Lord! We were only too happy to tell them that God had sent them to us for another installation, which they were happy to do on their "vacation" at our Guest House.

X-Ray Machines

Two used X-ray machines arrived in a shipment from the US and were installed in the renovated X-ray department. These second-hand units had been completely reconditioned before being sent to us. Fred S., an X-ray machine technician, came to Bangladesh for two weeks to set up the X-ray machines and get them working. He hand-carried a new X-ray tube for the smaller unit, which had stopped working about two months earlier. The tubes were delicate and required special handling. He got the small X-ray machine working the very day he arrived. Then he started working on the mysterious problem with the big machine. After several days of troubleshooting, he got that one working, too. We were elated to have the large X-ray machine operational.

Fred also had time to work on other laboratory and surgical equipment while he was at Malumghat and put many things back into working order. His visit was extremely helpful. However, only two weeks after Fred returned to the US, the large X-ray machine again refused to operate. Dave F., our X-ray technician, checked it thoroughly and believed it to be a faulty vacuum tube. We ordered the tube and hoped that Fred could make long-distance diagnoses and give instructions for the repair.

Running a complex hospital facility in the jungle was like operating a battleship on the ocean. We had to be self-sustaining in every respect. However, the big difference was that battleships were stocked with spare parts and technicians who knew how to repair complex machinery. We had to rely on God to keep things working properly or to send us people and equipment to put things back into working condition. It was remarkable how many things did work, considering the adverse climate, the inexperienced personnel operating them, and the lack of routine maintenance. However, we became experts at improvising and were constantly reminded that we could not expect to run a modern hospital in a jungle station in a third-world country without God's help and provision.

Emergency Trip to Mayo Clinic

For several months, I had been experiencing tiredness and very low energy. Routine lab tests at our hospital did not reveal anything unusual. However, in April, I had a sudden onset of chills, fever, and severe back pain. I was confined to bed rest for a whole week, and the symptoms slowly decreased, except for the back pain, which continued. Finally, after consulting with Dr. Olsen and doctors in the US by telephone, I decided to go to the Mayo Clinic in the US for examination and treatment as soon as possible.

At that time, doctor staffing in the hospital was at an all-time low. We expected two short-term doctors to help while I was away.

Dr. Harold A., who had worked at a hospital in Ethiopia, was the brother of Bob A., the head of our lab department. The other doctor was a recent medical graduate. However, the assassination of the president of Bangladesh delayed their arrival.

Finally, we were able to leave and went directly to the Mayo Clinic. There, I experienced a "Rip Van Winkle" reaction as I was exposed to the most modern medical devices, some of which I had never seen before. I received a thorough examination, and the only abnormality detected was a small cyst on the right kidney. These cysts are not painful and are usually benign. They did a needle biopsy of the cyst, and it was negative for a tumor. I was told that these cysts are very common and typically do not require surgery. No specific treatment was advised, and I was allowed to return to Bangladesh. My kidney function was not impaired. It was possible that my problem could have been related to "Chittagong Hepatitis," which continually plagued us at MCH.

Delayed by God's Design

Our return to Bangladesh was delayed because our visas had expired during our time in the US. While we waited for the visas and entry permits, we attended a one-day visit to a church conference in Winona Lake, Indiana, where we met a young couple that we thought might be God's choice to fill the need for a maintenance supervisor on our station. The husband was an experienced mechanic, and this couple was looking for a place to serve God with their skills. As we shared with them the need for a maintenance supervisor to maintain the hospital and compound facilities at MCH, we realized our return had been delayed by Divine design. They eventually came to Malumghat, and he became our workshop and maintenance supervisor at the hospital compound. Soon after this meeting, we received our visas and entry permits and returned to Bangladesh.

Shipment Lost

During our furlough year, we collected and packed many donated items to be shipped to Bangladesh by the Home of Peace, our shipping agency in Oakland, California. These included donated items from church women's ministry groups and equipment we had ordered from various medical manufacturers. I was responsible for ensuring that all the items got safely to Home of Peace. Some items were of considerable value. I felt prompted to take out marine insurance on that shipment, which we had never done before.

In our November 1982 prayer letter to our supporters, we reported that "your gifts to us for return to the field are packed, shipped, and heading for Bangladesh now." We rejoiced that these things included a large supply of hospital uniforms. I had carefully packed some special surgical tools in our hand-carry luggage to take on the plane.

When we arrived in Bangladesh after furlough, we learned that a strong hurricane had ravaged Hawaii before Christmas, sinking several ships. One of them was an Indian vessel, the Jalamorari, and one sailor on board lost his life. Our entire hospital supply shipment went down with that ship. This news came as quite a shock. We had been counting the days until the shipment would come. I applied to the insurance company and received a large settlement that allowed us to reorder most of the expensive items. Donors in the US promptly began working on replacing the things they had contributed. Isaiah 55:8 reminded us that "the Lord's ways are not our ways," and God was in control of events like storms and the sinking of shipments. Though we did not understand His ways, we could trust Him.

One of my medical school colleagues, Dr. B., had donated the working parts of a Spinalator machine for use in our PT Department. When he learned the ship had sunk and the parts were lost, he ordered a replacement mechanism and decided to come to Bangladesh for a short-term ministry. Dr. B. provided valuable training for our physical therapy workers.

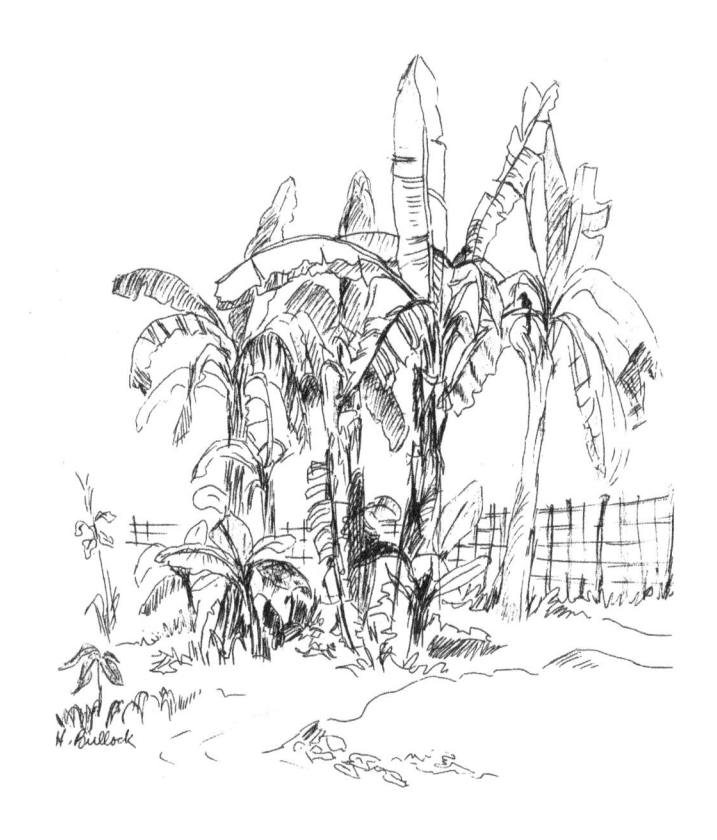

CHAPTER 36

God's Plan for Man

Pillow Speakers

After completing our language study, Tense and I became more active in the Audiovisual Department (AV) at the hospital. Tense spent many hours upgrading the materials, organizing the files, and teaching Bangladeshi Bible teachers how to make visuals and use the materials.

At that time, we replaced cassette players with a new system that allowed patients to listen to Bible programs from the AV Department through individual "pillow speakers" during their hospital treatment.

For this new system, we constructed small boxes that held a speaker with a fixed low volume and could be held up to the patient's ear to hear the program. One of our Bible Institute men supervised the programming and taping of the Bible messages in the two local languages, Bengali and Chittagonian. A patient could select the language of his or her choice and choose to listen. This way, no one could say they had been forced to listen to the Bible messages, as only the person holding the box could hear it.

Each morning, the AV technician would offer patients an opportunity to receive a speaker box. He would show the patients how to hold the speaker box up to their ears to hear the program. The patient's visitors could also choose to hear the Bible messages. Almost every speaker box was accepted by patients wanting to listen. Christian music and Scripture readings were broadcast to over fifty patients' bedsides for eight hours daily. This was an effective way to reach many listeners privately with the gospel message. The pillow speakers had a profound spiritual impact on the hearers in the patient wards.

"What Does the Holy Bible Teach About God's Plan for Man?"

In the mid-eighties, Memorial Christian Hospital was a very busy place with patients rapidly coming and going. There were only a few personal workers and many patients. The personal workers who visited the patients on the wards had difficulty finding quality time with patients because of the rapid turnover. It was entirely possible for a patient to be admitted to the hospital, treated for a few days, and then discharged without a clear understanding of the teachings of the Holy Bible. Patients who could read could be given gospel booklets and literature, but these were of no benefit to patients who were illiterate. Our team became increasingly burdened for our illiterate patients. They might have seen a filmstrip or flannel graph Bible story or heard a gospel message on a cassette tape. But they might not have understood the message and been able to put it all together. We realized that they would have to be reached through pictures and the spoken word. But with so few personal workers and so little time, how could this be accomplished?

After consulting with our teammates at MCH, we concluded that we should find a program in a format that patients could listen to and watch simultaneously that clearly presented the simple gospel message of salvation. At that time, film strips were commonly used. These were half-frame 35 mm. slides, shown with projectors, and the audio was on a cassette. We searched worldwide for such a program. We found programs on topics such as the Genesis flood, creation, and the story of Abraham, but nothing that gave a biblical overview of God's plan of salvation. We would have to produce it ourselves. Our task was to develop a narrated script with slides illustrating Bible principles and the gospel message.

First, we had to devise a suitable script that would not offend patients of various religious backgrounds. It would be a factual presentation of what the Holy Bible teaches, regardless of anyone's disagreement with the content. After consulting our co-workers in Bangladesh, we finally came up with the title "What Does the Holy Bible Teach about God's Plan for Man?"

The narrative begins by commenting on all the troubles that are in the world today and asks the question, "Are there any answers?" It then explains what the Holy Bible is and its origin, followed by the biblical account of Creation, the Fall of Adam and Eve, and the entry of sin into the world. Next, a careful explanation of the message of forgiveness of sin and salvation through faith in Jesus is given, along with an invitation to receive this message.

Tense and I made illustrations and photographs to accompany the narrative. We presented biblical characters with featureless silhouettes to make them culturally appropriate. The script was sent to the NGO team for their comments and suggestions. Finally, when we had agreed on the script and had suitable illustrations, we commenced production. We used a half-frame 35 mm camera to produce the slides, which was perfect because the image size was exactly right for the filmstrip projector. However, not far into production, the camera ceased to work. We had to shift to a full-frame 35 mm camera. We sent the exposed films to a laboratory in Cox's Bazaar, and the results were often faulty. We began to wonder if this was satanic opposition.

After many months of frustration and trying, we brought the slides with us when we went to the US on furlough to have the filmstrip produced by a professional audiovisual laboratory. The owner said he could easily produce it and told us to return in three weeks. When we returned, he informed us that he hadn't been able to work on it because his expensive camera had broken down. He would try to find a used one and asked us to return in six weeks. I asked him if he was a Christian, and he replied, "Of course." I told him that Satan did not want that program produced.

"Well, don't sic him on me!" he cried.

"It's too late," I said. "Consider what happened to your camera."

He got a far-away look in his eyes and said, "Oh yeah. Well, I'll do the best I can. Come back in six weeks."

When we returned in six weeks, we learned that his new camera had arrived, and he had produced the images. However, when they were sent to the lab for development, they were cut into individual images rather than leaving them as a continuous strip. The process had to be repeated. When we returned the third time, he said he had done the slides and sent the strip to Los Angeles for production. It came back with a big scratch right down the center.

"They said I did it," he commented. "But I said they did it. I will have to do it again. Come back in a few weeks." When we returned the final time, he had the film strip in his possession. We asked him to make three master copies for us. We would take one copy to Bangladesh ourselves, send another copy with a returning teammate, and leave one copy in the US as a backup, in case neither of us made it back to Bangladesh. Ships can go down, airplanes can crash, and people can die. The satanic opposition was obvious, and we wanted to be very careful.

When we finally returned to Bangladesh with the completed filmstrip, we had the major task of putting the script's narration into various languages and dialects. We began with Bengali, Muslim Bengali, Chittagonian, and Muslim Chittagonian, the most frequently used languages in our area. Later, we also produced translations in English and tribal languages to make the program available to others. One of our supporters composed and donated original background music for the filmstrip.

The program was divided into two fifteen-minute parts. We showed Part One and Part Two of the finished filmstrip in the hospital on successive days. This heightened the suspense, and patients were eager to see the second part. When the film strip was shown in a manner that made it impossible for patients in the hospital to avoid seeing it, some patients objected. To address this issue, we decided to show the filmstrip only to viewers who would wear earphones to listen to the soundtrack. We had purchased a device that could accept six sets of earphones at a time. Other patients could see the pictures without sound, which intensified their determination to hear the soundtrack as soon as it was their turn.

The filmstrip helped the personal workers have something to discuss with the patients during visits. After the patients had seen part two, the personal workers would ask them if they had any questions. One man lying on a cot at the end of the male ward saw the film strip and then asked to see both parts again. When the personal worker asked him if he had any questions, he asked, "Is there any way you can bring this to my village so my family can see it? They have never heard these things!"

When Tense and I turned 65 and retired from our work at MCH, the filmstrip had been converted to DVD and was constantly used at the hospital. We wanted to have it translated into other languages since it is a very simple but effective way of presenting the plan of salvation. As we visited our supporting churches and individuals, we showed the program in the churches and explained what we were hoping to do. After one church service, a boy about twelve years old came up to me in the foyer and said, "Thank you for showing that. I have heard many stories in Sunday School, but this is the first time I have understood how they all fit together."

One pastor asked if we could arrange to translate it into German. His parents were German, and he was anxious for them to hear and see it. We discussed this with the head of the translation committee of ABWE, and together, we laid out some guidelines for these translations. With the help of a friend who had recording equipment and many narration volunteers who were fluent in other languages, we were able to translate "What Does the Holy Bible Teach About God's Plan for Man" into German, Vietnamese, Manipuri, Brazilian Portuguese, Mandarin, Arabic, and Latin American Spanish.

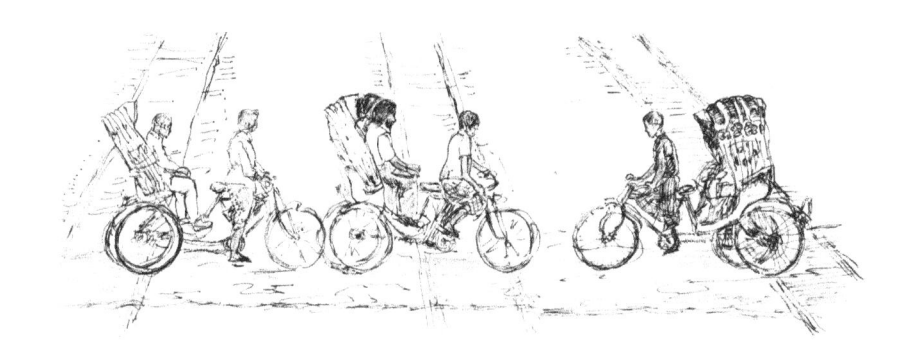

CHAPTER 37

To Catch a Plane

It had been a great summer with our youngest son David who was home from college during his summer break to spend time with us on the hospital compound. He helped me with a large backlog of projects that I had not had time to do (nor probably ever would). David managed to get many of the projects crossed off the list. Most of these involved hospital-related work, so his help made everything run smoother.

David had a reservation on British Airways from Dhaka to the US on August 5th at 8:30 p.m. to return to college for his fall semester.

We planned to accompany him to Dhaka to see him off and meet a short-term medical student and his wife and infant daughter at the airport to travel with them to Malumghat.

The summer months are the rainy or monsoon season in Bangladesh. The road from Malumghat to Chittagong winds through five river valleys, which originate from the Hill tracts and flow toward the Bay of Bengal. During the monsoon season, heavy rainfall in the hills can cause flooding in any of these valleys, sometimes making the roads impassable. We planned to go to Chittagong early, allowing plenty of time to deal with bad weather or unexpected problems. Several years before this, we had a near-disaster experience when taking David to the airport to fly to Manila for his senior year at Faith Academy. Our Volkswagen floated slightly as we attempted to cross a flooded stretch of road. We did not want to repeat that situation. We also needed plenty of time to purchase traveler's checks and get our plane tickets from the travel agent in Chittagong before flying to Dhaka on Thursday morning. That plan would give us a little time for last-minute shopping and a meal together in Dhaka with David before he needed to be at the airport to check in for his flight at 6:30 p.m. on Friday.

We did not have very much rain that year, but as August approached, the rains became more frequent and heavier. The staccato beat of rain increased to a constant roar on the asbestos-corrugated roof of our house on Monday, August 1st, causing some concern about the trip. It had been raining heavily for several days, and although we had not heard any bad reports about the road, we were glad we had planned to leave early Tuesday.

As we began our drive on Tuesday morning, we encountered some flooding in the fields just north of the hospital, but there was no water on the road. We were truly thankful that the road was dry almost all the way to Chittagong. It had started to rain again before we arrived at the city. The rain continued all night as we stayed at the ABWE guest house, and we heard reports of flooding to the north, where the rivers drain through Bangladesh.

Early Wednesday morning, we started downtown in the drenching rain, expecting difficulty getting to the American Express bank in a low-lying part of the city. Sure enough, we had to try several streets before finding one passable. Even so, we were in six-inch deep water.

Arriving at the bank, we pulled into a driveway at the side, and David and Tense went "ashore" to do David's banking. I cast off and cruised to the other side of the street, where I could watch the bank door from a slightly higher place. Getting the traveler's checks took about forty minutes. During that time, the rain continued to pour down. Finally, when Tense and David came out of the bank, I crossed the flooded street, docked the VW alongside the bank, and took them aboard.

Next, we went to the travel agency about two blocks away to settle a question about the plane fare—that is, we tried to go. It soon became apparent that this would be impossible by car, as the water was nearly two feet deep in front of the International Travel Office. Parking about a block away, I hailed a rickshaw, which ferried Tense and me to the travel agency, leaving David in the car. After our meeting, there was no return rickshaw handy, so we tried to wade back to where the car was parked. Suddenly, Tense went down into the muddy water. She had stepped with one leg into an unseen manhole and went in up to her hip. I pulled her back up, and she recovered her footing. She was unhurt, but her shoulder bag, holding the valuable tickets, passports, and traveler's checks, had gone underwater with her! Thankfully, she had placed them in a plastic bag inside her purse. We waded across the street to the car and jumped in out of the rain, which had increased in intensity.

Concerned about the high water, we tried to return to the guest house. We retraced our route, but the water had risen higher. The avenue had become impassable, even for trucks. We pondered what to do as we sat in our car surrounded by rickshaws, trucks, and other vehicles, all stranded by the high water.

At last, we decided to go to the Bible Literature Center (BLC) and talk with our Chittagong teammates while we waited for the water to go down. We thought it best to try to get our luggage from the guest house, if possible, and spend the night at the BLC to be nearer the airport in the morning. By 4:00 p.m., the water had receded enough to allow the BLC van to reach the guest house. We quickly packed our belongings and returned to the BLC.

On Thursday morning, one of our teammates took us to the airport in his van. We thanked him and checked in for our 7:30 a.m. Dhaka flight as we looked out on gray skies across the airport runway. The men at the counter assured us that the plane would fly. We went through pre-boarding clearance, entered the inner waiting room, and sat down to wait.

Seven-thirty came, but no plane. There would be a delay. David and Tense got out books to read, and I started a conversation with an Englishman, Mr. A., who said he had come up the road from the hospital area on Wednesday. He said that two bridges had been washed out and that he and his companions had had to leave their car and travel by boat, rickshaw, and bus.

As Mr. A. and I were talking, the rain spattered against the windows of the waiting room. He began questioning why we had come to Bangladesh to work at MCH. He asked me many questions and showed a keen interest in my answers. Tense looked up from her book and, seeing his interest, began to pray. The rain was coming down in sheets, and Mr. A. and I walked over to the window to watch it. I shared my own story about how I had trusted in Christ for salvation. I pointed out that the starting point is for a man to understand and admit that he is a sinner and that because of his sin, he is separated from a Holy God and will someday face God in judgment.

"But God has provided a way for man to be freed from the penalty of his sin through the sacrificial death of Jesus Christ on the cross for all mankind," I explained. "He can have a relationship with God by believing this and placing his faith in Jesus." Mr. A. listened hungrily to all these things and nodded in assent at each point.

The rain continued, and it became evident to us and the other passengers that the plane would not come that day. The airport officials had made many trips out to the runway by jeep but had returned each time shaking their heads. The standing water on the field made it impossible for planes to land, so the flight could not leave Dhaka until it was cleared to land in Chittagong. Giving up our flight plans, we retrieved our tickets and luggage and telephoned the BLC, asking them to send a car for us. It was almost noon. Mr. A. rode back into town with us. He appeared pleased that we had been delayed at the airport and that he had the opportunity to speak with me.

We decided to take the train to Dhaka instead of attempting to drive our small Volkswagen. I went to the train station to buy tickets for the night train, but they were all sold out. The only other option by train would be to sit up all night in a second or third-class coach, which was not a safe option. So, we decided to take the morning bus instead and returned to the BLC for a second night. Realizing that we would most likely not be in time to meet the medical intern's plane, we called our teammates in Dhaka and asked them to meet the short-termers at the airport if we arrived too late.

At 5:00 a.m. on Friday, August 5, we boarded the first bus to Dhaka, and the bus left the depot promptly, with an estimated arrival time in Dhaka of 12:00 noon. We started a conversation with Dr. M.S. and Dr. S.K., two educated Bengali men sitting in the seats in front of us who spoke fluent English. We were unaware of how important our meeting them would be to us in just a little while.

The bus stopped several times to pick up more passengers until it was overflowing with people inside, on the top, and clinging to the sides and back bumper. Reaching open country, the bus picked up speed, and we settled down for a long ride. At about 7:30 a.m., however, we reached an area where the fields were flooded on both sides of the road. Sometimes, the water came right up to the edge of the roadway. Finally, at about 8:00 a.m., we reached the tail end of a long string of trucks parked on the left-hand side of the road. The bus pulled into the right-hand lane and passed the trucks until it could go no further because the road was blocked by a stalled vehicle mired in mud.

We found ourselves in a tiny business section of a small village amid hundreds of parked trucks, buses, and rickshaws. People milled about. They had been stopped there since the previous night because the next six miles of road were under five feet of water! The rain was still falling, and the water was still rising. We were eight miles south of a town called Feni, where the ground was higher, and there was more likelihood of catching a bus to Dhaka. However, there was no hope of our bus driving through to Feni soon, and no boats were available.

As we sat in the bus trying to discern what to do, we prayed silently for an answer. Dr. M.S. and Dr. S.K. were concerned for us, knowing David was supposed to catch the plane from Dhaka to London that evening.

After considerable discussion, it seemed best to retrace our steps for twelve miles or so to a place where the railroad tracks crossed our road. Near there was a train station, and some people standing nearby informed us that a mail train to Feni was due later in the morning. We thought there might be a chance that we could get on the mail train and get to Feni. Perhaps we could get to Dhaka on time—or at least get there! Our bus was going nowhere, so we got off, put on our orange rain parkas, and, carrying our luggage and umbrella, managed to crowd onto a bus going in the reverse direction. Apparently, many other people had the same idea, as the bus resembled a tin full of sardines. As we retraced our path along the highway, we noticed the water lapping over the road in several places.

We arrived at the railroad crossing but saw no sign of a station. Miraculously, our new friends found two rickshaws for us and another for themselves. We set off in the rickshaws to find the station about four miles down the tracks on a side road. The heavy rain continued steadily. Wrapped in our orange ponchos, we clutched our carry-on bags and tried to keep a small plastic tarp over our suitcases as we slowly rode to the station. Tense noticed it was just after 10:00 a.m.—tea break time. She couldn't help but think how good a cup of tea would have tasted just then. As the rickshaws approached the station, we could hear a loud hum coming from a huge crowd of chattering people covering the platform. We climbed out of the rickshaws with all our luggage and made our way onto the crowded platform. Our friends inquired of the station master and learned that a mail train was expected at 11:25 a.m. The station master also assured them he would try to stop the train and get the conductor to take on passengers.

As we waited for the train in the small first-class waiting room, people kept arriving by rickshaw and on foot until several hundred people were crammed onto the platform and milling about. They all wanted to get on that mail train. We could easily predict what would happen when that train pulled into the station—a stampede! We also realized how slim our chances were of getting on the train with all our luggage and not being schooled in the fine art of functioning in a mob scene.

Our friends again approached the station master and explained how important it was for us to get onto that train so that David could catch his overseas flight. They asked him to assist us so that we could get on despite the crowd. He considered the matter carefully and said he would help us but didn't say how. He told us to return to the waiting room and wait. It seemed hopeless to think that we and our belongings would ever be able to get onto that train.

Suddenly, the porter made his way through the crowded waiting room, snatched up our luggage, and motioned for us to follow him. He guided us to the locomotive of that overloaded train. We managed to climb up the tall, slippery ladder attached to the side of the cab and joined about a dozen other passengers inside the cab. The engineer climbed down from the locomotive and conferred with the flagman while studying the swollen river. Then, the engineer climbed back up into the engine. A few moments later, the engineer again climbed down to consult with the flagman and then returned to the locomotive and stared at the river.

Finally, he decided to cross the submerged and, hopefully, still intact bridge. He released the brake and moved the throttle forward a little, easing the locomotive onto the bridge. The train lumbered forward and crawled slowly onto the bridge. The bridge was only about 100 feet long, but it seemed like it was taking an eternity to cross it. There was silence in the cab as every person held his breath and thought how quickly that heavy locomotive would sink if the bridge collapsed.

After what seemed like a lifetime, the train reached the other shore. An enormous cheer went up from the passengers all over the train as the locomotive finally eased off the end of the submerged bridge and onto solid ground, and there was a palpable release of tension inside the cab.

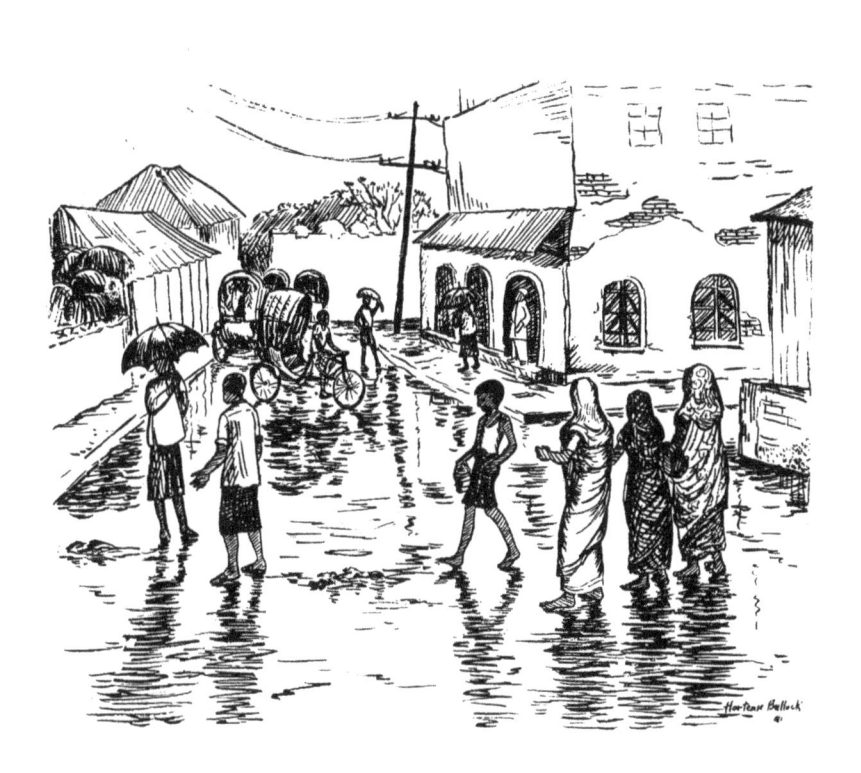

CHAPTER 38

Safe!

The train continued its slow pace toward Feni. We prayed silently but realized how helpless we were in the face of all this. The train stopped several more times at the sight of red flags, but the engineer soon discovered that these flags were actually red shirts being waved by would-be passengers. At long last, we pulled into the Feni station. It was then 2:00 p.m., and Dhaka was still 100 miles away. Was there a chance we could still get David to the airport on time?

We thanked our engineer, clambered out of the locomotive cab and then tried to find rickshaws to take us and our luggage to the Feni bus station. To our dismay, the streets were full of ankle-deep water, and no rickshaws were available. We picked up our luggage and waded toward the center of town, thankful that the rain was still holding off. Finally, with the help of our two Bangladeshi traveling companions, we were able to hail three rickshaws. Tense and I jumped into one, and while the two men got in another, we called to David to get the empty rickshaw coming toward him. Then we set off for Feni Bypass Road, where we expected to board a Dhaka-bound bus if they were running.

Some months earlier, Tense and I had made an official hospital visit to Dhaka and had stopped briefly in Feni to visit Southern Baptist NGO workers R.T. and Fran. Their house was only a short distance from the Feni Bypass Road. As our rickshaw drivers pedaled through hub-deep water, we realized we would soon pass directly in front of their house. We watched carefully for the Baptist compound. Suddenly, we were right in front of the gate, and I ordered the driver to stop. Jumping out of the rickshaw, I ran to the front gate. Fran saw me coming and emerged from the house to meet me. Explaining the situation quickly, I asked if we could use their car to get to Dhaka, knowing that a bus could never get us to the airport on time. At that moment, R.T. came out the door and said, "There's a van leaving for Dhaka from here in a few minutes! Come on in!" He said an auditor had driven from Dhaka that morning to work on the station audit and was preparing to return. Excited about God's timing at the precise moment, R.T. said we could ride with the auditor to Dhaka in the mission van, which was large enough to accommodate all of us, including our new Bangladeshi friends and our luggage! David quickly showered and changed into clean travel clothes.

It seemed unlikely that we would be able to drive from Feni all the way to Dhaka airport in the remaining time, but the driver said he would try. We would have to cross two large rivers on ferries. The driver reported waiting two hours that morning to cross one river by ferry because of the flooding. He drove as fast as he dared on the flood-damaged road.

We stopped once briefly to pick up another passenger from the Baptist Mission station in Comilla. He was a Bangladeshi engineer who was a Christian. The new passenger climbed into the back seat and greeted our Bangladeshi traveling companions, who were both Muslims. On the way to Dhaka, they quizzed the engineer about his faith, and he was quite willing to share his testimony with them. They continued to carry on a lively conversation for the rest of the trip. At one point, I heard one of the men ask, "Do you mean to say that you feel that your sins are forgiven?" The engineer replied that he was absolutely certain. As we listened to their continuing discussion, we were struck by the realization that the events of that day and our "change of course" seemed to have been orchestrated by God for the purpose of getting the message of salvation through Jesus Christ to our two traveling companions.

As we approached the river, we could see the first ferry next to the dock, as if it were waiting for us. We were almost the last vehicle to board the ferry, which shoved off moments later. After a speedy crossing, we disembarked quickly without waiting and tore down the road toward the next ferry landing a few miles away. That ferry, too, was at the dock as if it was waiting for us. It was almost like driving onto and off a bridge. When we reached the opposite side of the river, we began the last lap of the journey to Dhaka. Only then did we begin to think we might make it on time.

Arriving in Dhaka, we dropped off our Bangladeshi friends at their destination. I gave each of them a Bengali New Testament, which they graciously received, and thanked them for their excellent assistance to us. Then we went directly to the airport. We could hardly believe our eyes when we looked at our watches as we pulled up in front of the international entrance. The time was 6:40 p.m., only ten minutes past the start of the check-in time for David's flight. Gratefully praising God and thanking the mission driver, we entered the crowded airport. As we looked at the check-in sign, "British Air, BA 144," we realized it was time to say goodbye, and we had not had time to savor our last few hours together leisurely. Yet, we had shared a tremendous demonstration of God's faithfulness and power. David said several times during the trip, "If God wants me to catch that plane tonight, we'll make it. Otherwise, we won't. Only He can do it. Jehovah Jireh!"

After getting his boarding pass and checking his luggage, David suggested we go to the coffee shop for a few quiet moments together. We ordered some tea and looked out at the giant British Airplane on the wet tarmac, discussing the events of the miraculous day. We prayed and thanked God for our safe and timely arrival and His provision and protection. Finally, it was time to hug each other and wave goodbye to David as he checked through passport control and boarded the flight on time.

Daylight was fading as we arrived at the Mission guest house in Dhaka by rickshaw and were greeted with relief by our teammates who had traveled to Dhaka ahead of us and had been searching for us. Thankfully, they had picked up the short-term medical intern and his family, and we all traveled to Malumghat together as soon as the roads were passable.

> "But now, thus says the LORD, who created you, . . . Fear not, for I have redeemed you; I have called you by your name; You are Mine. When you pass through the waters, I will be with you; And through the rivers, they shall not overflow you." (Isa. 43:1-2)

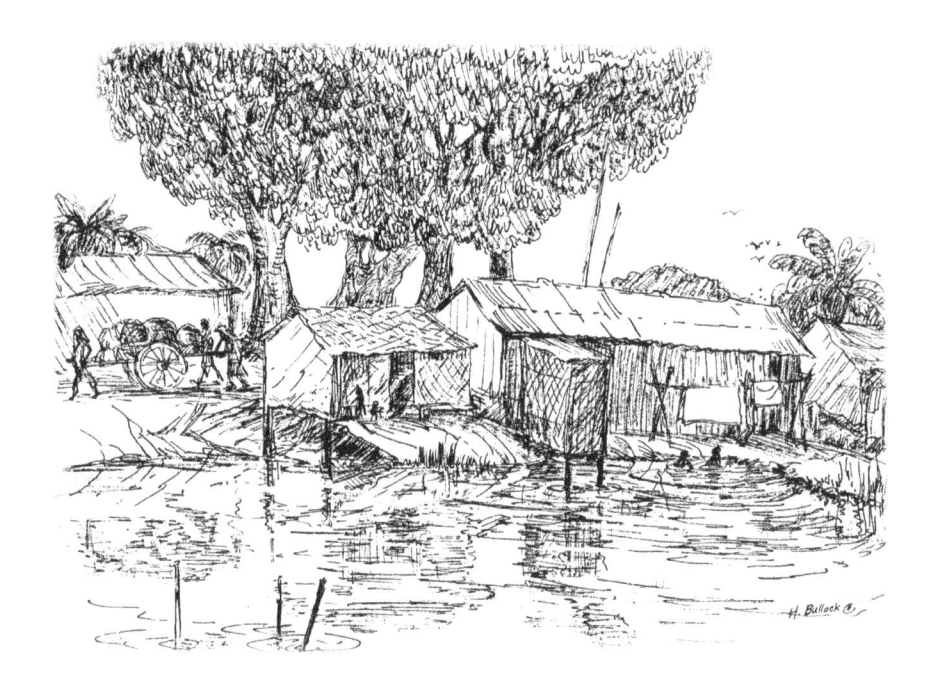

CHAPTER 39

Improvisation

External Fixation

Many orthopedic cases that we handled were complicated because there often were other issues that had to be resolved before we could treat the injury. It may have been an open fracture, where the ends of the broken bones were poking out through the skin. It was necessary to have some way to immobilize the fractured ends of the bones so they would not interfere with blood circulation. Plates and screws could not be used in such a situation. The wound may have contained dirt, rocks, sticks, cow dung, or other debris and had to be thoroughly cleaned before treatment.

Multiple fractures in one or more extremities are often treated by "external fixation." This was done by inserting multiple threaded stainless-steel pins or rods through the bones or bone fragments and then attaching them together by a rod while the deformity was pulled into the best alignment possible. It was held in that position until the fracture united or the skin and soft tissues were cleaned up enough to allow internal fixation. We did not have the commercially manufactured external fixation devices usually used to care for such cases. They were expensive and generally unavailable in Bangladesh. We often improvised and made our orthopedic equipment to treat the patient from items we had on hand. I read an article that taught me how to make this type of external fixation using multiple pins and rods.

First, I had to import threaded stainless-steel rods and pins with screw threads on them and cut them to suitable lengths. Then, I sharpened one end of the shortened rods. After the rods had been sterilized, they could be driven into the bone fragments like a screw is driven into wood. Next, the unsharpened ends were connected to another 1/4" or 3/8" steel rod, which did not have to be sterile because it would remain outside the body. It was connected to the threaded rod with nylon thread, and then the joint was reinforced with methyl methacrylate paste (bone cement made for use in dentistry), which did not have to be sterile. The fractured bone ends were manipulated into an acceptable position and held immobile while the bone cement paste solidified. The soft tissues of the wound could then be treated and cleaned. We could even apply a skin graft with the fixation rods in place if necessary. The limb could easily be moved about without causing pain to the patient. This fixation could be continued until the bone had healed. The whole assembly cost pennies compared to the expensive commercial external fixation devices that we would have had to order.

When the apparatus had served its function, it could easily be removed, and the threaded rods and pins could often be used again multiple times. This sort of external fixation served us well at MCH. In later years, we received donations of unused parts of commercially manufactured external fixation sets from hospitals in the US. Once the sets were opened, hospitals were required to dispose of unused parts, but they could donate them to MCH. We happily received any donated supplies.

One case where we used external fixation was for a woman who had fallen out of a tree three days before she came to the hospital, resulting in an open fracture of both bones of her forearm. Her husband brought her to the hospital from Sandwip Island, 69 miles north of our hospital. When she fell, the fractured bone ends were driven deep into the dirt. She also had a fracture of her shoulder and pelvis. Her husband had taken her to the local "hospital" on the island, where the staff sewed up the wound on her arm without cleaning out the dirt and sent her for an X-ray. The X-ray revealed the fracture of the arm, as well as of the pelvis and shoulder. He was told to take her to the government hospital in Chittagong. Instead, he decided to bring her to our hospital. That trip took two days of travel by boats, rickshaws, and buses. By the time they arrived at our hospital, they had spent almost all their money on travel and food.

The woman had gas gangrene on her forearm, and her condition was serious. We admitted her to the hospital immediately and did an extensive fasciotomy of the forearm. For this, the skin of the forearm was slit from the wrist to the elbow. Then all the fascial envelopes of the muscles in the forearm were slit, allowing them to expand. Dirt was found impacted into the bone cavities. We cleaned it out as much as possible, then suspended her arm by skeletal traction to the overhead frame and administered antibiotics. Four weeks later, her forearm had been saved, and skin grafting could be started to close the massive defects from the fasciotomies. We were unsure how well her arm would function, but we thought it would probably be much better than an artificial arm. Her hospital bill had become very large, but she qualified for financial assistance from the HOPE Fund.

We were humbled when patients came to us because they wanted expert care, and we did our best to treat each patient. During her prolonged hospital stay, she and her husband were able to learn about salvation, as taught in the Holy Bible. The seed had been planted.

Truck Crash patient

A truck loaded with soldiers who had been building a road near the hospital went off the road and hit a tree. Many injured soldiers were brought to the hospital. One man had a serious fracture of his tibia and fibula. The bones had been shattered into pieces, and we could not feel any pulses in the foot. We were worried that the arteries in the leg might have been severed. I immediately did medial and lateral extensive fasciotomies of his swollen leg. He still did not have pulses in his feet. We did not have any Doppler equipment to check the circulation. We were considering trying to do an arteriogram. Then I remembered that I had an ultraviolet light and some ampoules of Fluorescite, a preparation that becomes fluorescent under ultraviolet light. We administered it intraarterial to determine if he had circulation in the injured leg.

We took him into a darkened room to examine the leg under the ultraviolet light. Unfortunately, brown skin does not fluoresce like white skin. However, he did develop fluorescence in the toenails of both feet, so we knew he did have circulation. Arterial repair at that level would have been difficult without an operating microscope, which we did not have. Attempted exploration in the face of the many bone fragments could have worsened the situation. We put a large stainless-steel rod in the medullary canal of the tibia to stabilize the fragments and elevate the leg high. The pulses returned after a few hours, to everyone's relief, and he recovered well. His fluorescent orange urine impressed everyone as he excreted the fluorescein from his body.

The tibia fracture was not very stable and tended to rotate. As he had large open wounds on both sides of the leg, I could not apply a plaster cast. Since we did not have a commercial external fixation apparatus, I had to improvise external fixation. To do this, I inserted long bone screws into the bone proximally and distally and connected them with another rod held in place by methyl methacrylate bone cement, as used in total hip procedures. The patient made a good recovery. His friends and officers were impressed by this display of "ultramodern" technology, which formed a good rapport with them.

Forearm Rescue

A middle-aged man came down from Chittagong with severe osteomyelitis in his forearm that involved the entire shaft of the radius. Doctors in Chittagong had told him that he would require amputation, and he came to our hospital as a last resort to try to save his right arm. He knew if he lost it, he would be considered an outcast.

In my residency training in orthopedics, it was emphasized that we must avoid putting any metal, like screws or plates, into an infected site. However, while I was on furlough, I was privileged to attend a seminar on recent developments in trauma surgery involving wartime injuries. At that seminar, I learned that it was acceptable to insert an intramedullary steel rod through an infected site to maintain alignment and allow the healing process to progress as God had intended. When the bone was sufficiently healed, the rod would be removed. In osteomyelitis, the body tries to form a protective shell of new bone called an involucrum, bridging the infected area. When the involucrum is sufficiently developed so that it can maintain length and alignment, any residual dead bone, which is called a sequestrum, can be removed.

This man's arm was in terrible shape. There was drainage from the infection the entire length of the forearm. X-rays showed an early layer of new bone growth forming, but the infection occupied the entire radius bone. I explained to my patient what I intended to do and told him it would take a long time to heal. Even after the involucrum was fully developed, it might still be necessary to do another operation to remove any remaining dead bone. I also told him that I could not promise to save his arm but could only promise that we would try our best to avoid amputation.

He eagerly accepted our offer, and we proceeded with the insertion of the rod, followed by intensive antibiotic treatment and dressings. He was a cooperative patient and motivated to follow our instructions strictly. The result was remarkable. A few scars showed, but the forearm was straight and functioning normally. The sequestrum had dissolved, and he required no further surgery.

Cases like this were very rewarding and life-changing—to help someone to that extent and avoid deforming surgery. Most importantly, during his prolonged hospital stay and treatment episodes in the cast room after surgery, this man heard the message of God's great love for him and the gift of salvation. The seed of the gospel was firmly planted, and we hoped that he accepted salvation along with the healing of his body.

Acupuncture

At MCH, we used narcotics to manage postoperative pain. We typically received a supply of narcotics from the government pharmacy supply office on a regular schedule, but sometimes, the process took longer than usual. One time, the officials responsible for issuing the required permit were withholding the papers for unknown reasons. We suspected they were hoping we would pay a bribe. The situation became so serious that we had to tell patients who were coming into the hospital for surgery to bring pain medication with them for their postoperative pain control. They could purchase narcotics from the street-side pharmacies without a prescription, but we could not get permission to stock them in our hospital.

Nancie, one of our NGO nurses who had worked with me in San Luis Obispo before she came to Bangladesh, told me about a surgeon we both knew who used acupuncture to alleviate the pain of his terminally ill cancer patients. He had completed a two-week course in acupuncture in China and a one-week course in London, England, from a doctor who specialized in acupuncture for pain relief. After taking these courses, the surgeon performed acupuncture on one of his patients who was suffering excruciating pain from terminal cancer. Following the procedure, the patient became pain-free and slept for many hours. Nancie had observed the procedure and the results that she thought could be helpful in our hospital. She suggested that I contact this doctor to inquire where I could receive training on using acupuncture for pain control.

I contacted the doctor, and he recommended the one-week course in London taught by Dr. Felix Mann. Dr. Mann had studied acupuncture in many countries and had written books about his experience and training. He offered a course in pain treatment for doctors. Since Tense and I were scheduled to go to the US for a short furlough, I registered to take the course in London on our way home. We had friends in Dhaka who had a second home in London, and they kindly invited us to stay with them to help us save on our travel expenses.

There were 26 doctors in the class. At the beginning of the class, we introduced ourselves as we sat in a circle around Dr. Mann. He then pointed to three class members and asked if they were teachers. They all said they were.

"You don't believe in acupuncture, do you?" he asked them. They admitted that they did not believe in it but had come out of curiosity. He then asked this question, "Why is kissing nice?" They were startled. "If you can't explain that, don't knock acupuncture just because you don't understand it," he continued. This was certainly an unusual way to start a class, and I could see that it was going to be very interesting. He told his patients who were already scheduled for the week of the course that if they would be willing to be used to demonstrate the acupuncture technique, there would be no charge for that day.

Dr. Mann called on me because I had identified myself as an orthopedic surgeon. He seated me in the front row of the class so I could examine the patients when they came in and verify their orthopedic problems. We saw a random assortment of cases. After he administered the needle treatment, he asked me to examine the patient again. I was astonished to see the significant improvement in the condition of those patients from the simple insertion of a few needles!

On returning to Bangladesh in November, I immediately called in some patients who had been having severe pain before I left on the trip. They were still in so much pain that some of them were unable to work. I explained that I wanted to try a new treatment method, and they were agreeable. Amazingly, the pain decreased or vanished after only a few treatments. One patient was an X-ray technician in our hospital who was unable to work because of severe back pain. He was able to resume work after only two acupuncture treatments. I continued to use acupuncture as much as I could for any pain, including postoperative pain.

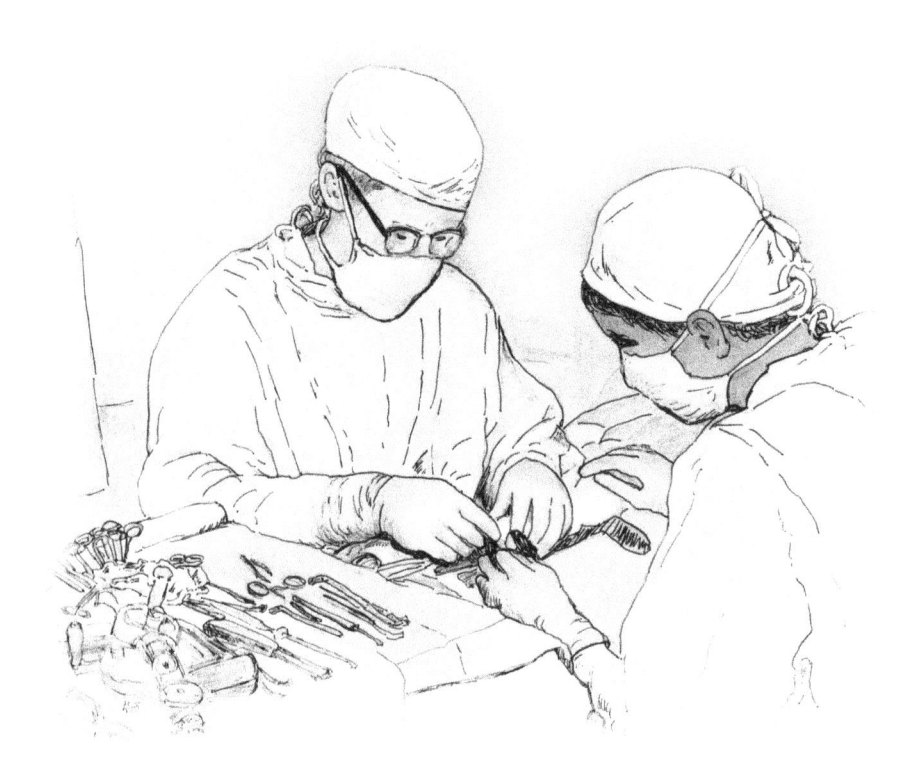

CHAPTER 40

A "Typical" Day in a Doctor's Life

People have often asked me, "What was a typical day like for you in Bangladesh?" I would chuckle when asked this question. There was no typical day. Every day was unique in the challenges, victories, and defeats. It seemed that there was at least one new crisis every day. There used to be a sign in the business office that read, "A day without a crisis is a total loss!"

I remember the events of one particular Saturday. I anticipated it would be a great day because I was not on call. Of course, there was one left-over surgery that I needed to do on a boy with a twenty-day-old fracture of his elbow. He had arrived the day before from the hills, a journey that took a whole day. I decided to operate on him that day, even though it was Saturday.

At 6:00 a.m., I heard a tap on my bedroom window. It was Dr. Joe DeCook, our OB/GYN. He was on call but didn't like to take care of trauma cases. He had been up since 2:00 a.m. taking care of two victims of a shooting that took place during a home robbery. The two sisters had been sleeping on top of the trapdoor in the attic of their house. This was a common measure for protection against burglars. However, when the burglars arrived, they shot through the trapdoor with shotguns. One of the shotguns was loaded with small-sized buckshot, catching one woman in her pelvis. The other woman, G.B., was shot in the back with six large-sized slugs, about 3/8 inch in diameter. One of them had penetrated her lung, and she had air in one side of her chest. Another slug had penetrated her spine, and she was paralyzed from the waist down. Joe wanted me to care for G.B., and he said he would treat the sister. And so, the day began.

After a quick breakfast, I went to the hospital to see the paralyzed woman. G.B. was a young married woman in her twenties with several small children. Her father was destitute after the robbery and was unable to pay for her care. However, she qualified for financial help from the HOPE Fund, and we could extend to her the full services of our rehabilitation team and provide her with the necessary surgical and medical care.

We did an examination and concluded that the spinal injury did not completely sever the cord. I decided I should try to get the slug out of the spinal canal to relieve pressure on the cord. Her condition was not very good, and I had to wait until we could get some of the air out of her chest and get blood ready to give her. Her relatives were reluctant to give blood but were willing to buy blood from the blood bank. There was no time to argue with them today, so we let them buy blood.

While waiting to operate on G.B., I made rounds in the wards to check on my current patients. On Saturdays, we tried to make rounds quickly to save as much time in the day as possible for any emergencies that might arise.

In the female ward in bed #4 lay an eight-year-old girl who came from one of the off-shore islands with a six-day-old open fracture of her wrist. The bone was sticking out of the flesh, and her arm was enormously swollen from infection. A complicating factor was that she had tetanus. I treated her by putting pins through the bones so we could hang the arm from the overhead frame to allow the swelling to go down. She was being treated for the infection, and her tetanus spasms were under control. Her fever had also come down. When the swelling decreased, we discovered that she also had a dislocated elbow joint. We would try to operate on her elbow in another week or so.

Next, I went to bed #7 and saw a boy who was about seven years old. He had a two-month-old dislocation of one of his hips. We had put him in traction and were waiting to see if surgery might be necessary. We saw a lot of these neglected dislocations.

My next patient was a woman in bed #9, about thirty years of age, with severe tuberculosis of her fourth and fifth lumbar vertebrae. The bodies of the vertebrae were nearly completely eaten away, and she had chronic drainage from her groin.

When I got to bed #15, I checked on an elderly lady with compression fractures of her spine due to osteoporosis. She had a back brace and was learning to function while wearing it. She was about ready to go home.

Next, I moved to the male ward, which was always busier for me. The elderly man in bed #2 looked like a skeleton with brown plastic stretched over it. His general condition was extremely poor, and he had gangrene in his foot. He had undergone a partial amputation of his foot a few days prior at another location, and we were waiting for the infection to subside before completing the amputation.

In bed #3 lay the little boy who was waiting for an elbow operation.

The man in bed #4 was in traction. He had fallen from a five-story building in Chittagong and had broken both legs and his arm in two places. He had developed a deep-space hand infection from a laceration on his wrist and had to be taken into surgery to have this opened and drained. He told me he could read, so I gave him some books and tracts. However, he couldn't hold the books.

Bed #5 held a small boy with a chronic hip disease. I had put him in traction for a few days before applying a cast.

The boy in bed #6 had a severe contusion of his brain from getting hit by a truck. This was a common accident on the highway in front of our hospital. We didn't think he would live, but he survived, and he was about to be released to go home.

The man in bed #9 had fallen from a tree, fracturing his hip on one side and breaking five ribs, his collar bone, and his pelvis on the other side. He had undergone surgery for his hip and was about ready to go home.

Another small boy, about eight years old, lay in Bed #10 with deformities from severe rickets. He was knock-kneed so badly that his knees were bent sideways at a 45-degree angle. I had done several osteotomies, cutting the bones and straightening them. He was in a cast and was preparing to go home.

In bed #14 lay an elderly gentleman with a relatively straightforward fracture of his hip. I pinned his hip but had technical problems in surgery, and the operation was a failure. The pin broke through the neck of the femur, and I had to treat him with traction. Was this a failure? Not exactly. I discovered he could read, and we became good friends. But there was a problem—he couldn't read without glasses. I obtained some donated glasses from the godown and found a pair that allowed him to read the Bible literature we had given him. He showed interest, and I was able to talk with him more during the remaining weeks of his recuperation.

After completing my rounds in the wards, it was time for the elbow surgery on the boy in bed #3. The surgery went smoothly, and I finished in about an hour.

Next, I went to the OPD to see a couple of patients who had not been treated the day before. The OPD is usually closed on Saturday. However, today, there were a lot of emergencies to be seen, and the OPD looked like the triage center of a war zone. One man had gangrene on his forefoot so bad that the front two-thirds of his foot was missing, and the rest of his foot was in poor shape. He was admitted for an amputation.

Another patient who had come to the OPD was a fourteen-year-old boy who had a huge tumor on his upper thigh. Upon viewing the X-ray, I determined it looked like a chondrosarcoma, which is a malignant tumor. Because the cancer extended far up into the thigh bone, it was necessary to do an amputation through the hip joint, taking the entire leg. This is called a hip disarticulation. I told him what needed to be done, and he agreed to that surgery and was admitted. I would have to do his surgery another day.

There were several other minor situations to address in the OPD—an infected ankle, a broken arm, and a few others. After that, a man was brought in who had fallen out of a rickshaw when it was hit by a truck. He dislocated his hip. I sent him to get an X-ray. Next, I saw a man who had been shot by robbers the night before. Part of his hand was missing, and he needed emergency surgery to amputate one finger. I scheduled him for surgery at 1:30 p.m.

I went home for a quick lunch and returned at 1:30 to see the X-rays of the man with the dislocated hip. I scheduled him for a closed reduction surgery to follow the hand surgery. I checked again on the woman with the spinal injury from gunshot wounds. She seemed improved enough to allow surgery, so I scheduled her for surgery that day following the hip dislocation case.

I began my surgeries that afternoon with the hand surgery case. I amputated one finger and repaired a digital nerve on another finger. Then I moved to the hip surgery. I reduced the dislocated hip but found he also had a fractured acetabulum, and that would need to be operated on in a week when his condition improved.

Then, I received a call from the male ward to check on the man in Bed #2. About that time, his blood pressure took a nosedive. I worked on him for about half an hour and got some temporary improvement. He seemed to have an adrenal crisis but may have had gram-negative septicemia. It was a poor prognosis, and I was doubtful of his survival.

My next surgery was for G.B., the woman who had been shot in the back. I discovered the bullet had shattered the back parts of three vertebrae, but the spinal cord appeared to be intact. There was considerable pressure on the spinal cord from the bone fragments. I did a decompression laminectomy at three levels and took out two other bullets. She withstood the operation quite well, and I thought she might have a chance to regain function in her legs.

While G.B. was in recovery, I returned to the OPD, where another patient had just arrived. He was a nineteen-year-old man who looked to be about ten years old. He was severely deformed from a disease known as Osteogenesis Imperfecta. His trunk was quite short, and he had a barrel-shaped chest. His arms and legs were grotesquely distorted, and it was almost impossible to tell where his elbows, wrists, knees, and ankles were because his bones were bent like pretzels. A friend had been carrying him and dropped him, which resulted in a fractured humerus on one side and a fractured femur on the other side. Knowing how to put him in a cast was quite a challenge.

I discovered one of our short-term doctors, Dr. Dan D., had seen this young man for a fracture six years before I came to the field. At that time, Dan had given him a Bible to read. This young man had gone to school through class six, with his father carrying him to school every day. He earned a living by tutoring young children. I was happy to tell the father that we might be able to straighten out his distorted arms and legs so that the young man could function better. The father sadly replied that he was a very poor man and couldn't afford any treatment. I told him we would work something out. What a wonderful feeling to know that I could treat cases like this through the financial assistance of the HOPE Fund! I put the young man on a gurney and said he would have to wait to be treated until after the surgeries were completed.

At 6:30 p.m., I finally finished the last surgery and sent a note to my wife to bring some food because I still had the complicated cast work to do. I praised God for my two orthopedic technicians, who were hardworking, conscientious young men. Tense arrived shortly with snacks to sustain us all, which were much appreciated. While we rested and ate, I sadly learned that the man in bed #2 died while I was in surgery. I was sorry that we could not help him.

At 8:00 p.m., I finished the cast work and went home to rest after this very non-typical day. As I reflected on the events of my "day off," I was sorry that I missed out on my Bible class with the Limb and Brace Shop technicians. I wanted to teach Bible classes, work on AV recordings, witness in the wards, and preach in the Chapel, but when could I do that when I desperately needed to do medical work at the hospital?

It was impossible to measure the spiritual effect of the medical and surgical work. But we did see evidence that the medical care we rendered softened hearts to the truth of the love of God and gave them time to consider the message from the Bible as they healed.

G.B.

After G.B.'s surgery, she was still unable to walk without assistance. Our Limb and Brace Shop workers made leg braces for her, and a wheelchair was obtained from a shop in Chittagong. Intensive physical therapy was required to teach her how to use the braces and wheelchair. G.B. spent many months with our skilled technicians, who trained her to care for her personal needs. They also taught her how to sew and do other handicrafts that would allow her to support herself. She learned to cope and to do simple household tasks in spite of her disability.

G.B. showed the usual response to such an injury. At first, there was a deep depression and rejection of nearly everything. Her husband divorced her because she was no longer useful as a wife and mother. He took another wife and also took the children. Slowly, however, the depression disappeared, and a cheerful and pleasant personality emerged. She once again hoped that life might be worthwhile and that she had something to look forward to. During this time, she listened carefully to the personal workers, listened to Bible messages on cassette tapes, read the Holy Bible and other Christian literature, and showed some interest. However, she would not indicate that she had made any decisions.

Surgery was performed for serious bedsores she had developed during an ill-advised short trip home that turned into a near disaster. Finally, we determined that she could go home to her father's house because she was proficient enough in using her appliances, and her various bedsores had healed. Our hospital Limb and Brace Shop crew had made the necessary changes in her house that she needed to be able to function—ramps, parallel bars, and a special bed. Just before she was discharged to go home, one of our female personal workers had a serious talk with her to ask her what she had learned while in the hospital. G.B. told her that she believed what the Holy Bible said about salvation and had become a true child of God.

When G.B. arrived home in her village, curious neighbors crowded around her to see what she could accomplish. They were astonished that she could get around and be helpful in the usual household activities. Sadly, she faced much opposition in her village and with her family.

After returning from furlough the following year, we eagerly asked about GB's condition. We were heartbroken when we learned that her family had neglected her, and G.B. died from pneumonia one month before we returned to Bangladesh. When she knew she was dying, she told everyone that she was going to be with Jesus.

Bone Cancer Patient

I operated on the boy with the bone cancer of his thigh bone and amputated the entire leg and hip joint, including the entire femur. Under ordinary circumstances in Bangladesh, this would mean the patient would have to use crutches for the rest of his life. No one in Bangladesh had been able to build a Canadian hip disarticulation prosthesis, which was the necessary kind of artificial leg for this type of amputation. I gave our Limb and Brace Shop the assignment of building this prosthesis. They had never built one either, as this type of amputee is rare, but they said they would try. The patient's family had run out of money due to the expenses connected with his surgery, so they appealed to the HOPE Fund for help, which was granted.

The prosthesis consisted of a fiberglass bucket in which the patient sat. This was connected to a special hinge that fastened the bucket to the artificial leg. Altogether, the leg had two separate joints—hip and knee. These were both flail joints, meaning the patient had no active control over their movements except through gravity, inertia, and momentum. Learning to walk with such a prosthesis was difficult and required much practice. Production was delayed because our supply of fiberglass resin was unpredictable, causing the process to take longer than expected. We had to purchase the resin from a boat manufacturer in Chittagong, who had to import it from Japan. The shelf-life of the resin is short, so the boat manufacturer could not import large amounts at any one time. We had to wait until he had some excess resin to sell.

After ten months, the prosthesis was finally completed. It was thrilling to see the boy's excitement as he tried his first hesitant steps with his new prosthetic leg and discovered that he could walk without crutches. It would require a lot of practice before he could walk safely and confidently, but he was determined.

Two years later, the boy came to see me. He had outgrown the artificial leg and needed a new one. I was surprised he had lived this long, as this disease had a poor prognosis, especially without cancer treatment. I was pleased with how well he walked with his Canadian hip prosthesis.

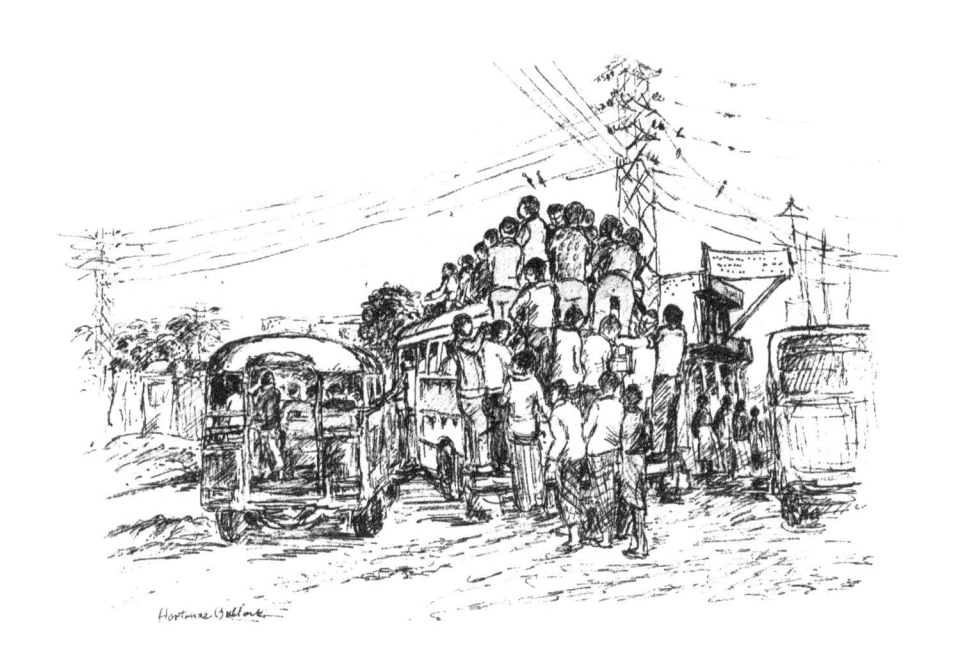

CHAPTER 41

Teaching Jungle Orthopedics

A Larger Orthopedic Department

The orthopedic practice grew to where we saw up to sixty patients per day. We had to put benches outside Room 13 where patients could sit until they were called for examination or treatment. These waiting patients blocked traffic in the hallway, making it increasingly difficult for our Central Supply staff to deliver supplies throughout the hospital. The nurses' office near the X-ray department was at least twice the size of Room 13 and opened directly to the Central Supply Room. I thought it would make an ideal orthopedic room. The nurses agreed to move their office to another room that had become available so we could use their room to make a larger orthopedic department.

I was excited that the new orthopedic room was large enough to have two examining tables for better patient flow. We also could move the fracture table into this room, as needed, for applying body casts. This room also had two cupboards on wheels that could be rolled to the wards—one for setting up or taking down traction, and the other cupboard contained casting materials. There was also plenty of room to give orthopedic training lectures to my staff.

Jungle Orthopedics

After working at the hospital for over seventeen years, it was evident to me that the demand for orthopedic care would not stop when I left the scene. However, I realized that many short-term general surgeons and the other doctors at MCH had little training or experience in orthopedic surgical techniques and procedures. In their residency training, these general surgeons rotated through various surgery divisions, such as neurosurgery, gynecological, and pediatric surgery. They did much observation but got minimal hands-on experience, as the cases were usually handled by the full-time residents in those specialties.

Orthopedic problems are common at mission hospitals, especially at MCH in Bangladesh. The doctors are often pressed into handling orthopedic emergencies. I could see a need for a simplified treatise on handling orthopedic problems in such a setting.

In 1994, I wrote an instruction manual about the tools, principles, and overall management of orthopedic surgery in a primitive setting. I called it "Jungle Orthopedics" and used this for training doctors and orthopedic technicians at our hospital. The articles were very basic, assuming no knowledge of orthopedic terms, equipment, or procedures on the reader's part. The major emphasis was on handling trauma cases, as well as non-emergency orthopedic problems that were quite simple to care for. This manual covered various types of traction and materials used for traction, and orthopedic tools, such as screws, fixation rods, and pins. This instruction booklet also covered infections, wound care, x-rays, and fracture treatment.

I also made several PowerPoint presentations on DVD called "Orthopedic Nuggets" about diagnosing and non-operative treatment of orthopedic-related conditions. These presentations proved helpful to the short-term general surgeons who came to work at our hospital. Later, I used PowerPoint as a resource when training orthopedic technicians. To further aid visiting orthopedic surgeons, I made a notebook of photos of all the orthopedic surgical instruments we had and organized them into a three-ring notebook. This also aided our operating room staff and technicians in identifying the equipment.

The Shipment and the Knee

Dr. Robert Goddard completed his two-year language study in Dhaka and then came to MCH to take over the care of patients while I went to the US for furlough. He was an excellent general surgeon but had limited orthopedic surgery experience. I asked the medical committee for their approval to train Dr. Goddard in orthopedics for three months. I wanted to instill in him as much knowledge of orthopedic surgery as possible before we left. Dr. Goddard would have to handle the orthopedic patients while I was gone. The short-term general surgeon at MCH covered general surgery while I trained Dr. Goddard in orthopedic surgery.

The medical committee approved the plan, and Dr. Goddard quickly absorbed the teaching I gave him. I did not doubt that he would be able to handle the orthopedic responsibilities he would face after my departure. Still, it was possible that he would have to refer some cases to hospitals in Chittagong. I decided to take him there to meet physicians and learn about the hospitals and other medical facilities.

Meanwhile, a shipment of laboratory items for the hospital had arrived in Chittagong and was on the dock awaiting customs clearance. The shipment also contained personal items for Bob Adolph, the head of our hospital laboratory, who had just returned from furlough. Bob learned that Dr. Goddard and I were going to Chittagong, so he asked if he could go with us to clear up a matter with the customs agent and pick up the shipment with the hospital truck.

The bill of lading for the shipment said there were 21 crates of items, but the inventory submitted by Bob Adolph had only claimed 18 crates. There were three crates of items for which there was no inventory or explanation. The clearing agent said that someone from the hospital would have to come to Chittagong to speak with the Chief Collector of Customs and explain what was in those three mysterious unknown crates. Since Dr. Olsen had obtained a special agreement with the government that we could import items for use at the hospital without having to pay duty on them, we did not want to do anything to jeopardize that agreement.

We passed around an inquiry to see if anyone at the hospital had any idea what might be in them. A short-term worker from Canada had come to help at the hospital workshop. He informed us that he had been asked to include three boxes of supplies for the hospital in the container with Adolph's shipment, which he did. Various churches had collected the contents of the boxes, but they did not supply an inventory, which was critical for customs clearance.

We traveled in the hospital truck to Chittagong and reserved rooms at the ABWE guest house. While Bob was at the customs office, Dr. Goddard and I visited hospitals and met doctors. While visiting the medical laboratory in Chittagong, the laboratory director asked if he could show us some X-rays. He put an X-ray film up on his view box, and I was shocked at what I saw. It showed a horribly fractured upper end of the tibia at the knee with numerous fragments of bone. This is technically known as a comminuted fracture. I asked how this had happened and was told that the young man had been driving a motorcycle when he was forced off the road by a speeding bus, causing him to strike a cement post with his knee.

The patient had been in the Chittagong Medical Hospital for about two weeks without treatment. His doctors were attempting to obtain the necessary documents to send him to India, hoping he could get a total knee replacement there because that procedure was not being done in Bangladesh at that time. The director then explained that the patient was his nephew.

I told the director that it would not be possible to put a total knee into a bone so severely fractured that it was only mush. There had to be some bony stock on which to place the total knee implant. This young man needed treatment to allow his body to congeal the multiple fragments into some sort of solid base, and then, if necessary, the total knee implant procedure could be performed. There was one more complication—the patient was diabetic.

I was scheduled to leave for furlough in only three days. I told the director I would be willing to treat his nephew if they could send him to our hospital that day and if Bob Adolph could get the customs matter cleared up so we could leave as soon as possible. Dr. Goddard and I would do the surgery. I assured the director that I would carefully explain to Dr. Goddard how to handle the patient's post-operative care. Then, I notified our hospital to make room for him so we could begin treatment immediately upon our return to MCH.

A possible way to handle that situation popped into my mind as I looked at the X-ray image. Somehow, those multiple fragments had to be collected into a mass that the body could heal into a solid block of bone that could support a metallic total knee device. I reasoned that we might be able to run multiple stainless-steel pins through the mass of bone fragments from multiple directions, hoping to spear enough of them to form a solid bony plate. Then, the plate could be manipulated into the proper position, using the end of the femur as a mold and held there by a plaster cast attached to the pins. I tried to explain to the director what I planned to do, and he seemed to understand. I considered that the procedure might be called a "porcupine treatment," but I did not tell the director that. We then left for one more appointment before returning to the guest house, hoping but doubting that the shipping confusion had been resolved and the truck would be ready to return to MCH.

Later, when we arrived at the guest house, we were surprised to find the truck parked there, loaded with the shipment that Bob Adolph had come to clear from customs. Sometimes, we experienced customs issues that took several days to clear up. He told us that when he sat in front of the Chief Collector of Customs, he had explained that he did not have an inventory for the three crates but was sure that the contents were meant for use at the hospital. To Bob's amazement, the usually stern collector said, "No problem. We will just change this from 18 to 21, and you may take the shipment." Bob wondered what had happened.

We did not know that the laboratory director had a connection with the Chief Collector of Customs, who had a connection with the patient. Perhaps they were from the same family group. Word had traveled from the laboratory director to the Customs Collector that we would accommodate the patient on an emergency basis, and the Customs Collector had done his part to expedite our return to the hospital. The "bamboo telegraph" is astonishingly rapid and effective in this part of the world. We returned to the hospital, the patient arrived that same day, and Dr. Goddard and I did the surgery the following day. The surgery went as planned, and I left the patient in Dr. Goddard's hands when Tense and I left for our furlough.

Upon our arrival at MCH one year later, the young man who had been treated for the knee injury returned to our hospital to see me. I was amazed at the result of the surgery. He had no pain and an acceptable range of motion in the knee. He was delighted with his results. A total knee replacement could be postponed indefinitely. The patient expressed his appreciation and said his uncle, who lived in Dhaka, was eager to meet me. His uncle asked that I contact him the next time we went to Dhaka so he could take my wife and me to lunch. We made a note of his contact information for our next trip to Dhaka.

Connections in High Places—God's Provision

Several years later, when we were getting ready to retire and return to the US, Tense's sister and her family came to visit us in Bangladesh, and we met them in Dhaka. Thinking they might enjoy riding from Dhaka to Chittagong on the train rather than flying, I had made reservations for train tickets for the seven of us. It was about an eight-hour trip by train and about an hour by plane.

While in Dhaka, we remembered that my knee patient's uncle had invited Tense and me to have lunch with him. We contacted him and had an enjoyable visit over lunch at the Intercontinental Hotel while our visiting family members rested at the guest house. During our conversation, I mentioned that we planned to take Tense's family to Chittagong on the train the next day.

"Oh, Dr. Bullock," he exclaimed, "you must not go on the train." At that time, there was severe political unrest in the country, with frequent general strikes, often accompanied by violence. He told us there had been train attacks and said we must fly instead. I said I appreciated his advice but that it could take as much as three weeks to get plane tickets, and our guests did not have that much time.

He handed me his business card and told me to show it to the Reservations Desk at the airline reservations office. I noticed the title after his name was "Secretary of Communications." That meant that he was a cabinet minister in the government. Communications included all forms of transportation! We thanked him and immediately went to the airline reservation office.

I told the clerk we needed seven tickets from Dhaka to Chittagong for the next day. He looked at me and then began to laugh. The laughing spread through the reservation office. These Americans were asking for seven tickets on one day's notice. How amusing! Then, an astonishing thing happened. As I took out the business card and handed it to him, I told him the card owner had said we should be given the tickets. He looked at the card, and his eyes widened in amazement. He picked up his phone and made a quick call. Upon hanging up the phone, he produced seven tickets and handed them to us. Once again, it was amazing to experience God's protection and provision for us through a series of connections only He could have orchestrated.

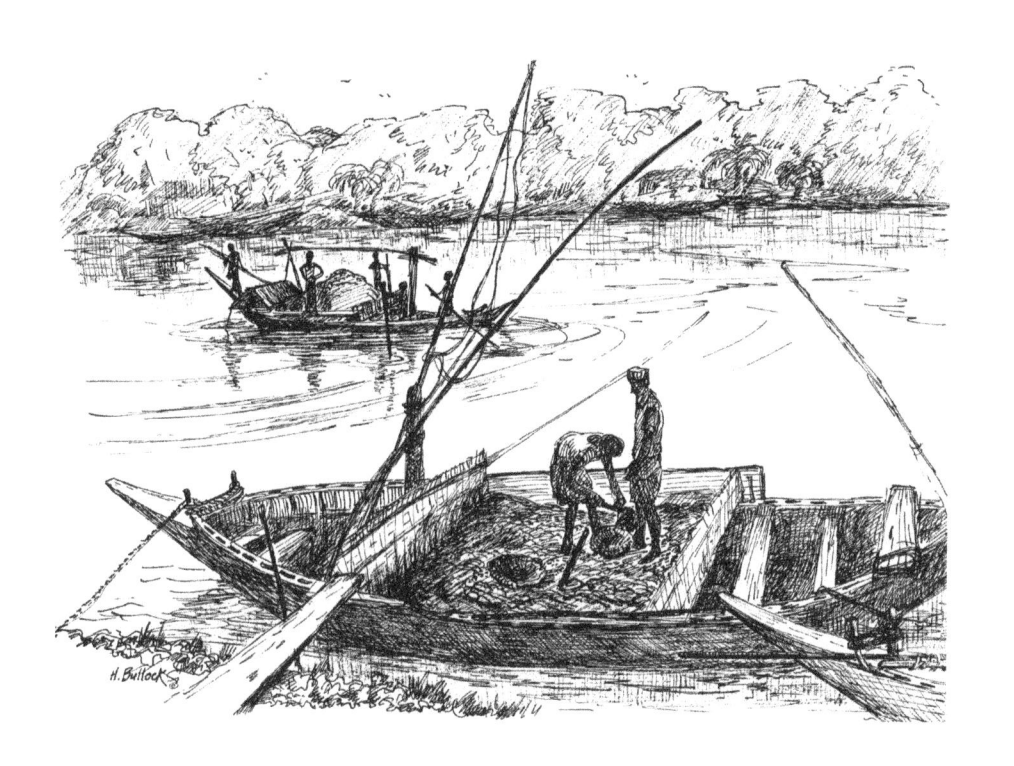

CHAPTER 42

Challenging Cases

Facial Injury

When we first arrived in Bangladesh, many boats coming and going in the Khal behind the hospital were powered by sails, with perhaps a small motor, for windless days. Later, they were mostly powered by diesel motors with heavy flywheels.

One day, a local fisherman was brought to the hospital with severe facial injuries. He had been attempting to start the engine of a small boat that had a flywheel. The weather was cool, and the man wore a scarf around his neck as he attempted to start the engine. He had leaned over the flywheel as the engine started, and the flywheel began to spin. The wheel caught the man's scarf, which jerked his face sharply downward into the metal structures surrounding the engine. It broke every bone in his face. I had never seen a fracture like this. The facial structures were floating.

God would often send a short-term doctor just in time with special skills needed to care for patients with specific injuries. On this occasion, a plastic surgeon, Dr. Steve Morris, had just arrived to work with us on a short-term assignment. He previously worked at the hospital as a medical student when I had just arrived in Bangladesh. I was relieved that God had brought Dr. Morris back to our hospital at the exact time I needed his help.

Dr. Morris examined the patient and told me this type of injury was called a "Le Forte" fracture. He said he knew how to treat it. Usually, it was treated with an Oxford External Fixator, which we did not have. Therefore, we had to construct one out of screws, pins, and wires. First, the patient's fractured jaw was wired back into as close to an anatomic position as possible. Then, the upper facial bones were stabilized by putting screws into his eyebrows and wiring them to the floating facial bones, which were also wired to the reconstructed jaw. This wired his jaw shut, so we also did a tracheostomy so his airway would not become obstructed if he should vomit. We worked on him for three hours and brought his teeth and bones back into place.

The patient made an uneventful recovery, and we were pleased with the result. We did not know what he looked like before the accident, but his appearance after treatment was acceptable and functional. Most importantly, the patient heard the plan of salvation from the Holy Bible many times during his postoperative recovery.

Dental Care at MCH

Dental problems were usually sent to dentists in the city. Although I did not do regular dental care, there were times when I had to wire teeth together to treat a fractured lower jaw. One night, I was faced with a problem for which I had no solution. I was called by a medic to come to the hospital to see a patient who had multiple fractures. The woman had been walking and meditating on the roof of her third-story apartment with her eyes closed. She stepped off the roof's edge and fell three stories to the ground. She landed on her feet, and the impact caused her knees to slam into her jaw, breaking it and shattering her facial bones. She also broke both tibias and fibulas and both femurs. The upper teeth were impacted into the cheekbones, and the lower teeth impacted into the jaw. Miraculously, the two upper teeth were still anchored in solid bone and could be wired to the lower teeth still attached to solid bone. I wondered what to do with the multiple floating fragments of bone that still had teeth attached to them. Would they stand any chance of surviving? I surely did not know.

The recent typhoon had caused much damage in our area. A relief team had come to help with the typhoon recovery problems and was staying in one of the empty houses at the hospital compound. I learned there was a dentist on the team and sent a message asking him to come to the operating room to advise me on how to treat this patient. I especially needed to know what to do about the floating fragments of bone with multiple teeth still in them. While waiting for him, we addressed the multiple bone fractures in the long bones of both legs. We stabilized them as well as we could with implanted metal rods.

The dentist poked his head into the operating room door and asked what I wanted him to do. I asked him to come in and look at the X-rays and give me some advice. He looked at the X-rays and came closer to the table to see the teeth. I heard him say, "I have never seen anything like that," as he fainted and fell backward onto the floor. He was dragged out of the operating room, and we returned to the multiple problems before us.

I had to try to simplify things as much as I could. I decided not to try to reattach the loose fragments of bone that still contained teeth. I reasoned that there would be multiple sources of infection if I did. We wired the upper attached teeth to the lower attached teeth, stabilizing the facial structures and the jaw. We performed a tracheostomy so that the patient would not drown in vomit. She withstood all the procedures well, and her overall condition stabilized enough to transfer her to a bed. Her postoperative course was difficult, as could be expected, but she lived through it. After about six weeks of recovery at our hospital, she was transferred by ambulance to be seen by a regular dentist in the city. We sent the bone fragments that still contained teeth with her.

My Most Challenging Case

I knew before I came to Bangladesh that I would be seeing some patients with problems that were either beyond or at the very limits of my expertise. I pledged to try my best to solve them. One of those cases involved a young boy who was about six years old when he was brought to the clinic and was seen by a doctor filling in for me while I was home on furlough. The boy had been seated on a stool at his home when his father, for whatever reason, cuffed him on the back of his head. The boy fell from the stool and was momentarily paralyzed. He soon regained consciousness but began to experience increased difficulty in walking, so they brought him to the hospital.

X-rays revealed anterior dislocation of the first cervical vertebra on the second vertebrae, causing pressure on the spinal cord. The doctor who was seeing him in my absence applied traction and then a brace. The traction did not help, and dislocation recurred. The boy was put into a holding brace until I returned from furlough.

On my return, X-rays were repeated and revealed an absence of the upward spike of the second vertebra, called the odontoid process. That spike serves to stabilize the position of the two vertebrae. We determined this was a congenital defect. Fusion of the first and second vertebra would be necessary to stabilize the situation.

While I was away on furlough, I was given an expensive set of orthopedic instruments called Vinke Tongs for use at MCH. This type of skeletal traction was much more effective than the older Crutchfield tongs. They were applied to the boy immediately, and traction was continued. This time, the correction of the deformity was not that easy. I ordered traction to be continued for seven weeks, hoping to gain reduction, which would make the surgical procedure much easier. Otherwise, a portion of the first cervical vertebra must be excised to remove the pressure on the cord. This would be a dangerous surgery because the first cervical vertebra was close to the vertebral artery and the spinal cord. Miraculously, the dislocation reduced during the seventh week of traction, so we prepared the boy for surgery. I had some training in cervical fusion, so I felt confident to proceed.

The seven long weeks of recuperation were difficult for the little boy as he lay flat on his back in bed with his head in traction. During this time, an extremely important event occurred in his life. He was from a Hindu family, but he had been attending the Bengali Christian school for children of our hospital workers, where he had received much instruction from the Holy Bible in his classes. In addition, he had also participated in the AWANA Bible-teaching program for young Bengali boys and girls. Participants received merit badges as they completed assigned tasks, which included Bible verse memorization.

After the boy had been put into traction, our hospital personal worker showed another patient the filmstrip entitled "What Does the Holy Bible Teach About God's Plan for Man?" The boy could not see the pictures as he was confined to his bed in traction. But he could hear the narration and wanted to see the pictures so much that he began to cry. Seeing this, the personal worker arranged a private showing for the boy the next day. The lessons from the scriptures he learned in school and his AWANA lessons prepared his heart to receive the message he saw on the film strip. That day, he trusted in Christ for salvation, which was a turning point in his life.

As I was making rounds in the wards the next day, I spoke with the little boy, who bubbled over with excitement as he told me his great news. He then eagerly began reading every piece of Bible-teaching literature we could put into his hands. A few days later, he shared the message of salvation from the Holy Bible with his younger cousin, who also trusted in Christ. The boy began telling his family about his salvation.

On the day of the surgery, the boy asked his family to be at his bedside as he prayed before the operation. His family was very moved by his prayer and his testimony. The surgery went well, and he was placed into a halo brace. He was soon able to leave the hospital, still wearing the brace, and it was then that he shared the gospel message with another child who also believed in Christ for salvation.

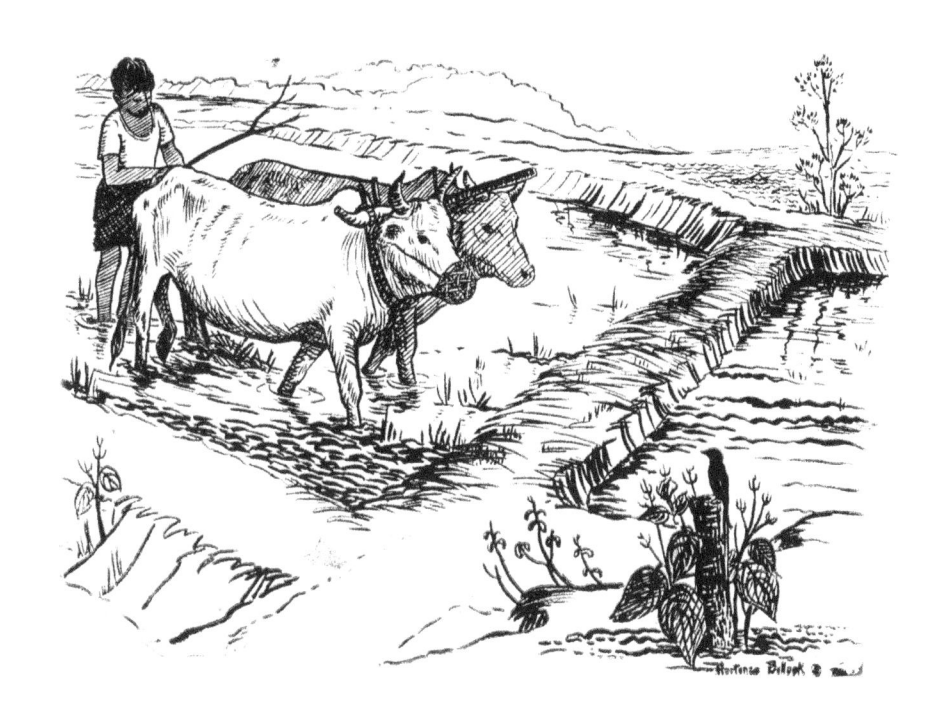

CHAPTER 43

Grateful Patients

Most of our patients were grateful for whatever treatment we could give them. They would often bring a gift after their discharge to show their gratitude. Some of these gifts became my most cherished possessions. Even though, in many cases, we might not have been able to speak the language well, our demonstration of compassion and concern for their physical needs gave us the opportunity to tell them what the Holy Bible teaches about God's great love for them and the salvation that is available through faith in Christ. Success in surgery was far less gratifying than spiritual healing for a patient and his or her family.

The Gift of Buffalo Doi

One winter day, a man presented at our hospital with a very difficult orthopedic problem. He was a farmer who had been tending to his water buffalo, which he used for plowing. This was an enormous animal with huge, curved horns. The farmer had tied a rope to the buffalo's neck and was holding onto the rope. The buffalo suddenly bolted and ran. The rope got twisted around the man's right index finger and hand, and the finger was pulled off at the base, along with a large piece of skin over the hand. His arm was wrenched in such a way as to produce a galeazzi fracture. This is a fracture of the lower end of the shaft of the radius bone and a dislocation of the lower end of the ulna bone.

The patient had come from Teknaf, which was 90 miles away down near the Burma border, to seek help for his difficult injury. Ordinarily, we would immediately operate on this sort of fracture, as it is quite unstable, but the accident had happened the previous day. When a wound is more than eight hours old, the risk of infection is too great to allow an open operation on the bone. We had no choice but to try to treat the fracture closed while we treated the open wound on the hand.

After a few days of wet dressings and antibiotics, we took him to surgery for a plastic revision of the traumatic amputation and a primary skin graft to the hand. At the same time, we did a closed reduction of the fracture and were able to improve the position considerably. His postoperative course was relatively smooth, and we were eventually able to send him home in a cast, with the hand exposed for dressings. During the time he was in the hospital, his attitude changed from worried anxiety to cheerful hope—hope that he would still be able to use his right arm in his farming occupation.

When he came back for his six-week recheck and walked in the door, I immediately recognized him because his ears stuck almost straight out from the sides of his head. He was dressed for the winter weather with a brightly colored stocking cap and scarf and was wearing a heavy sweater. Being from the US, we didn't feel very cold. But for the Bangladeshis, winter is bitter cold. He was grinning from ear to ear, and his eyes were shining. In his good hand, he was carrying a clay pot with a narrow neck wrapped in a banana leaf. I knew immediately that it was filled with doi, a sweet yogurt made from the milk from his buffalo.

This doi was the best kind of doi—a thick, creamy curd and very sweet. It is highly prized by the Bengali people. He brought it to me as a thank-you gift for his treatment. These types of expressions of gratitude from my Bangladeshi patients were extremely rewarding. I accepted his gift with thanks and proceeded with his treatment. The skin graft had healed just fine, and the bone had healed in an acceptable position. We removed the cast, and he was instructed to continue the exercises to restore mobility to the arm and hand, which had stiffened by the prolonged immobilization in the cast.

I went to my house and got some of our yogurt, made from a Canadian culture we brought from the US. I told him it was from Canada and that this was my exchange gift for him. He was delighted! Yogurt lovers enjoy sampling yogurt from other parts of the world. He hugged me in the Muslim fashion—first a hug on the right side and then on the left side of the head, and then he shook hands with me in deference to our custom. I hoped he would never forget the treatment he received at our hospital and the message he had heard about the gospel of salvation from the Holy Bible. The reputation for providing compassionate care at MCH had spread widely, attracting many people seeking treatment at the hospital. It was extremely difficult to function at MCH with all the restrictions and handicaps placed on us by the authorities, but compassion is free and cannot be regulated.

Grateful Mother

Every day was filled with surprises regarding the patients who came and their conditions. One day, a little boy of about six or seven years of age came to the hospital with his anxious and desperate mother. A year or so previous, he had developed osteomyelitis in his femur, and a section of the infected shaft had either sloughed out or had been removed by a quack doctor. This left a floppy leg with a three-inch missing part of the femur. There was no chance that this was going to heal by itself, and he was doomed to be handicapped for life. I did not know whether the woman's husband was alive, and this appeared to be her only child. They came from the island called Moheshkhali, which lies off the southern part of Bangladesh in the Bay of Bengal. Most of the people who live there are fishermen.

I had never seen a case like this in the US. In surgery, we removed the fibula from that leg and cut it into two pieces to the proper length to fit in the gap in the tibia bone. The wound healed, and the leg was put into a cast until the bone grafts could grow together. The treatment was successful, and he became able to walk again. This meant an altogether different future for him and his mother.

Several years later, the grateful mother returned to the hospital with a present for me for having helped her son become able to walk and work. She reported that the boy was walking well and going to school. I could not think of any time in the US when one of my patients or their family went to so much trouble just to thank me for the care I had rendered. She had traveled by boat from Moheshkhali Island and landed in Cox's Bazaar. From there she traveled by bus to the hospital. The country was under martial law due to political unrest, and there were many army checkpoints along the road.

The mother carried a paper sack containing a few eggs and a partially dried fish spread open like a butterfly. She started with a dozen eggs, but at every army checkpoint, the soldiers took one, and she arrived with only three left. She explained that the fish would need to continue to dry and instructed us how to accomplish this. We were to put it on a pole about ten feet in length and prop it up against the house in full sunlight above the reach of cats and other predators, but we had to bring it in at night to avoid the nocturnal predators. We did this for several weeks until the fish had thoroughly dried. We were extremely happy to have a screened porch to keep this fish at night because it was quite odoriferous. Finally, after about three weeks, the fish was dry and could safely be stored inside our freezer until it was time to use it.

That time to use the fish came when we had a khana for some of the hospital staff. A lady on the physical therapy staff was from the island of Moheshkhali and was fond of dried fish curry, so our cook used our gift to make fish curry for the feast. When she smelled and tasted that dried fish curry, she was delighted!

Osteomyelitis Girl Patient

One day, while working in the orthopedic department, we became aware of an immensely powerful and obnoxious odor. We thought a soiled dressing or a badly soiled cast might be tucked away somewhere, but a quick search of the department did not reveal such items. The stench was increasing steadily. I looked out the door of the cast room into the hallway and saw a teenage girl slowly walking toward us. As she walked, pus was dripping from her leg. Her garments were soiled, and her overall appearance was extremely dirty. She came directly into the cast room.

This drainage had been going on for several months, and as a result, she was an outcast in her village and had to sleep outdoors. An X-ray revealed severe osteomyelitis involving the entire tibia bone. A large chunk of dead bone was surrounded by a shell of attempted new bone formation as the body tried to wall off the infection. We admitted her to the hospital and cleaned the draining leg. In surgery, I removed a large piece of dead bone and carefully removed the infected tissue with curettes down to clean, bleeding bone. Rubber drains were placed in the wound, and it was packed with a dressing. She slowly made an uneventful recovery and was able to leave the hospital with the leg in a plaster cast, using crutches to walk. When the cast was removed, the drainage sites had all healed, and the leg was dry. This was a remarkable change for this girl! During her recovery time in the hospital, she heard the truth about God's plan for man's salvation as taught in the Holy Bible.

Several years later, a young woman in a white bourka came to the orthopedic department. She was beautiful, wearing makeup and gold jewelry, and smelled of perfume. When my staff questioned her, they discovered that she was the girl who had terrible osteomyelitis. She had come to the hospital to invite us to her wedding! Unfortunately, I was about to leave on furlough and could not attend the wedding, but I was overjoyed to see the remarkable change our treatment had rendered in this girl's life.

Tea Estate Visit

When we first arrived at the hospital, Sunday was our official day off, and the hospital was closed that day. Many years later, the closed day was changed to Friday, the Muslim holy day, and Sunday became just an ordinary business day and the start of our work week. On Sundays, people passing by on their way to the beach resort at Cox's Bazar would often stop at the hospital to try to be seen as outpatients. They reasoned that they had come all this way and might as well try to get some medical treatment.

One Sunday, while I was enjoying my day off, a hospital peon came to the door with a note saying a man at the front gate wanted to see me. Along with the note was the business card of the man, Mr. A., who was the manager of a tea estate in the Sylhet district. I usually refused such requests on my day off, but something about this seemed unusual. So, I sent a message to let him inside the gate and went to the hospital to see him.

When I arrived at the hospital, there were two men waiting to see me. They spoke excellent English and politely apologized for disturbing my day of rest. I felt that was very unusual also. Then the man who was the tea estate manager explained that his small daughter had a problem that none of the doctors they had seen could diagnose. He asked if he could bring her to the hospital for me to see her. Her problem was a musculocutaneous complaint, so it seemed to be in my line of expertise.

Just then, an idea popped into my mind. My wife and I had been planning a short vacation to Sylhet, famous for its tea gardens. We thought we had made reservations at a guest house there, which we had seen advertised. I told the visitor about our impending vacation and that we had reservations to stay at a guest house. I suggested I could see his daughter then, which would spare him the inconvenience of bringing her several hundred miles to our hospital. When I told the men about the guest house, they told me it had not yet been built! The tea estate manager then insisted that we stay with him on the tea estate as his guests. We planned to stay for one week, and he said that would be fine. I gladly accepted his invitation. That began a great adventure and an exciting part of God's plan for us.

Our hospital van driver took us to Chittagong, and from there, we flew to Sylhet. We were met at the airport by a driver from the tea estate who took us by car to the estate, far from the city. After traveling about fifty miles and crossing one river on a ferry, we arrived at the tea estate and were taken to a large house on a hill.

On the way, Tense and I prayed silently as we wondered how God might open up an opportunity for us to share the gospel with our host. At supper that first night, our host began the conversation with a question.

"Well," he asked, "what do Baptists believe?" Wow! The door had been opened widely. I told him that we believed the Bible is true and is the very Word of God. We had brought with us a Bengali language version of the New Testament, and I gave it to him to read. He happily accepted my gift.

His young daughter, the patient, was a hyperactive child about six years old. It would have been impossible to examine her without her being under general anesthesia. She had a severe foot deformity and walked with a pronounced limp. I waited until she fell asleep that night to examine her. She also had a deformity of the ear, called a cauliflower ear, and a spinal curvature (scoliosis), along with her crooked foot and ankle. I told her father I would research her problem and let him know the diagnosis and proposed treatment.

The next day, Mr. A. gave us a grand tour of the tea estate. As the estate manager, he was like a king, completely in control of everything. Even the police wouldn't enter the estate without his invitation.

The hills were covered with tea bushes. We watched the women tea pickers loading their baskets with tea leaves. They brought the loaded baskets to the collecting stations. From there, it was taken to the tea processing area and prepared for sale. It was a fascinating experience to see his operation.

Upon returning home, I searched my medical books and was able to determine that the little girl had a condition called diastrophic dwarfism, which I had never seen before. She was going to require surgery on her foot and ankle and then surgery for scoliosis. I sent a message to the father, informing him of the diagnosis and the recommended treatment. I invited him and his family to be our guests at our residence while the girl had surgery on her foot and ankle.

Mr. A. and Mrs. A., their three children, two ayahs (nursemaids), and one driver arrived at our home a few days before the scheduled surgery for their little girl. We had a lot of curry cooking in our kitchen, and they were thankful to have our home to use as headquarters during their daughter's operation and early recovery time. She had to get used to the big plaster cast on her body and both legs. We planned to have them stay with us in October when they returned to have her cast removed and to be fitted for her foot brace. Our household helpers worked hard to make our guests comfortable and provide delicious meals to maintain our reputation as good hosts.

Satanic opposition was a common experience and no surprise to us when it happened. On the day before the scheduled surgery, I reached up to adjust the exhaust fan in the wall, and the fan blade struck my left fourth finger. The tip was fractured, and the skin was cut. Thankfully, a short-term surgeon was at the hospital. He dressed the wound and sutured the skin. Then, I made an aluminum splint for my fingertip. The next day was surgery day for the little girl. I put a sterile dressing on the finger and then covered it with a sterile finger cot. Over that went a sterile plastic glove and a sterile rubber glove. I was able to do her surgery despite my wounds.

The surgery went well, and eventually, she could walk without a limp and ride her bicycle. I advised her father to take her to England for spinal surgery. We did not perform scoliosis surgery at our hospital. God works in mysterious and wonderful ways. While they were guests in our home during their daughter's time of treatment and recovery at MCH, this family attended the Bengali national church and heard the message of salvation and God's plan for man from the Holy Bible.

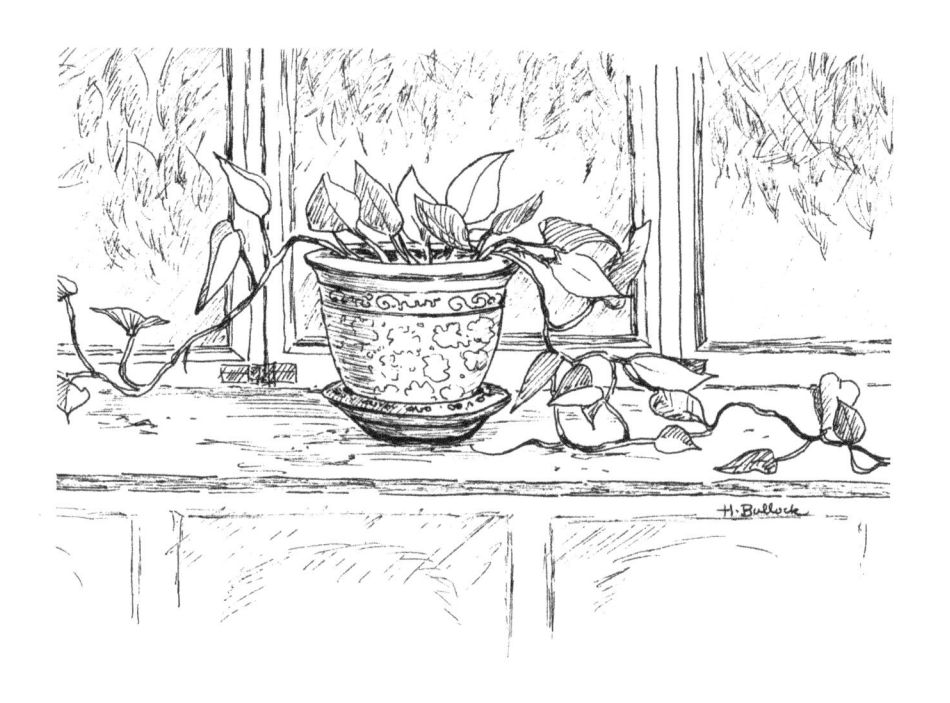

CHAPTER 44

Teamwork

Busy Surgery Day—the Usual Question

I frequently did not have time to see every patient in the wards on my rounds personally and also have time for surgical cases. Some of the other doctors had taught our surgical technicians advanced skills, and they were proficient. When patients came in with a strangulated hernia, an intestinal obstruction, or a cleft palate, I was thankful to be able to ask these trained technicians to do surgeries that were not in my field of expertise. I assisted these men as they operated and learned from them.

I quickly learned that the NGO nurses who had been at MCH for many years had acquired knowledge and skills about the culture that I had yet to learn. I would ask the nurses to do everything they could to manage the patients for me and to make a list of those that I needed to see.

We had to plan an extra surgery one day because we had not been able to finish all the surgeries from the previous day. Cases already planned for that day included surgery on an ankle fracture, surgery on a knee joint, a large skin graft on a leg, and another open knee surgery.

One day, a member of Parliament called and said he was planning to visit the hospital the next day before 10:00 a.m. That probably meant he planned to go to Cox's Bazar and stop at our hospital en route. His exact arrival time was uncertain. He might have been several hours late or may not have arrived at all. We did not know if he wanted to have a tour of the hospital or perhaps had one question about a specific matter. When a government official visited the hospital, we had to accommodate his request, so we planned to visit him between our cases.

At 7:30 a.m., Dr. Bob Goddard called me on the intercom to tell me my first surgery would have to start late because he had to take a patient into the only operating room for emergency surgery. Sometimes, the delivery room could be used as a second operating room. However, at that particular time, it was being used for a delivery. We had only one operating room crew, and they could not run two operating rooms simultaneously.

In the OPD was a man with a depressed skull fracture because his son hit him on the head with an object. We would probably also have to operate on him that day, but he had no money. Another patient waiting for treatment was a lady who was bleeding with possible placenta previa. The baby had died.

At the end of Bob's call, he said, "Come on over after breakfast, and we will get you started as soon as we can." Other than that, it appeared that it was going to be a fairly normal day.

Nancie D., our nurse in charge of the surgery department, sent me a note to ask her usual question. "John, you know we can't do all these things in one day. Which of your cases really must be done today?"

Managing Interpersonal Relationships

While working in cramped quarters under a huge workload with limited time and energy, we had to be very careful about managing interpersonal relationships with our coworkers at MCH. It was much like working on a submarine, and we could not let personal likes or dislikes interfere with the work we were trying to accomplish. Most of our personnel were skilled professionals who worked independently without supervision. Often, stressful situations would cause us to act or think irrationally. It was very important for us to heed Matthew 18:15-17.

> Moreover if your brother sins against you, go and tell him his fault between you and him alone. If he hears you, you have gained your brother. But if he will not hear, take with you one or two more, that 'by the mouth of two or three witnesses every word may be established.' And if he refuses to hear them, tell it to the church ... (Matthew 18:15-17a NKJV).

It was also very important to try to have a sense of humor and look for humor in almost every situation, if possible. I arrived at the hospital one day to make rounds but was a bit late. My orthopedic technicians had made rounds before I arrived. I had been teaching them how to make morning rounds in the wards to check on my patients. What they said or did must have upset the NGO nurses on duty because when I arrived on the ward, I was met with angry stares and comments such as "Your technicians did this and did that."

"Well," I said, "round up the usual suspects," and everyone laughed. The tension evaporated, and the situation was defused nicely.

Short Term Helper

In 1987, when we reported to one of our supporting churches in California, we stayed at the home of Don and Frances S., an elderly couple who were members of that church. Frances a retired nurse, asked if she could come by herself to spend three months living with us in Bangladesh to help with the work. We assured her that we would welcome her coming. When she came, Frances helped with packing and sorting instruments and organizing the orthopedic storeroom. She was an encourager to us and helped other members of the NGO staff. She reminded me of my mother. Having her come was like having a visit with my mother. After her visit, she continued encouraging us through her prayers and correspondence. She told us her short-term mission trip had been the highlight of her life.

Visit to Tense's Mother

For our annual month-long break from the mission station in 1989, we returned to Oregon for a planned family reunion to celebrate Tense's mother's 90th birthday. She had been having health problems, and shortly after our arrival, she received a cancer diagnosis. We were thankful we had come home to spend some time with her. Tense's brother and sister-in-law committed to caring for her when we returned to Bangladesh.

While in the US, I had an eye exam because my eyes had developed vitreous degeneration, with floaters and flashing lights in the visual fields of both eyes. This condition is not good for a surgeon as it interferes with close work. The eye exam revealed a retinal tear dangerously close to a complete retinal detachment. The doctor tacked down the loose area of the retina with cryosurgery so that I could return to Bangladesh, where I was desperately needed at MCH.

At that time, all the other doctors at the hospital had left the field for various reasons, leaving only me. Dr. Goddard planned to return soon for a brief time but then leave the field in May 1990, and Dr. Olsen was going to return soon, but he was primarily involved in Bible translation and would be working only part time at the hospital. We were expecting two new appointees to come soon, an OB/GYN and a family practitioner, but they would need to raise their full support and complete language study before joining the workforce at the hospital. We planned to continue to work at MCH until the new doctors could come on board full-time, maybe another three or four years.

Chrissa and Joshua Visit

When we returned to Bangladesh, we took our daughter Chrissa and her youngest child, Joshua, with us. This was Chrissa's first visit to the country, and she greatly appreciated the opportunity to see MCH firsthand and meet our teammates. She had spent years praying for the work at the hospital and helping us by handling some of our affairs while we were out of the country. Little blonde-haired Joshua was twenty months old, and he was quite popular with the Bangladeshis, making friends everywhere he went.

Death of Tense's Mother

When Chrissa and Joshua returned to the US, Tense went with them to care for her mother, who had cancer. Before Tense reached the US, she received word that her mother had died. Tense stayed six weeks in Oregon, helping tidy up her mother's affairs and closing up the family home.

Tense's mother had been a faithful supporter and had helped with our mail and the storage of our belongings, as well as sending care packages full of healthy snacks packed with love. She also kept us up to date on the financial and political scene. We knew we would miss her terribly, but we were confident we would see her in Heaven.

Granddaughters Visit

Because I was facing several years as the only full-time surgeon on duty, the field team sent us to the US for six months to rest and prepare for that big assignment after already serving a couple of months alone while Dr. Goddard had a break. After reporting to a few of our supporters and taking some time for family activities and rest, we returned to Bangladesh, taking our teenage granddaughters, Rachel and Sarah, for a three-month visit. They brought their homeschool materials and spent time each day studying, but they also received a broad educational experience through their trip. The girls taught English in the national elementary school and assisted the staff in the hospital. They especially enjoyed washing the newborn babies. Interacting with the Bangladeshis and their families gave them insight into the culture.

My Most Valuable Teammate

When I surrendered to the call of God to leave my orthopedic practice in San Luis Obispo, California, and go to the other side of the world to the country of Bangladesh, Tense willingly went with me and played a vital role in my service there. Life as a doctor's wife was good preparation for her busy life on the hospital compound. When I worked as a doctor in California, Tense's life was demanding. She never knew when I would come home and get something to eat. Tense had to arrange all the family events around my schedule while trying to meet the needs of all our family members. I did not get many days off, and since I was in a group practice, we had to coordinate my days off with the group calendar. If our family planned something and an emergency came up, we would have to cancel our plans. I often came home late at night after making rounds at the hospital to check on my patients.

Tense had to learn to be flexible and adapt to changing plans often. There were many events that got canceled at the last minute because of sudden conflicts. However, God used these things to teach her patience and to prepare her for our future service in Bangladesh. It seemed almost easy for Tense to adapt to our busy missionary life after 25 years as a doctor's wife in the US.

As my helper and wife, Tense took her role of keeping me alive very seriously, ensuring I received enough food and rest to manage the challenging schedule I was undertaking with all the surgeries and orthopedic cases. She assisted me with our correspondence and bookkeeping and coordinated our family schedule of activities, guests, and meetings. She oversaw our household employees, which included a gardener, a cook, a laundry worker, and a bearer (assistant to the cook). Additionally, she helped organize our orthopedic equipment storage at the hospital godown. She willingly and expertly accepted the challenge of packing and moving frequently while living in multiple homes on the hospital compound until we reached our final residence in House #12. Without her assistance in managing our home and supporting me in various ways, I would not have been able to navigate the demanding series of surgical and medical problems at the hospital. She was undoubtedly my most valuable teammate on the compound.

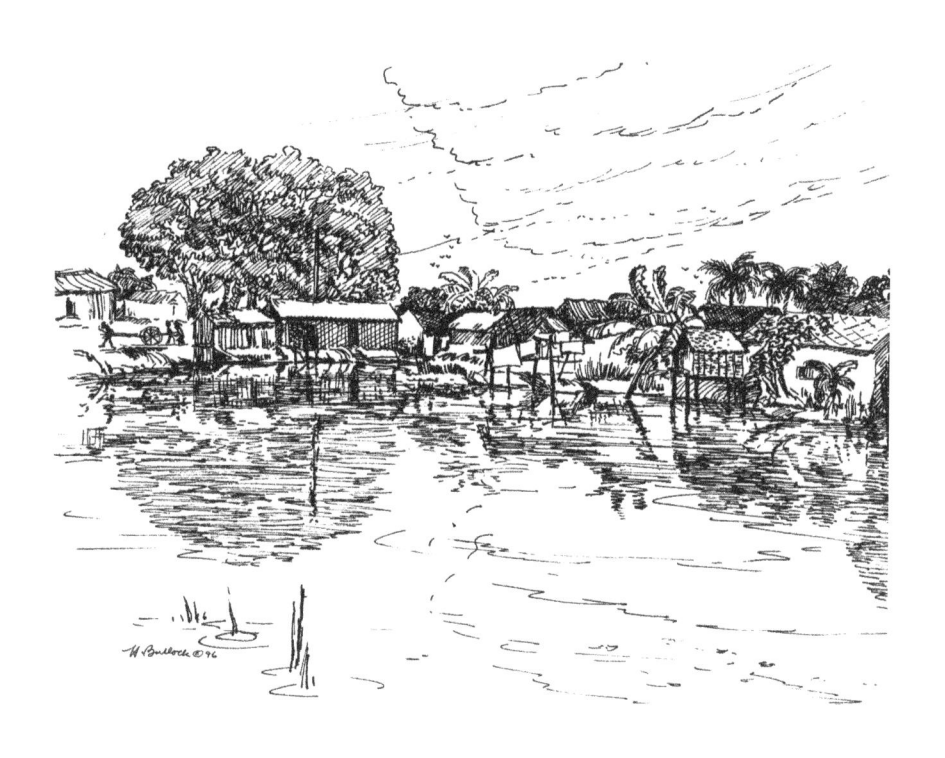

CHAPTER 45

Seventeen Years!

A Helicopter Adventure

It was a hot, muggy Saturday in August 1991, the first day of our work week. I was the only doctor on duty that day at our hospital and had finished my rounds. As I left the hospital, I noticed that a Bangladesh military helicopter had landed on the soccer field close to the tribal headquarters building. Then I saw George C. walking toward me with two men from the helicopter. George told me they were looking for me and introduced them. One was an official from Avia Export in Dhaka, a Russian helicopter export company. The other man was a Russian doctor from the Russian embassy in Dhaka.

Both men had flown from Dhaka to Chittagong the day before when they learned that one of the export company's employees had been severely injured in an accident. He had been running for exercise beside a lake on a sweltering day and decided to dive into the cool water. His head struck a submerged log. He sustained multiple fractures in his neck and was instantly paralyzed from his neck down. His rescuers took him to a hospital in Chittagong. The doctors there said they could not do any surgery on him because they did not have the training. They thought the patient was too seriously injured to be moved, so he had simply been put into a bed.

The two Russian men had commissioned a Bangladesh military helicopter to fly down to our hospital to find me and ask me to come back with them to Chittagong to examine the patient. They pleaded with me to bring all the necessary instruments and come to Chittagong to operate on the injured man. They also wanted to find out if I would be willing to transfer him to our hospital for treatment. They had not brought any X-rays with them, so I could not evaluate his injury or determine whether surgery was even indicated.

I offered to travel to Chittagong to examine the patient if they would transport me in a helicopter. It took over three hours to drive on the road, but the helicopter could arrive in twenty minutes. They agreed to return me to my hospital as soon as possible after I had examined the patient. I told them that even if surgery were indicated, I would not consider operating on him in Chittagong. If they wanted me to operate on him, he would have to be transferred to our hospital.

I asked Tense to quickly prepare a bag for me in case I had to stay overnight. I also arranged to have my senior orthopedic technician travel with me. We took a patient transfer litter, skull tongs, and emergency cervical collars.

Upon arrival in Chittagong, we were taken directly to the hospital, where I could examine the patient. He was conscious and was just lying in a bed. No treatment had been started. I determined that he had sustained a crush-type fracture of the 5th cervical vertebra and was quadriplegic. We applied the cervical tongs and put his neck in traction. It seemed to me that there might be a chance to remove any pressure on the spinal cord by surgery, but it would be necessary to have a CT scan of his neck to determine if this would be possible. At that time, there was only one CT scan machine in the country, and it was at the Army Hospital in Dhaka.

I determined that the best course of treatment would be to transfer the patient to Dhaka, hoping that a neurosurgeon there could perform surgery if the CT scan indicated it was necessary. The only other alternative would be to take him back to Moscow for treatment there. I told the Russian men what I recommended, and then we went to the Russian Embassy office in Chittagong to discuss the matter.

Sitting in the office, one of the Russian men asked me how long I had been in Bangladesh. When I told him I had been there for seventeen years, his eyes opened wide, and he exclaimed, "Seventeen years! Why?"

"I did not choose to come here," I replied. "God sent me." Then I explained to him that our purpose in coming to Bangladesh was to be part of the team trying to bring the message of God's love and salvation taught in the Bible to the Bangladeshi people.

I returned to Malumghat by helicopter and left my orthopedic technician behind to assist in transferring the patient to Dhaka and then back to Moscow. Watching the helicopter take off from the MCH compound, I thought, "Yes, seventeen incredible years of surprises, challenges, heartaches, and blessings."

PART FOUR

Reassignment

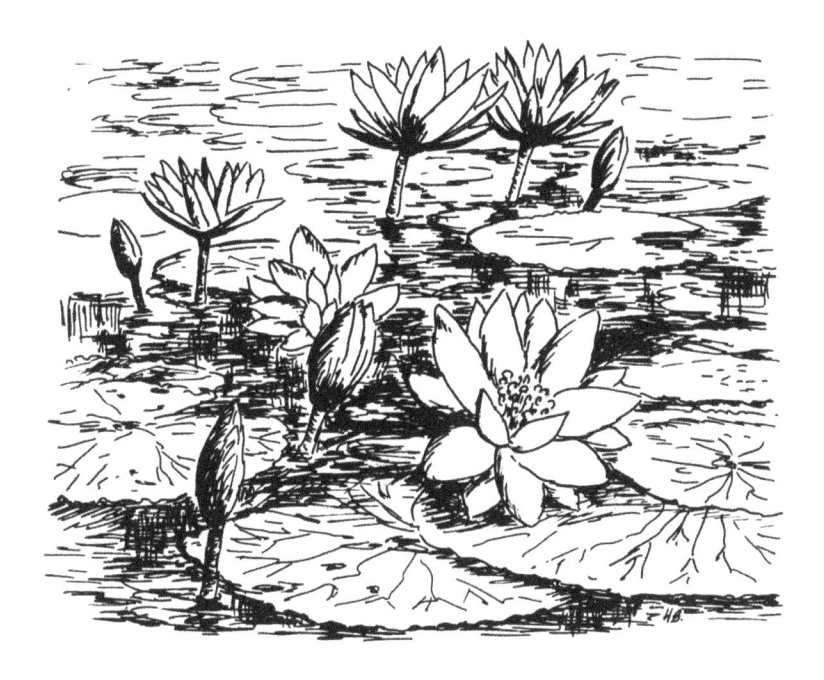

CHAPTER 46

Life More Abundant

Retirement

The policy of our mission board at that time was that NGO workers were required to retire at age 65. During our last three months at Malumghat before retirement we were furiously busy with packing, patient care, selling household goods, making special visits, and receiving many wonderful invitations to farewell dinners and Christmas teas. The final farewells were painful, as we did not know if we would return to Malumghat in the future for a short-term teaching ministry in the orthopedic department.

Short-Term Help for the AV Department

In 1991, a young woman who had majored in Cinematography came to help in the AV Department for one year after her college graduation. She reorganized the Audiovisual Department and trained the AV staff in video production. With her guidance and help, they produced a series of Bible-teaching videos for adults and children. They also produced health teaching and medical training videos at the hospital. Tense and I were actively involved with producing videotapes for health teaching and training orthopedic technicians and other medical personnel at MCH. Tense helped our short-term cinematographer with these video productions. They also produced a puppet drama video about the book of Esther.

The Longest House Call

A few months after our retirement while we were doing our final reporting to our supporting churches in the US, I received a message that the ABWE home office was urgently trying to contact me. Dr. Olsen had fallen from his motorcycle in Bangladesh and fractured his hip. He needed surgery. However, there was no doctor at the hospital who could do the hip surgery. He did not want to have a Bengali doctor operate on him in a Bangladesh hospital. The only other option was to evacuate him to either Bangkok or Singapore, where he could have surgery. To complicate matters further, he was over six feet tall. The hospital workshop crew had to make the hospital bed longer to accommodate him. If he was transferred by plane to Bangkok or Singapore, that meant getting him to Dhaka, where he could get onto a wide-body jet.

Taking him to Dhaka, 250 miles north, over bumpy roads in an ambulance, would be a painful ordeal. Secondly, getting enough seats for him to lie down for the flight would be exceedingly difficult on such short notice.

I was asked if I would be willing to return to Bangladesh on an emergency basis and perform the surgery at our hospital. I immediately answered, "Of course I will go. Just get me a plane ticket. I need to get Tense back to Utah, which will take a day or so, and then I can go."

When we got home, there was a message on our answering machine saying that I had a plane reservation for a flight scheduled to leave in two days. We hurriedly packed some clothes into a suitcase. I telephoned the Zimmer representative with whom we had dealt previously and asked him if he could find some Hagie pins for me. They are a workhorse pin, smooth on one end and threaded on the other, with a nut on the threaded end. They are very versatile and can be used in many applications. However, they were no longer being manufactured. I knew we had a few at the hospital but did not know how many.

The representative on the phone said, "John, they don't make those anymore. Why don't you use a compression screw, which has replaced the Hagie pins?"

"But we don't have any compression screws," I told him. I told him I was leaving Salt Lake City in just two days.

He said he would send me some to take with me. He said there was a Fed Ex office on the way to the airport and that I should stop there to pick up the things he would send me.

At the Fed Ex office, we found three suitcases filled with over $10,000 worth of equipment, a complete set of compression hip screws and the tools for applying them. I was only allowed two suitcases plus one carry-on for my flight. We repacked my suitcase, eliminating a few things, to the point where we could take only two of the new suitcases, plus my carry-on bag. Then we went to the airport.

When I went through security at the airport, the bells went off when they X-rayed my baggage. The agent asked me what was in it, and I explained to him that I was an orthopedic surgeon on my way to perform an emergency surgery in a foreign country and that the tools were essential. Picking up one of the packages, the agent asked me to open it. I refused, pointing out to him that it said right on the package, "Sterile unless opened." I needed to have it sterile when I got to Bangladesh. I also told him that he knew exactly what was in the package because it had been X-rayed. He then asked if my passport said I was a physician/surgeon. I told him that occupations are not listed on the passports. He finally agreed to let me board the plane. The same scene was enacted at each stop, but I finally got to Dhaka with all the unopened packages.

Upon arrival in Dhaka, I had to go through the customs line before I changed planes for my domestic flight to Chittagong. I knew that the medical equipment I was bringing in should be permitted. However, there was a risk that the customs officer might seize the medical equipment and put it into quarantine. Getting it out could take weeks. We didn't have weeks. The fracture was already one week old, and the surgery needed to be done as soon as I arrived.

As I approached the customs officer, another passenger was talking with him. The customs officer saw me pushing the cart bearing my three luggage pieces.

"Make way for the foreigner!" he exclaimed.

"Praise the Lord!" I whispered as I wheeled my cart past the customs officer and headed to board my in-country flight to Chittagong. The hospital van was waiting for me in Chittagong and took me to MCH.

The surgery went well, and Dr. Olsen made a good recovery. I had to leave to return to the US one week later because I was only given a two-week visa at the airport. My return trip was complicated, but I made it home with the remaining surgical equipment I had not needed for the surgery.

"That was the longest house call I've ever made," I told the Zimmer representative when I returned the unused equipment. That trip made me realize that I wanted to return to Bangladesh to help in any way I could, whether by training orthopedic technicians, assisting with the medical work, or helping with the Audiovisual Department.

Return to Help in the AV Department

The general surgeons did not have time to do cast work, set up traction, and do other orthopedic chores. It was necessary to have a staff of fully-trained orthopedic technicians to support their work. Some previously trained orthopedic technicians had died, some were fired, and some left for better pay elsewhere or a different line of work. New orthopedic technicians had to be trained to keep the orthopedic department functioning. We were willing to return to Bangladesh for short-term assignments during our retirement years if we were physically able so

I could teach orthopedics to general surgeons and train orthopedic technicians as needed.

When we left Bangladesh in 1992, no one was available to take our place in supervising the Audiovisual Department. I also felt a strong responsibility to help maintain the AV Department and realized that making frequent trips to accomplish these goals might be necessary.

In 1996, we returned to Bangladesh for three months to work in the AV Department. This seemed an excellent opportunity to take our teen grandsons, Tim and Steve, with us so they could see Bangladesh and learn about the work at MCH. Upon our arrival, we learned that the head of the AV Department had been discharged just two weeks earlier. The surviving staff was bewildered and poorly equipped to manage the department independently without leadership. Our teammates at Malumghat were heavily involved in their other responsibilities and could not spare the time to manage the AV Department.

Our being there at that time seemed to be God's perfect timing. Our experience and familiarity with this department enabled us to help them get reorganized. We taught them how to use and maintain the equipment and produce important ministry and public health productions. Tim and Steve quickly became involved in assisting in this department. Tim and Steve also helped with projects and chores at the hospital. The boys were a valuable help during the three months they were with us at MCH.

More Return Trips

Over the next nineteen years, from 1996 to 2015, we returned multiple times, training four groups of orthopedic technicians and teaching orthopedic surgery to general surgeons. It was often difficult to get the new general surgeons to realize that orthopedic-related conditions and injuries were something they would be dealing with almost every day. Other than obstetrics, orthopedic problems were one of the main reasons many patients came to the hospital. If our doctors could not care for them, they would have to be sent to another hospital in the country. Often, there would be times when our doctors were alone at the hospital for months and would be handling a variety of cases, including orthopedic-related conditions. They needed to be prepared.

Each time we returned, Tense continued teaching English classes to orthopedic and X-ray technicians and taught art to children and adults. During those years, she spent many hours creating Bible story illustrations for the AWANA program.

Our last visit to Bangladesh was in November 2014 for five months to train a new group of orthopedic technicians. It was becoming more physically difficult for us to return, as we were both 87 years old. During that term, our daughter Karen brought her family to see Bangladesh and the hospital where their grandparents had served for over twenty years. It was a delight to show them all that God had accomplished.

Veera's Hope

In 1997, I returned to MCH for several months to train another group of orthopedic technicians and train one of our general surgeons in orthopedic surgery. Three weeks before I was scheduled to return to the US, a young girl about eight years old, whom I will call Veera, was brought to the hospital by her father for surgery. Five years earlier, he brought her to the hospital for an examination to seek help for his little daughter. When Veera was two years old, she contracted poliomyelitis. Her hips and knees became stuck in a 90-degree flexed position, and she could not straighten them. She could only move about by crawling on her hands and knees. She had large callouses on her knees and the tops of her feet. Veera had no hope of any sort of useful life.

After examining Veera, we told her father that we could not restore full function to her legs, but we could straighten out the flexion contractures so she could wear weight-bearing braces and would be able to learn to walk with crutches. The procedure would allow her to move about in an upright position and to go to school. We explained that this would require four separate major surgeries to do the surgical releases at both hips and both knees so that her legs could be brought into full extension. Her recovery would require a long period of hospitalization, and she would be fitted with crutches and braces.

The father wanted to have this treatment for his daughter, but the total cost of her multiple surgeries would be more than the family could afford. I referred them to the HOPE Fund Committee, which evaluated the family's financial situation and recommended how much they would be expected to pay. The HOPE Fund could provide financial help for some of the cost, but there was still a large expense that the family would have to provide. Then, her father took his daughter home with plans to discuss the matter with the extended family and attempt to raise the money.

I did not see her again until I returned to MCH five years later, in 1997, in my post-retirement years, to do orthopedic training. When Veera's father brought her back to MCH, he informed us that the family had finally raised the necessary funds to pay for her surgery. This presented a huge dilemma for me. Usually, this surgery would be done in four sessions, with a few weeks of recovery time between each surgery. That way, if infection should develop, it would only involve one operative site and not all four sites. However, I did not have enough time to do those surgeries at intervals before my visa expired, and I had to return to the US. Also, I had not trained the general surgeon in the release of extensive contractures like this girl had, so I could not leave this operation for him to do by himself. I felt compelled to provide this child with these surgeries while I was at MCH. There was no one else there at that time who had the training to do these surgeries.

As I puzzled over how to handle this problem, I thought of possibly doing all the surgeries simultaneously. If I had seen Veera when I first got to Bangladesh, I certainly would not have done four surgeries in one day. There are guidelines to be followed as a certified orthopedic surgeon, and this was more than a stretch of those standards. But, realizing that her family had been willing to work and save for five years to give their crippled child a chance at a normal life, I felt there was no alternative.

Following the surgeries, it was going to be necessary to be able to turn her in bed to provide access to her back and front for dressing the incisions, bathing, toilet care, and preventing pressure sores. The only way this could be accomplished would be to suspend her body about six inches above the bed by ropes connected to stainless steel pins in each leg and in her pelvis. This would have to be continued for at least four to six weeks before she could be lowered to the bed and joint motion started for physical therapy.

I decided it was worth the chance, as there was no other way to solve her problem. Also, I did not know when or if I could return due to the precarious visa situation. Our nurses had much experience handling complex problems, and I was confident they could assist the doctor and carefully supervise Veera's post-operative recovery. I would leave detailed instructions for her care.

Her father agreed to the treatment plan, and we proceeded. With the patient under general anesthesia, I performed four surgeries and released both hip and knee contractures in one operation. After the surgery, I constructed the complicated positioning of the patient above the bed. Her post-operative course did not have any complications.

Veera remained at the hospital for several weeks after her surgeries. Also, she received therapy and instruction from our physical therapists to help her learn to walk with her braces and crutches. During this time, the personal workers shared with Veera and her family the great message of God's love for her and the spiritual healing available through faith in Christ. I received no communication from the general surgeon regarding Veera's progress after I returned to the US, so I assumed things were going well with recovery.

Three years later, I returned to give similar orthopedic surgery training to Dr. Stephen Kelley, the new general surgeon at MCH, and train new orthopedic technicians. Dr. Kelley was an accomplished thoracic and cardiovascular surgeon who had just finished his language study and was eager to accept my offer to give him orthopedic training. He soon became highly skilled in treating orthopedic cases.

While I was training Dr. Kelley, Veera and her father came to the hospital to get her braces repaired and to see me to express their gratitude. She had recovered well from her multiple surgeries, and I was pleased with her progress. She was walking with her legs in braces, which had been made for her by the Limb and Brace Shop at MCH. She was using Canadian crutches, which are gripped by the hands and do not extend above the elbow. The crutches were held in place by cuffs that clamped to her forearms. We gave her a Bengali language New Testament and hoped and prayed she would understand the message of God's love for her and decide to put her faith in Christ.

I last saw Veera and her father when I returned to Bangladesh in 2010 to train a new group of orthopedic technicians. Standing in front of the hospital one day, I noticed a nice-looking young woman with braces and Canadian crutches walking toward me. I was astonished when I realized it was Veera. She told me she was attending university and studying business administration and computer science. What a change her treatment in our hospital had made for this young woman's future. Instead of crawling around on all fours for the rest of her life, she was able to go to school, get a job, and have the possibility of getting married and having a family.

Then, she did something that brought tears to my eyes. Contrary to her culture, where a woman would never touch a man's hand other than her father's, Veera put her crutches against the adjacent railing, took my hand, and stood beside me for a picture. I will never forget that! Years later, I learned that Veera had finished college and was teaching school. She had gotten married and had one child. I thanked God for allowing me to be the tool He used to make a miraculous change in a young woman's life and give her hope for her future.

CONCLUSION

Only One Life

Before we were born, God had a divine plan for our lives. He chose and carefully molded us throughout our early lives, just as a potter molds clay to make a useful vessel. He prepared us for the important work we were called to do at Memorial Christian Hospital in Bangladesh. He orchestrated every circumstance we faced and guided us in the right direction to carry out His plan. From our arrival at the hospital in 1974 to the last trip in 2014 in our eighties, God sustained and enabled us to do His work.

Christ used physical healing in His ministry to draw people to Himself. Memorial Christian Hospital has served as a powerful magnet for many years, drawing people who came for physical healing to a place where they would be treated with compassion and shown the love of Christ by doctors, nurses, and other medical workers. While they were being treated at MCH for their physical conditions, they had the opportunity to learn of the message of salvation and spiritual healing as taught in the Holy Bible. Many have put their faith in Christ and have received the promise of eternal life.

Reader, we ask you the same question that was asked of us years ago: "When you are no longer alive, will it have made any eternal difference that you lived? Or will you simply leave this world?" You might accumulate great wealth, prestige, or notoriety during your lifetime, but these things have no eternal value. Only things that are done for God will have eternal value. Will you let God take control of your life and live according to His plan, whatever that might be?

> Only one life 'twill soon be past,
> Only what's done for Christ will last.[27]

~ C. T. Studd

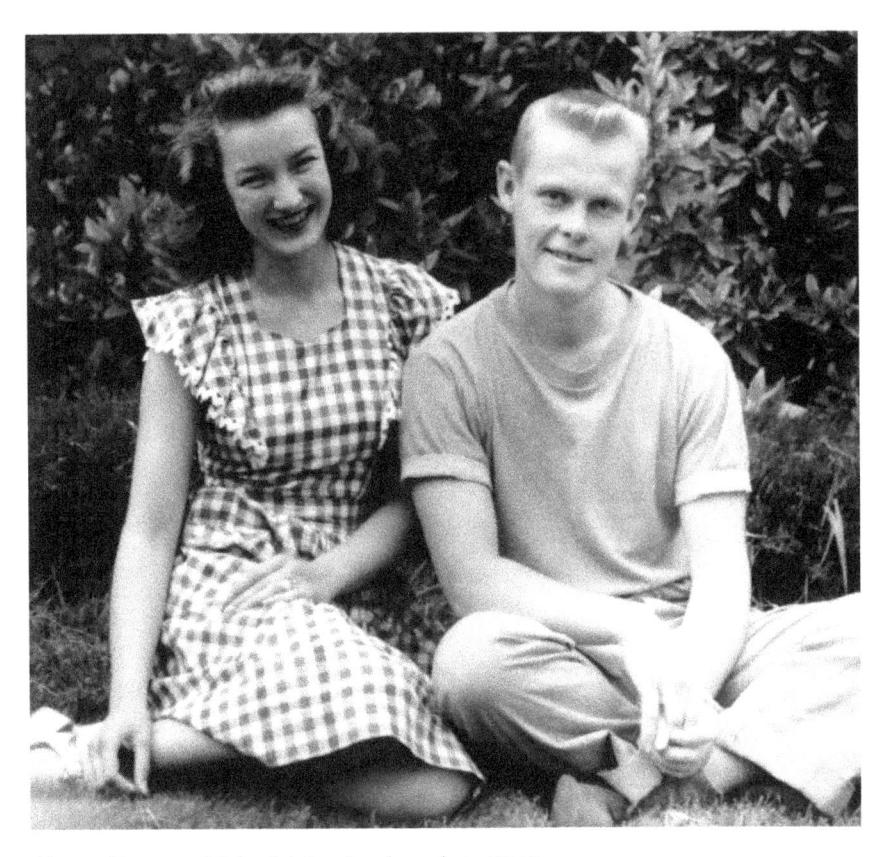

Above: Tense and John high school grads in 1945.

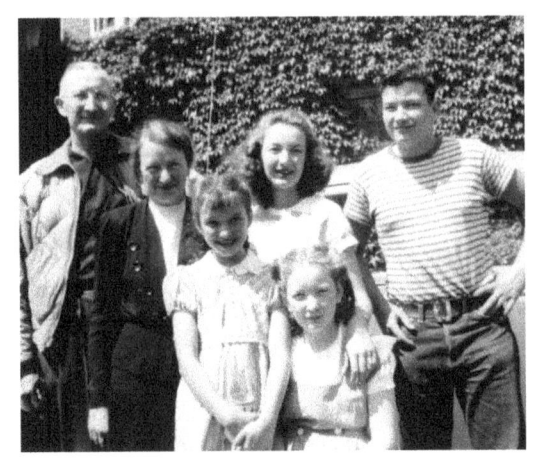

Left: Tense's family visited her at college.

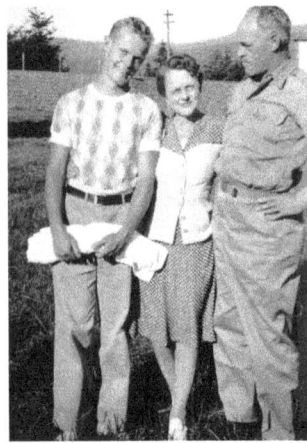

Right: John with his parents in Medford.

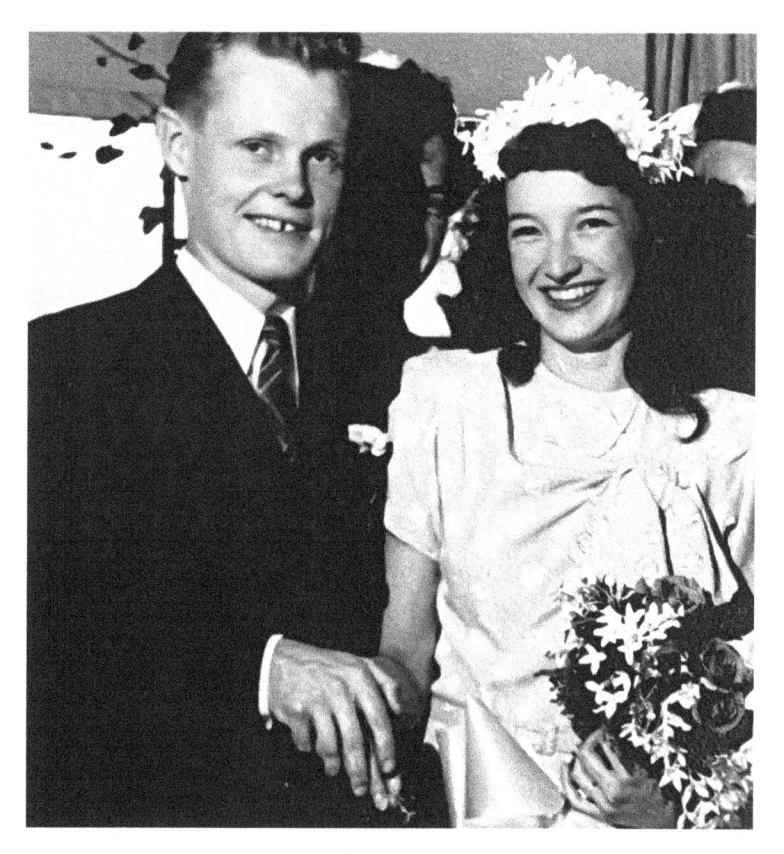

Above: John and Tense married June 1947.
Photo credit: Shangle Photography, Medford, Oregon.

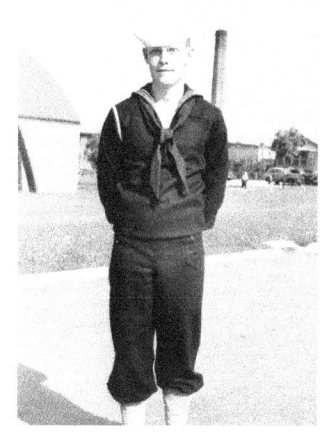

Left: John at the Great Lakes Naval Training Station in Illinois.

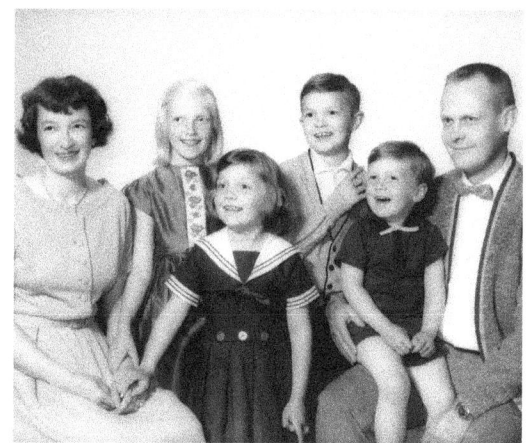

Right: Our family in 1962.

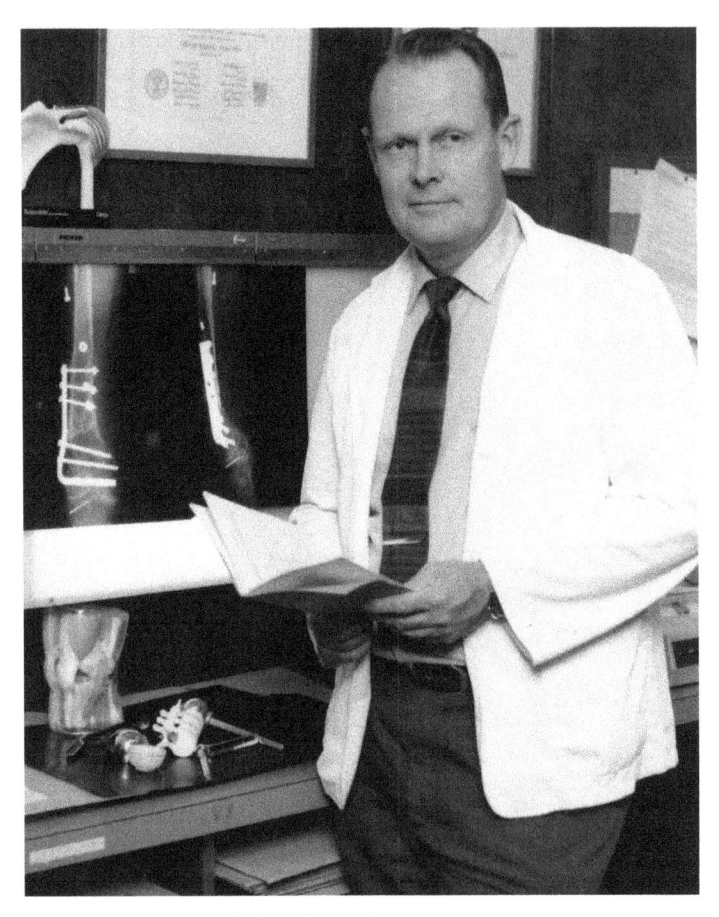

Above: Board Certified Orthopedic Surgeon, 1970.

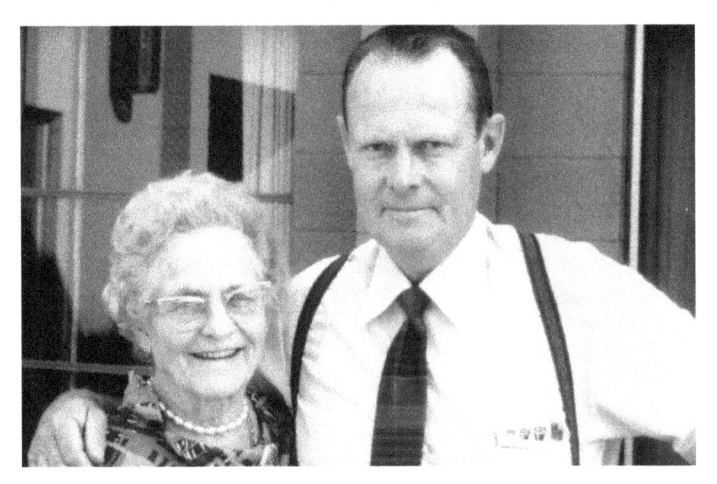

Above: John with his mother in May 1974.

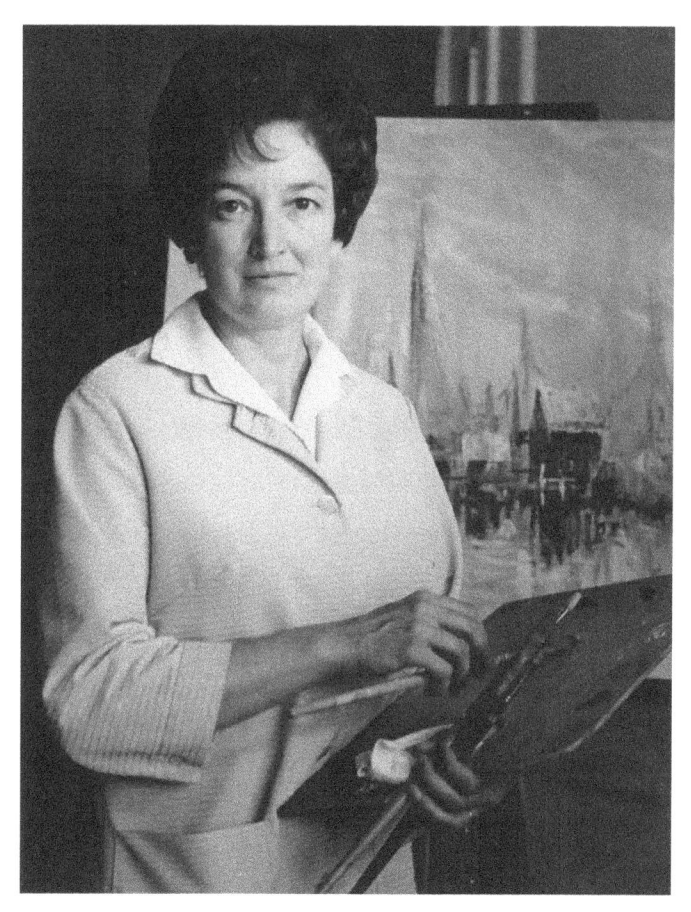

Above: Tense in her art studio (photo credit Jeanne Thwaites).

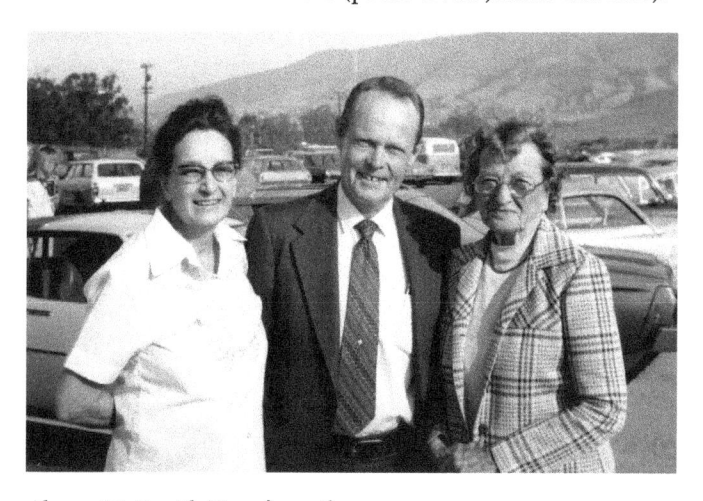

Above: Visit with Tense's mother.

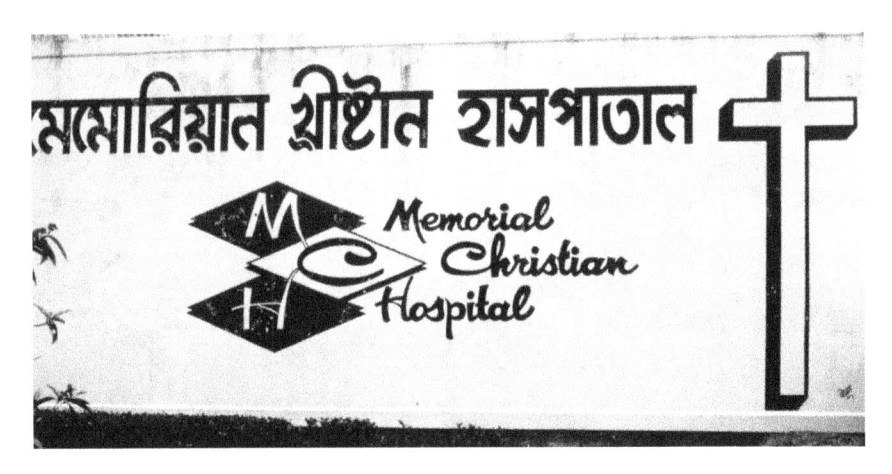

Above: Our first glimpse of Memorial Christian Hospital.

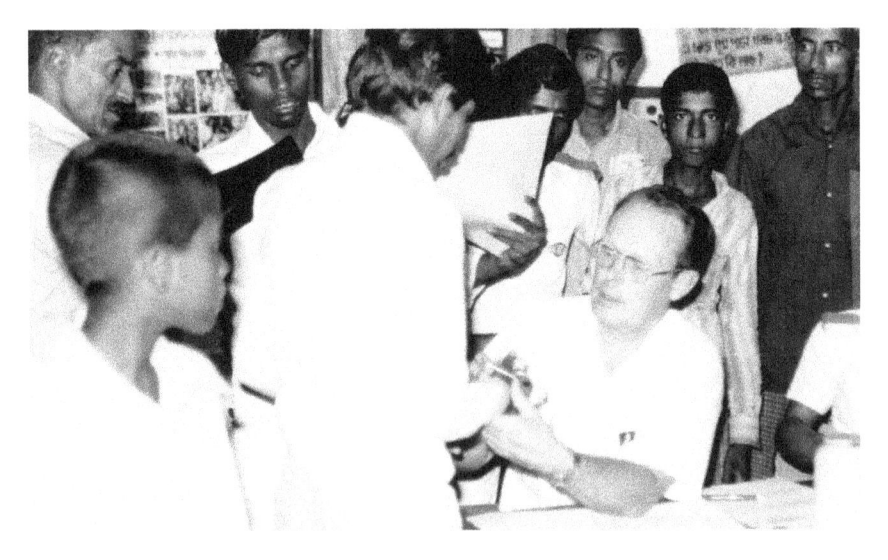

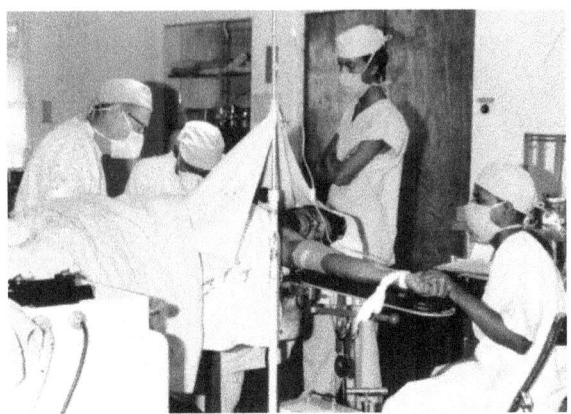

Above:
Dr. Bullock examines a patient in the crowded Outpatient Dept.

Left:
Surgical team assists Dr. Bullock.

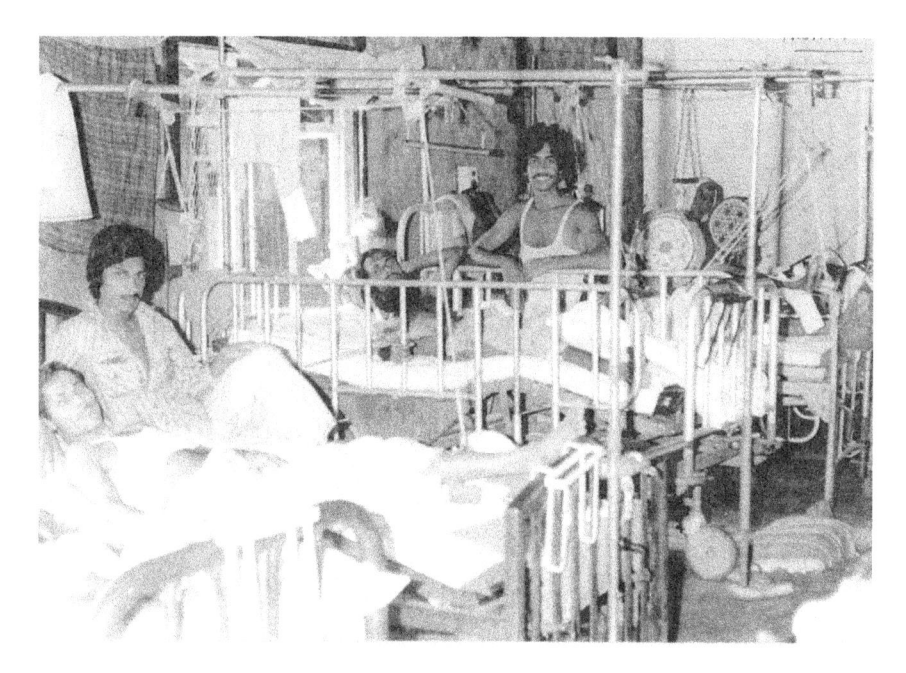

Above: The men's ward at MCH.

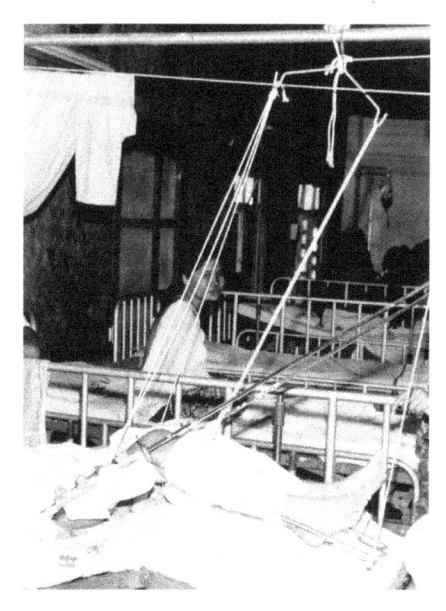

Left: Traction was a major part of orthopedic treatment.

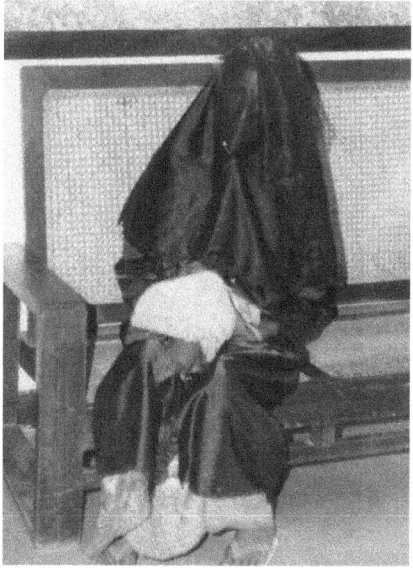

Right: Woman waits for her husband's permission to have hand surgery.

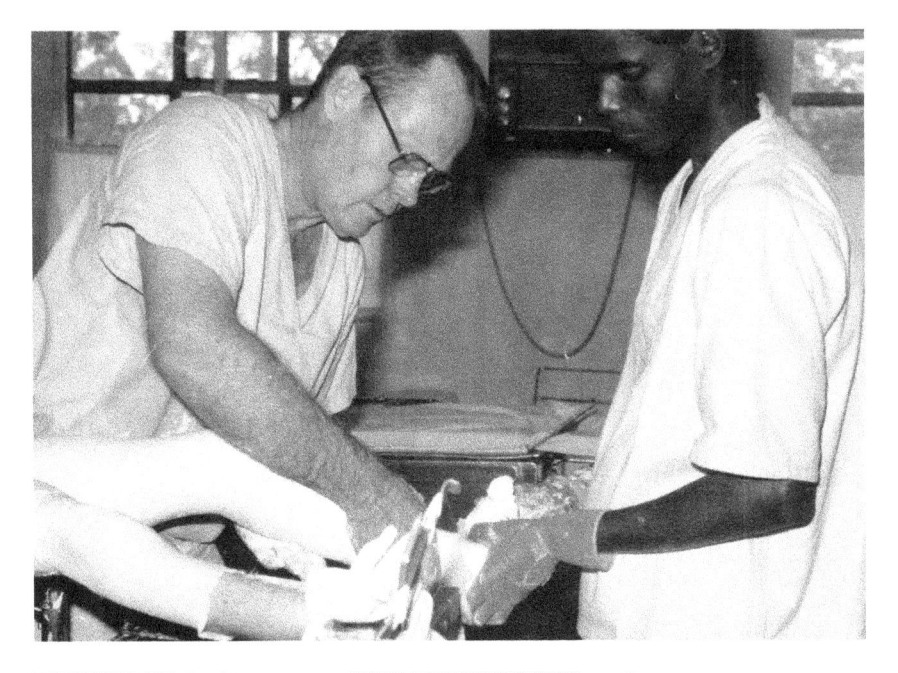

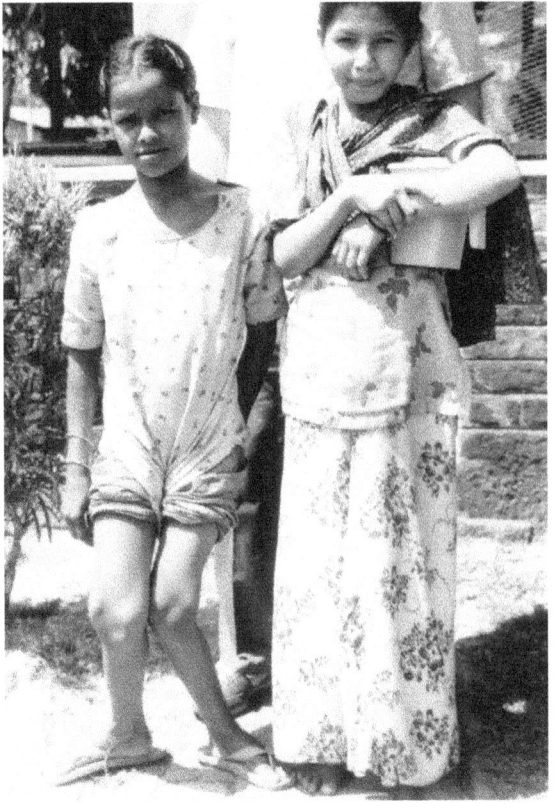

Above:
John teaches ortho tech to put on a cast.

Left:
Child with skeletal deformities caused by rickets.

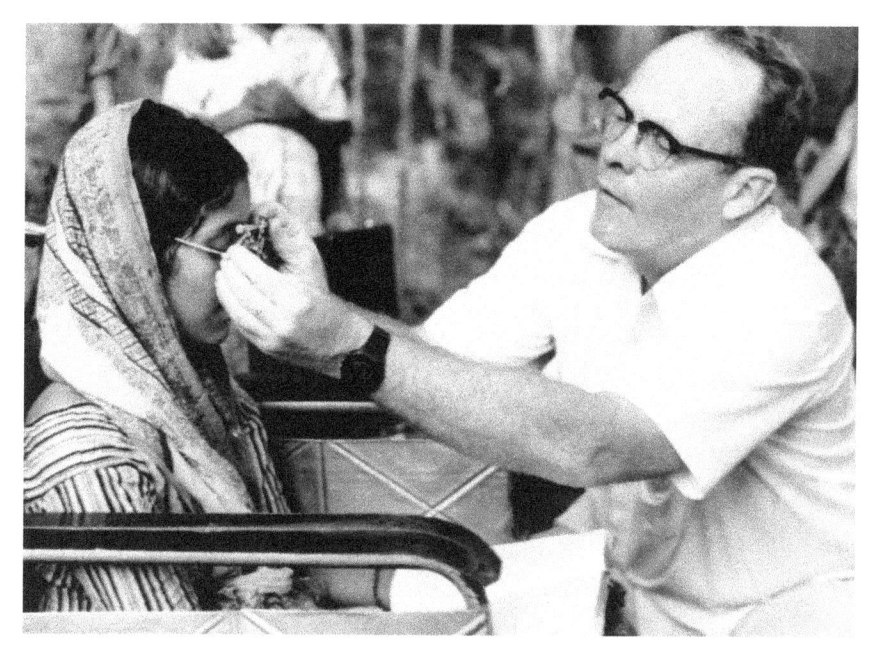

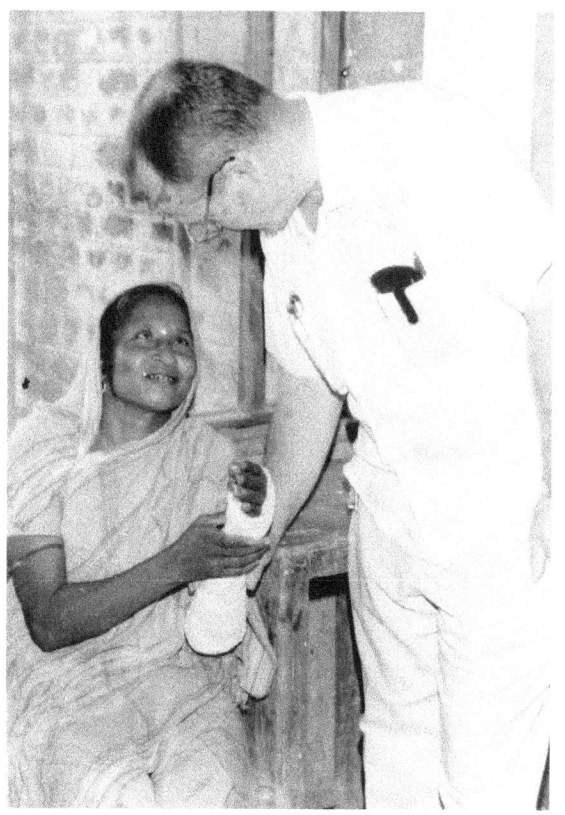

Above:
Donated eyeglasses help the patient read gospel literature.

Left:
Grateful patient.

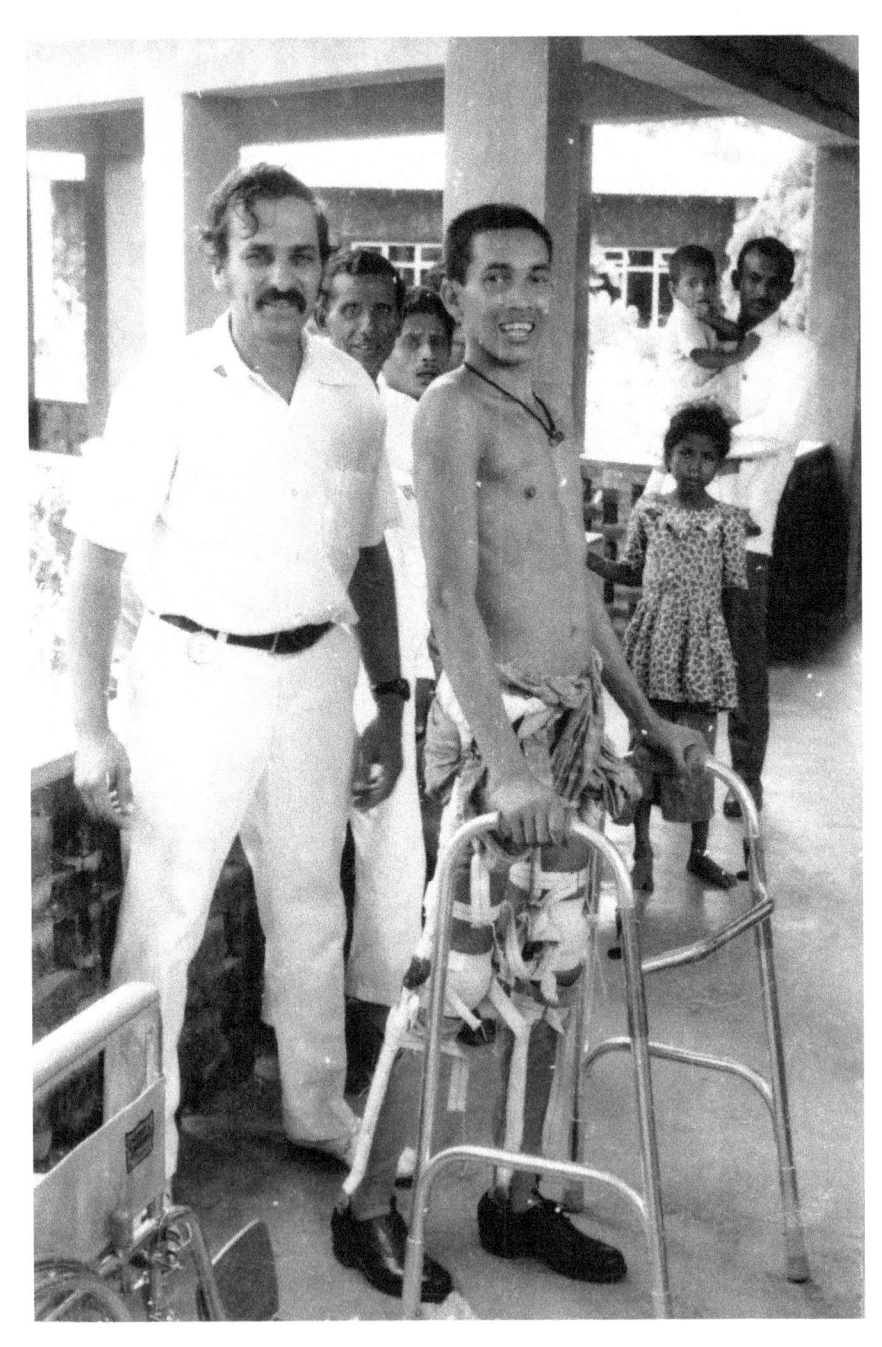

Above: Larry Golin, Physical Therapist, set up the PT Dept. and Limb & Brace Shop.

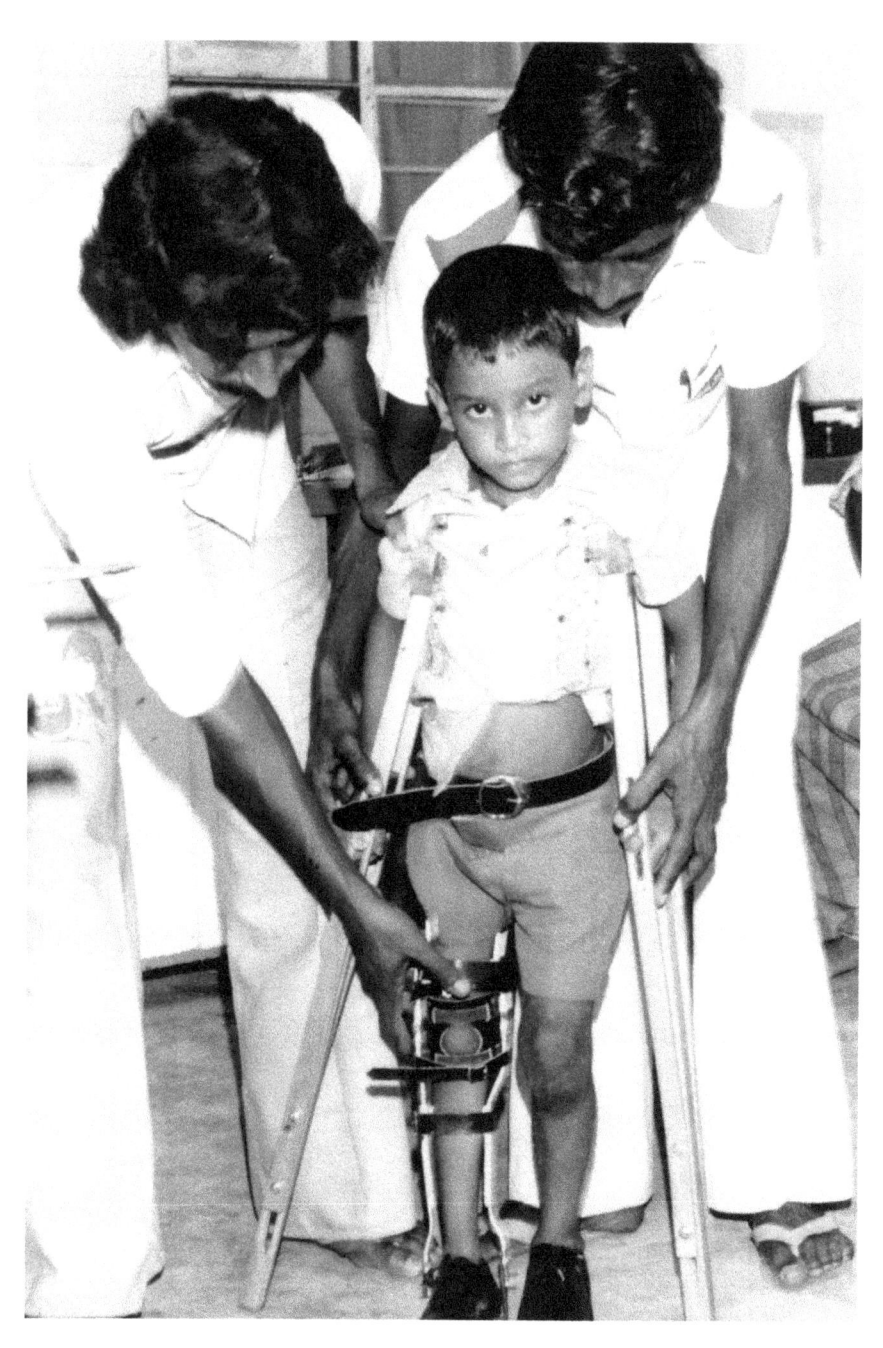

Above: PT staff teaches paralyzed boy to walk with leg brace.

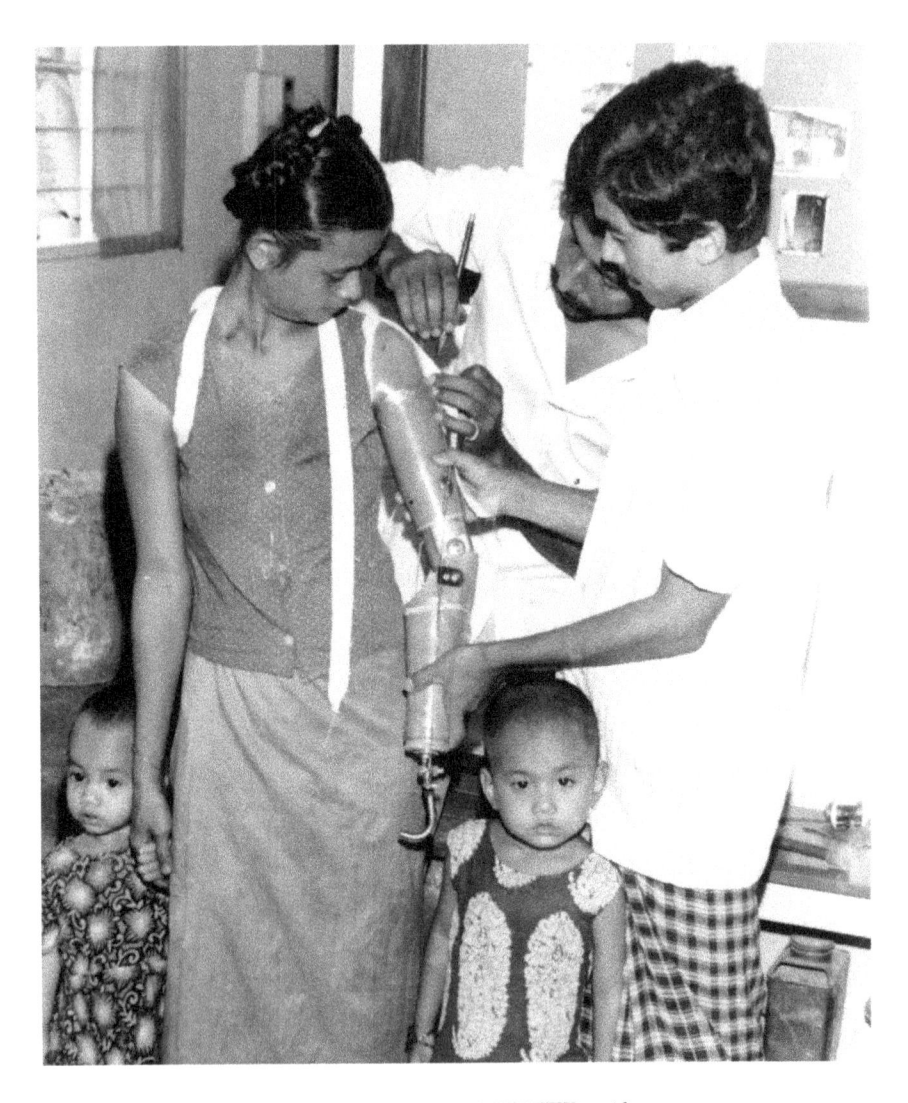

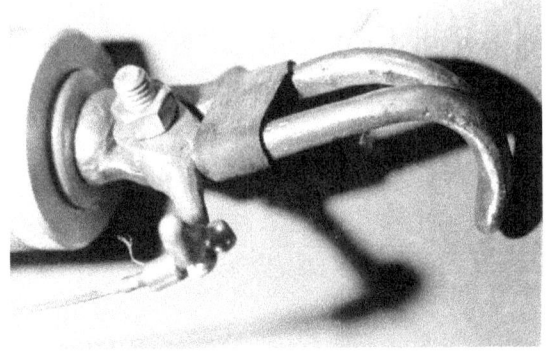

Above:
MCH nurse fitted with artificial arm made in our Limb & Brace Shop.

Left:
Brass hook for prosthetic arm.

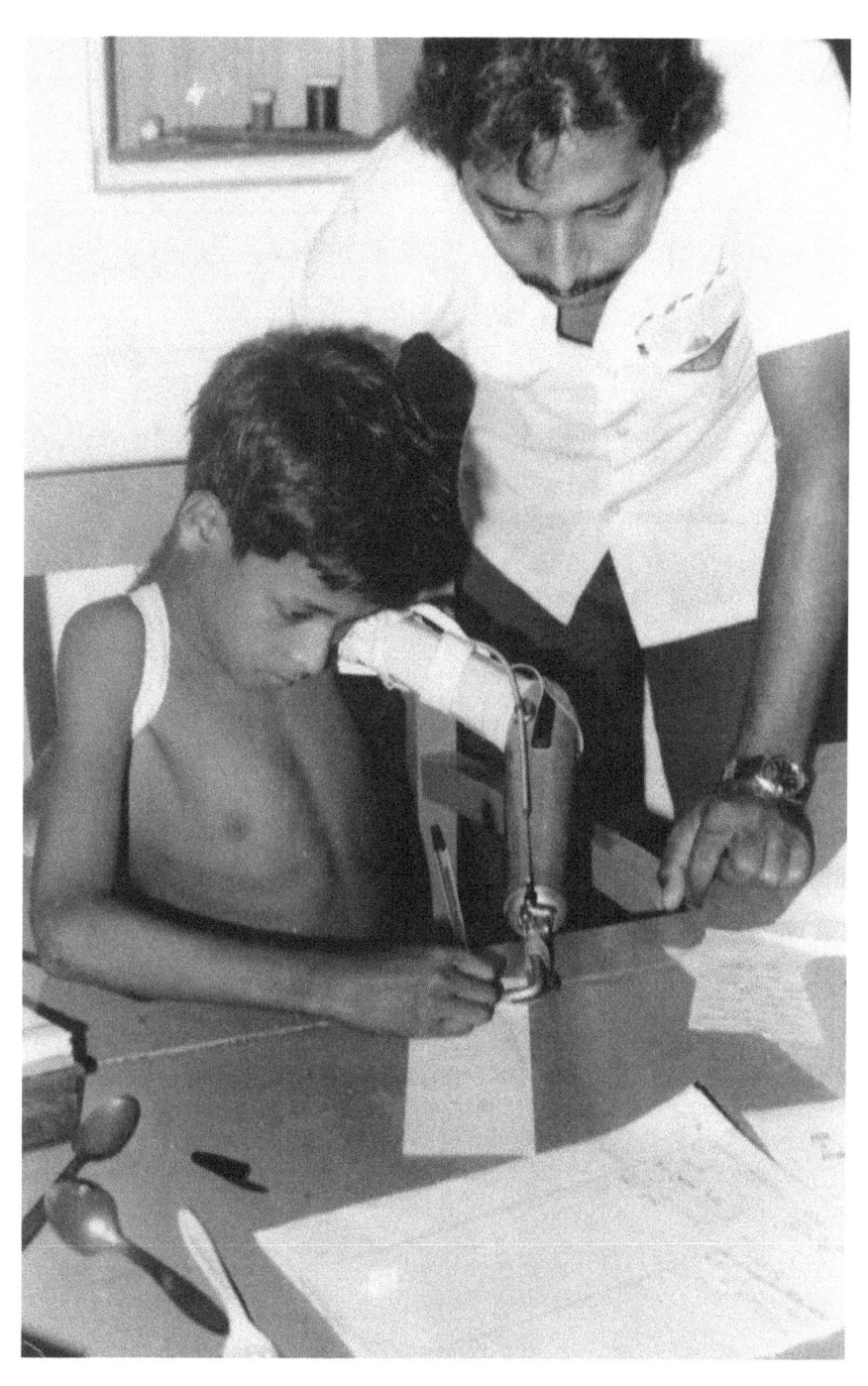

Above: Boy soccer player learns to use his prosthetic arm.

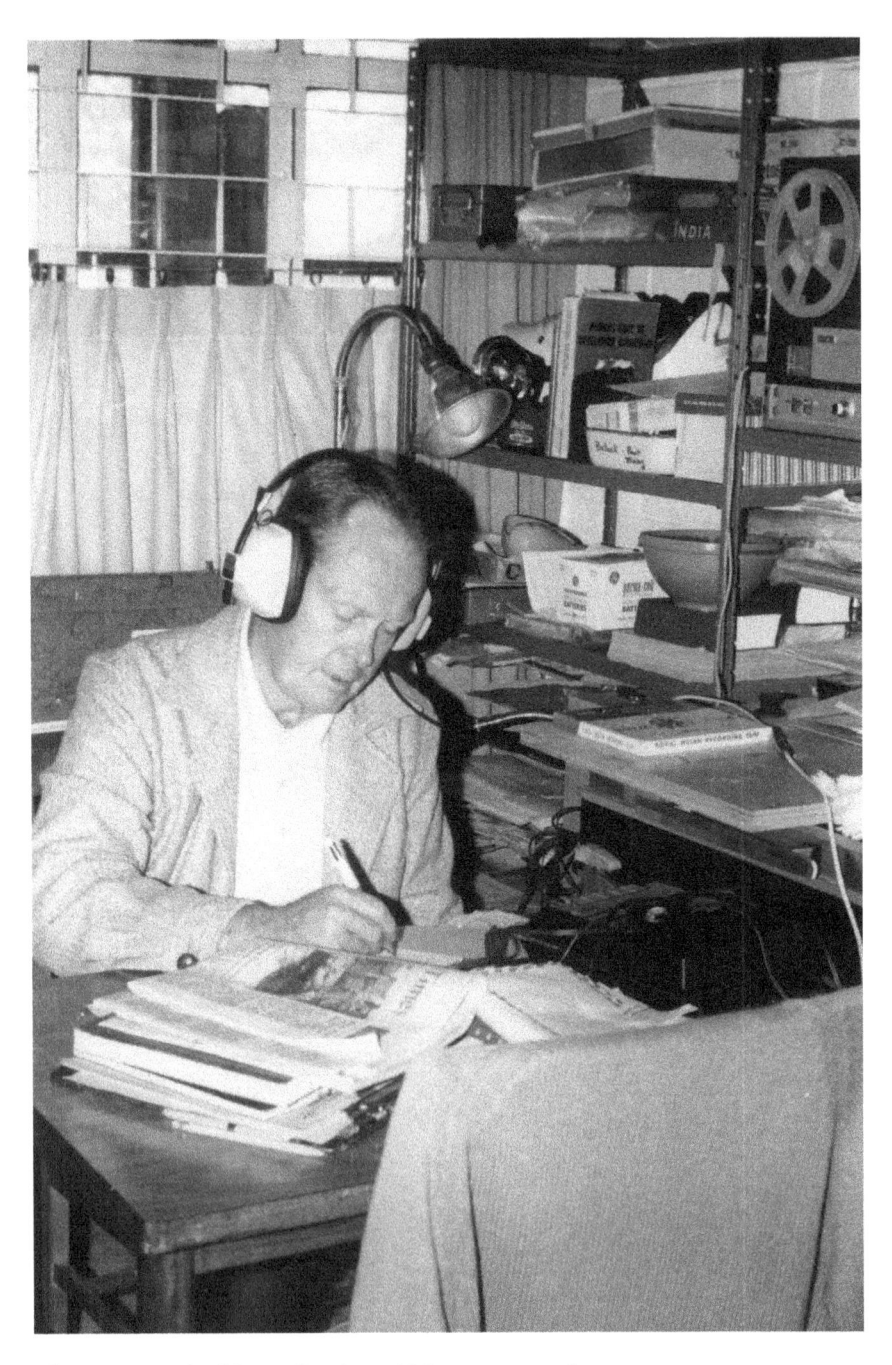

Above: We studied Bengali at least 30 hours per week.

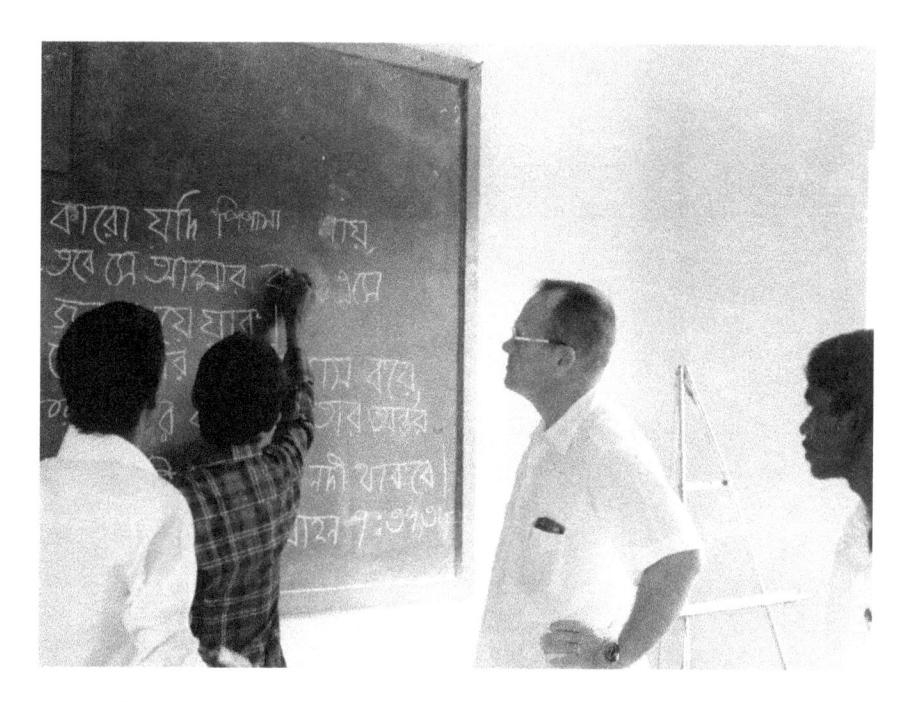

Above: John taught a Bengali Sunday School Bible class.

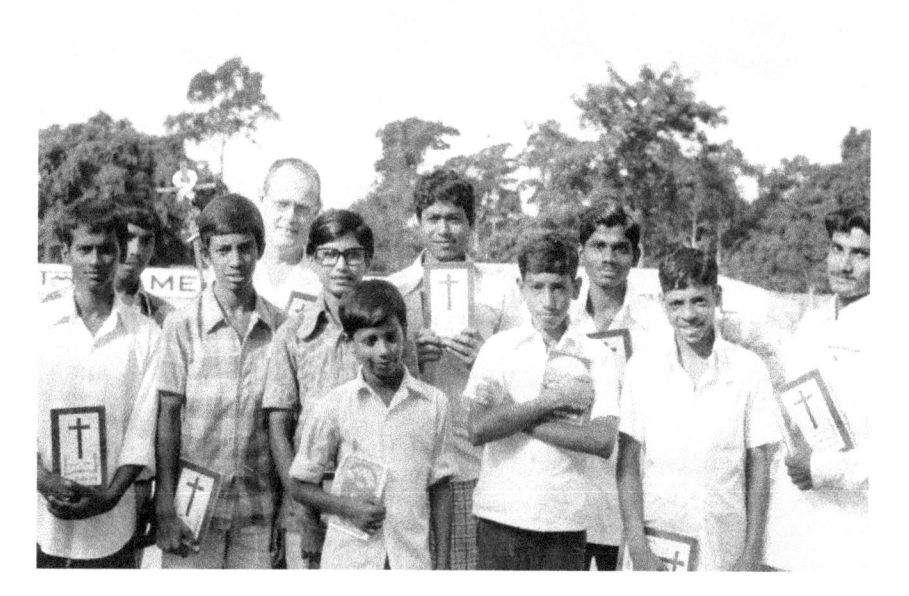

Above: John's Bengali boys Bible class.

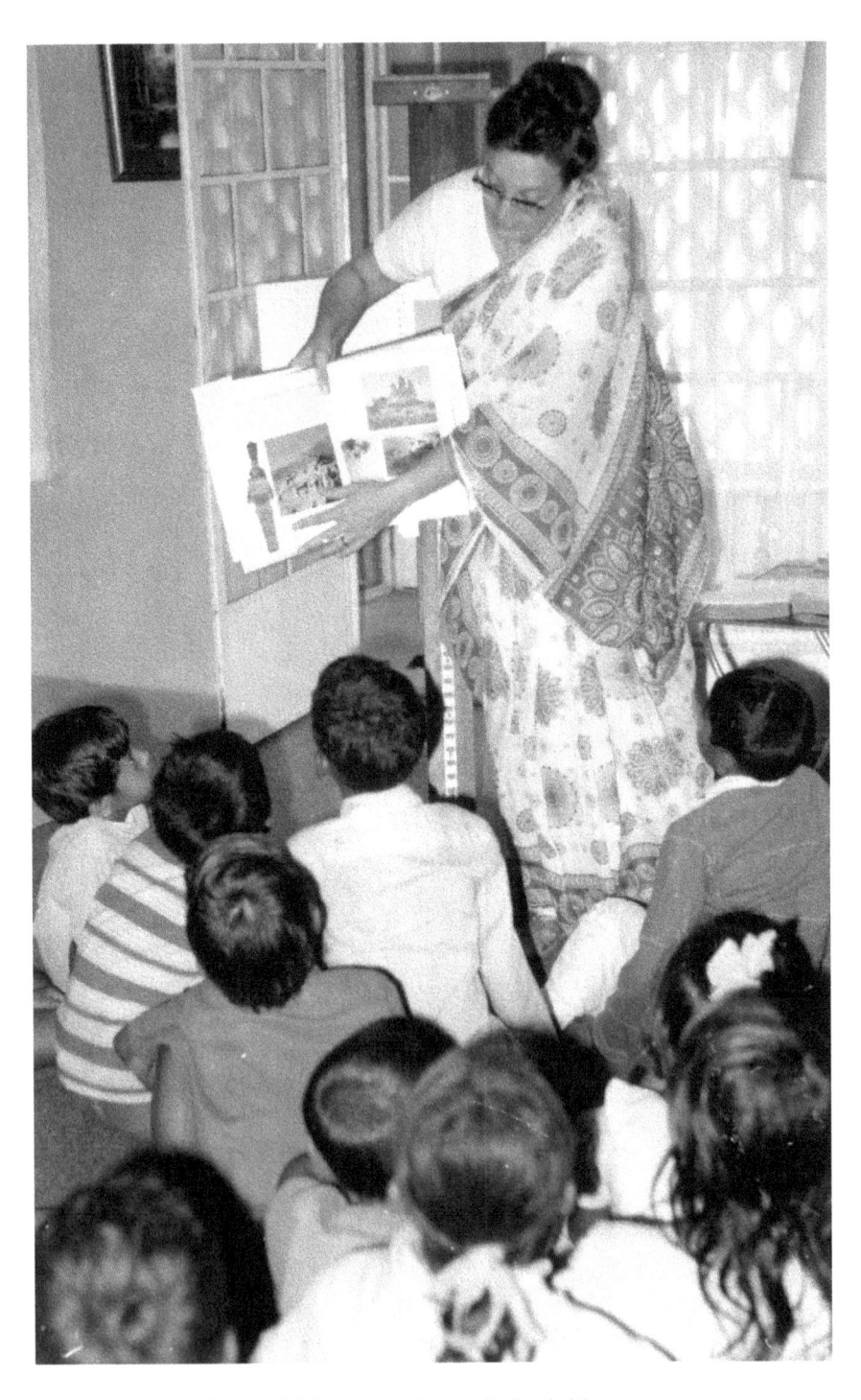

Above: Tense teaching Bible lesson to Bangladeshi children.

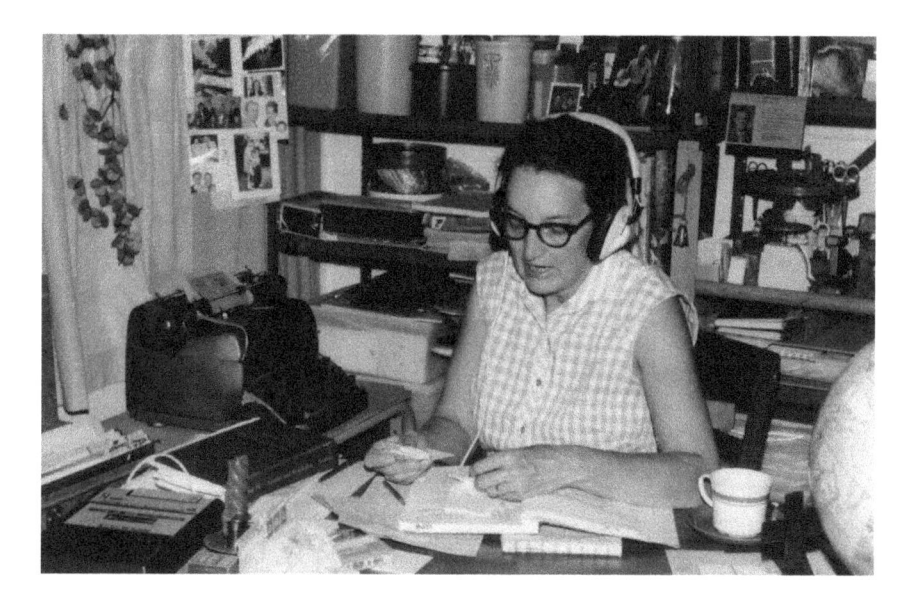

Above: Tense studying Bengali in our one-room apartment at the Guest House.

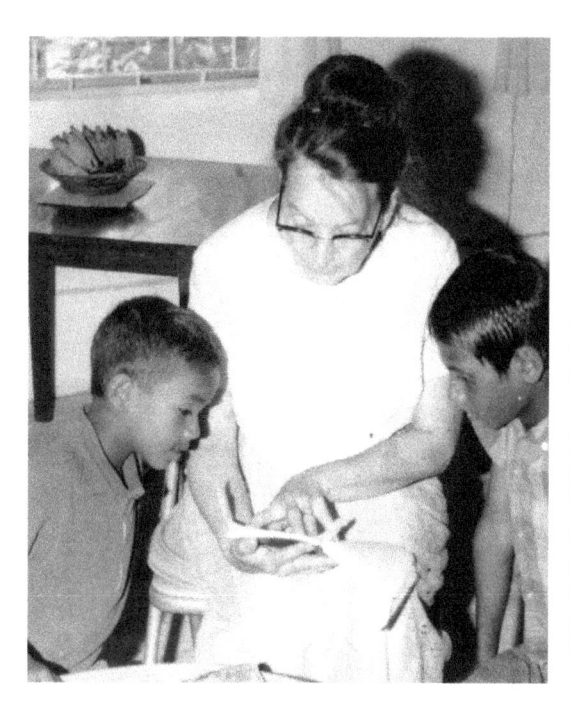

Left: Tense helps Bengali boys learn AWANA verses.

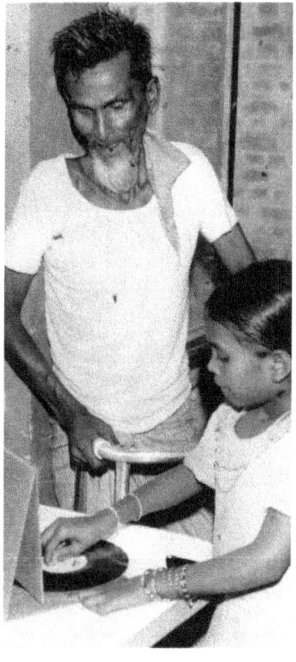

Right: Listening to Bible message on Card Talk cardboard phonograph.

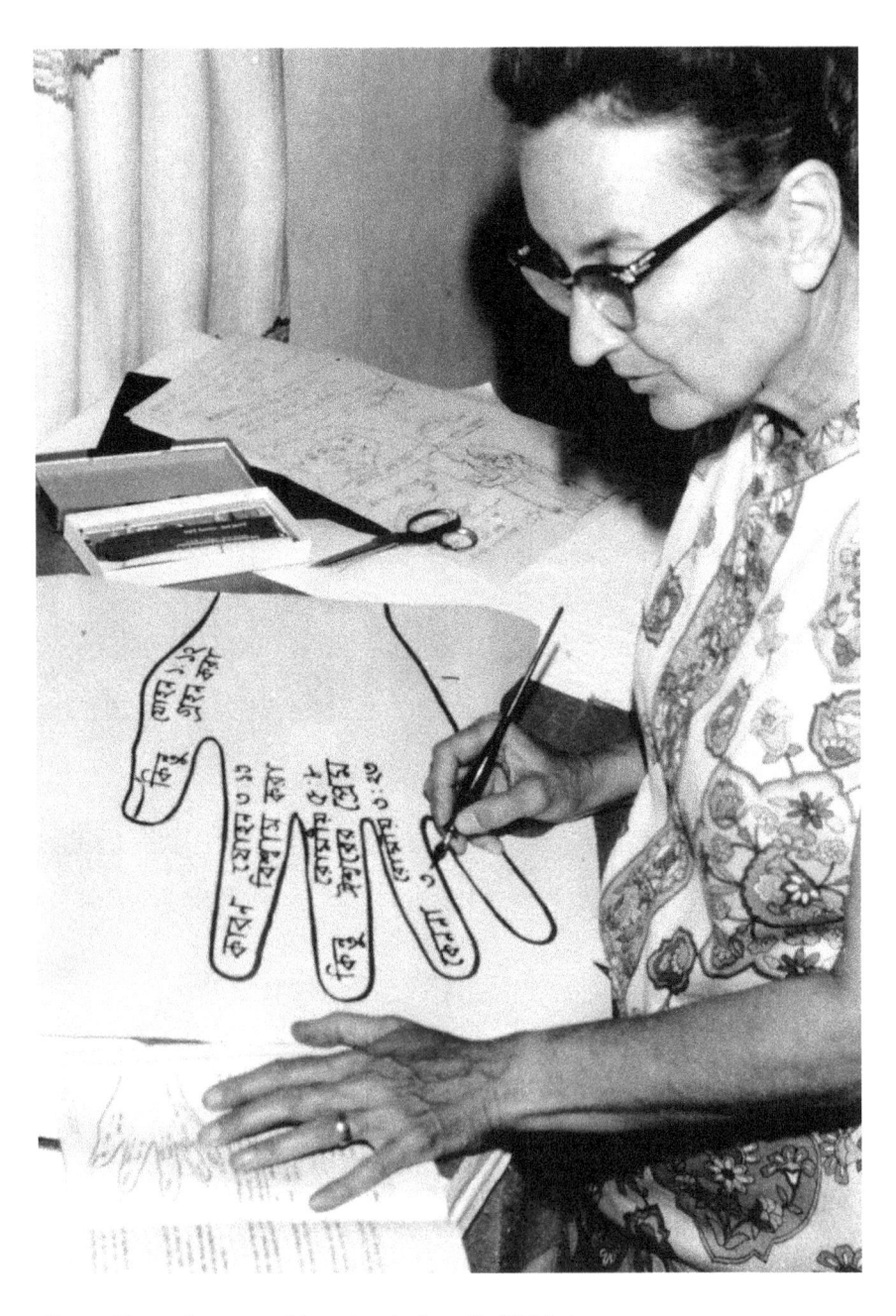

Above: Tense draws teaching visuals for tribal Bible lessons.

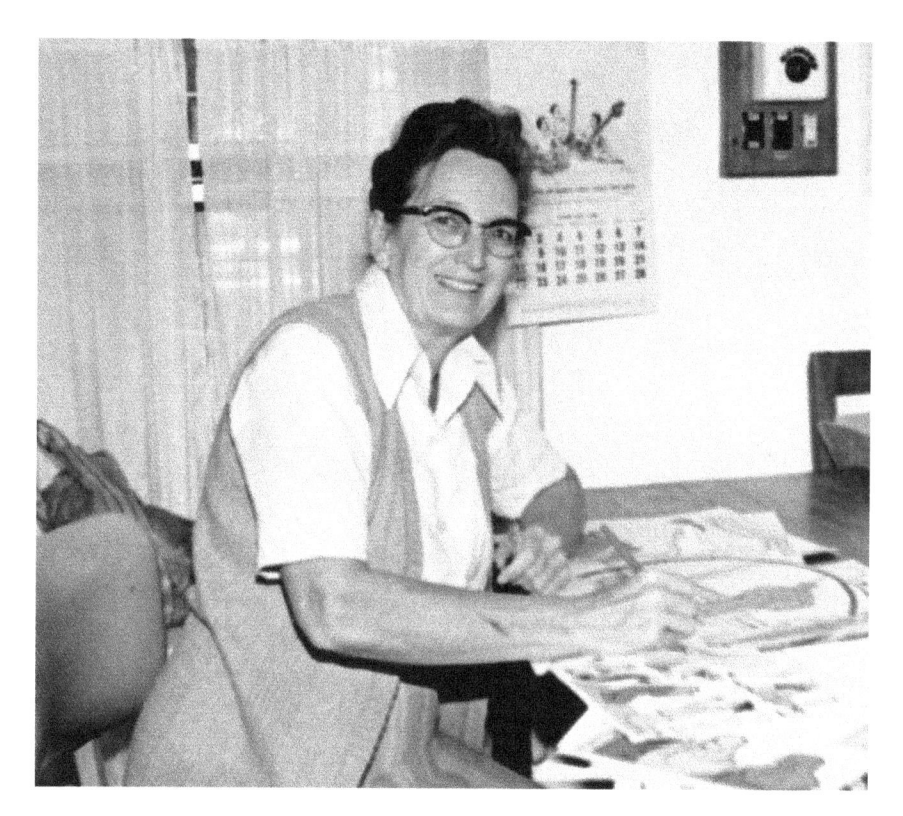

Above: Tense draws Bible teaching illustrations in AV office.

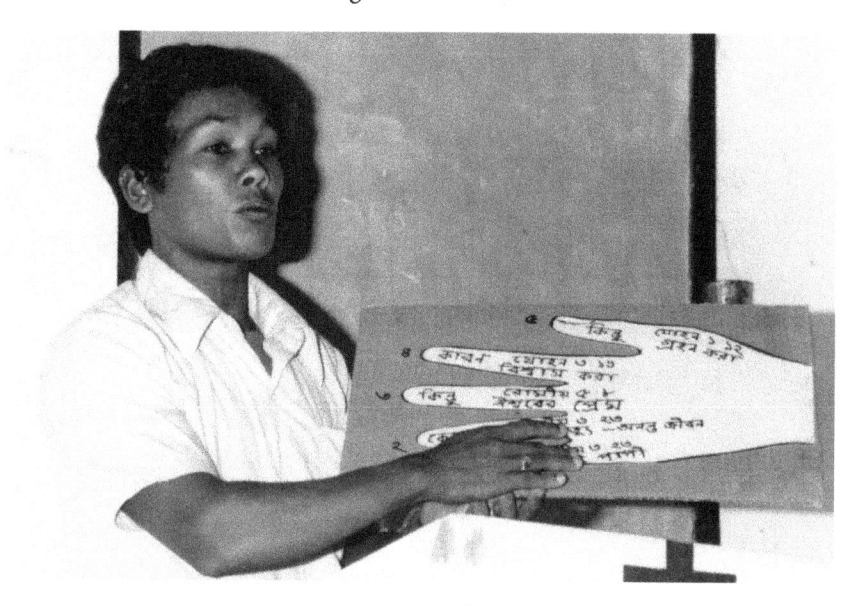

Above: Tribal Bible teacher uses Bible teaching visuals.

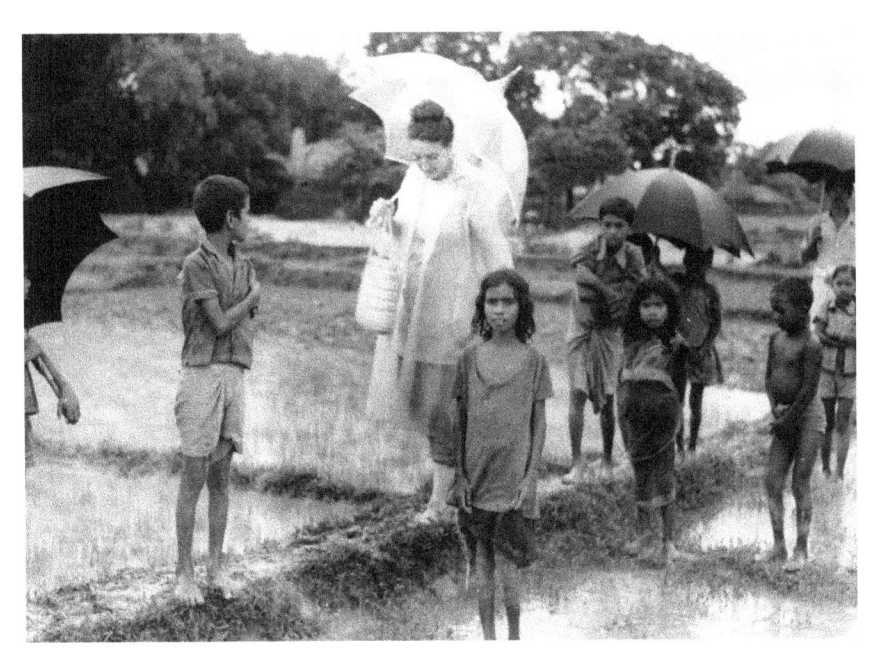

Above: Tense walks on the levee to the village.

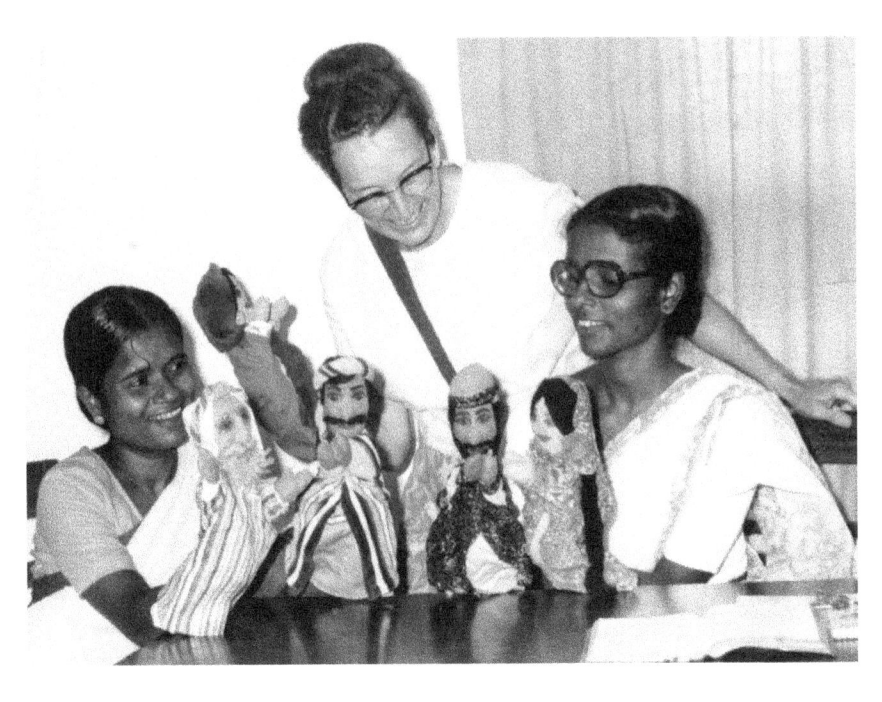

Above: Tense works with the puppet outreach team.

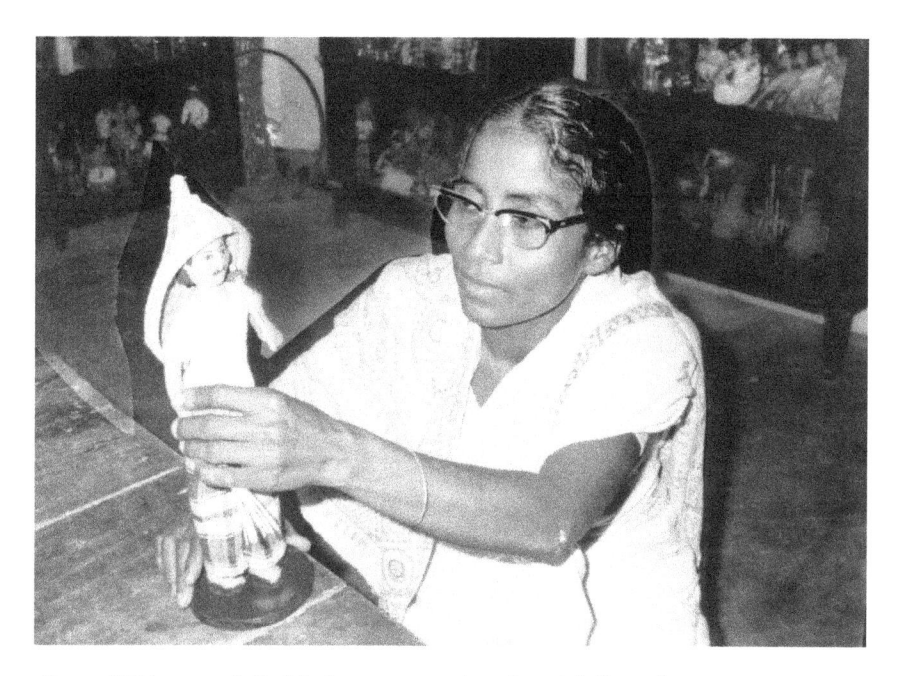

Above: Widows and disabled women made cultural dolls and handicrafts at Heart House.

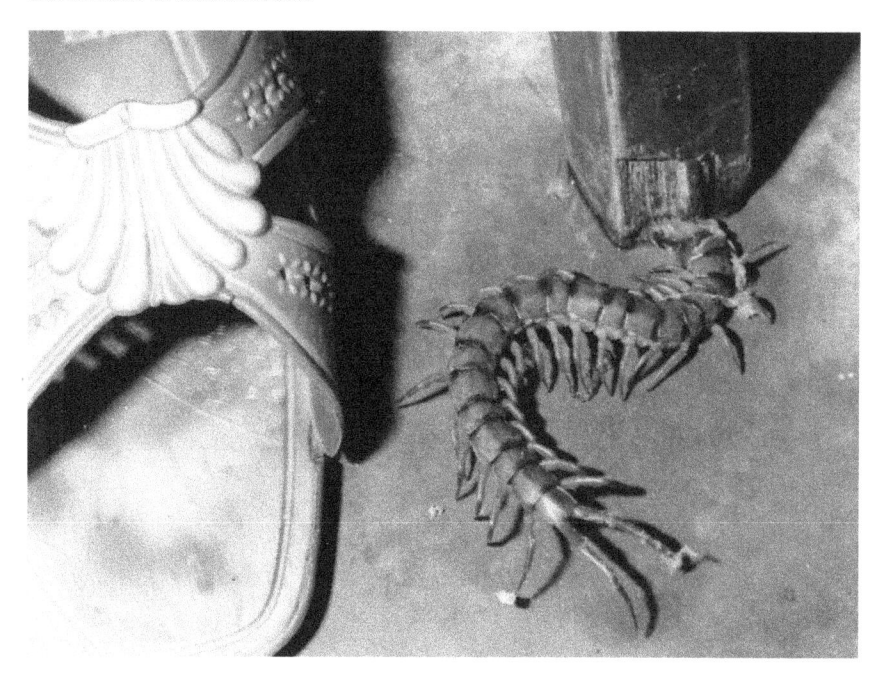

Above: Tense protected from a dangerous centipede.

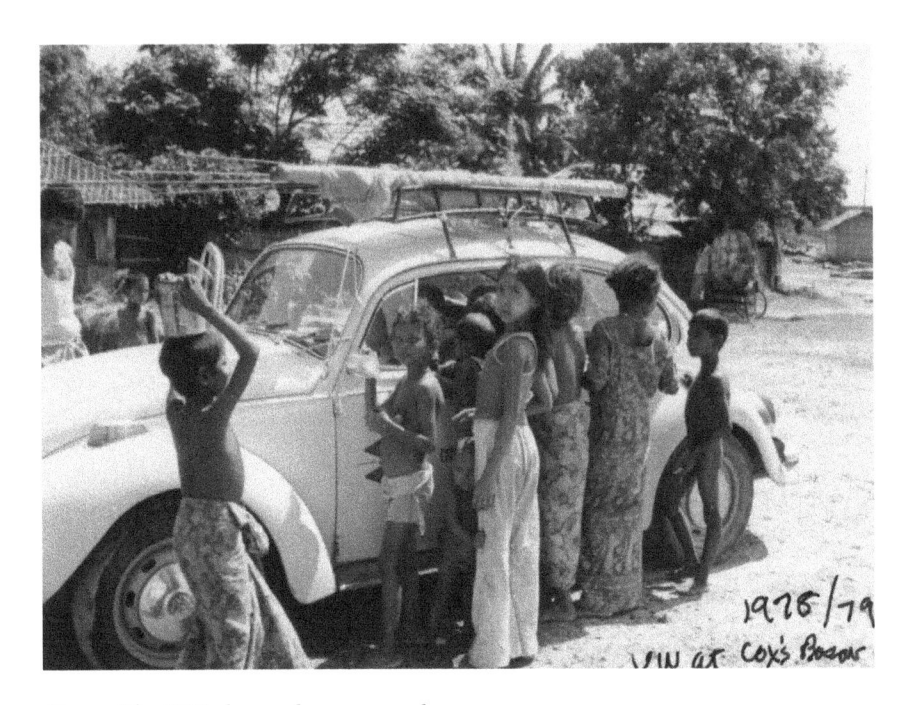

Above: The VW always drew a crowd.

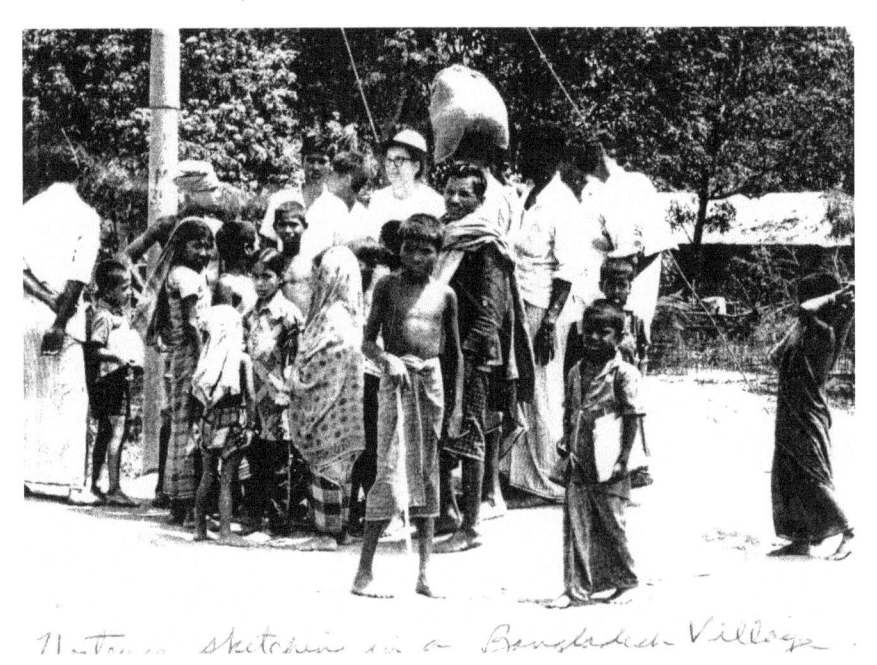

Above: Tense sketching in the village always brought curious observers.

334

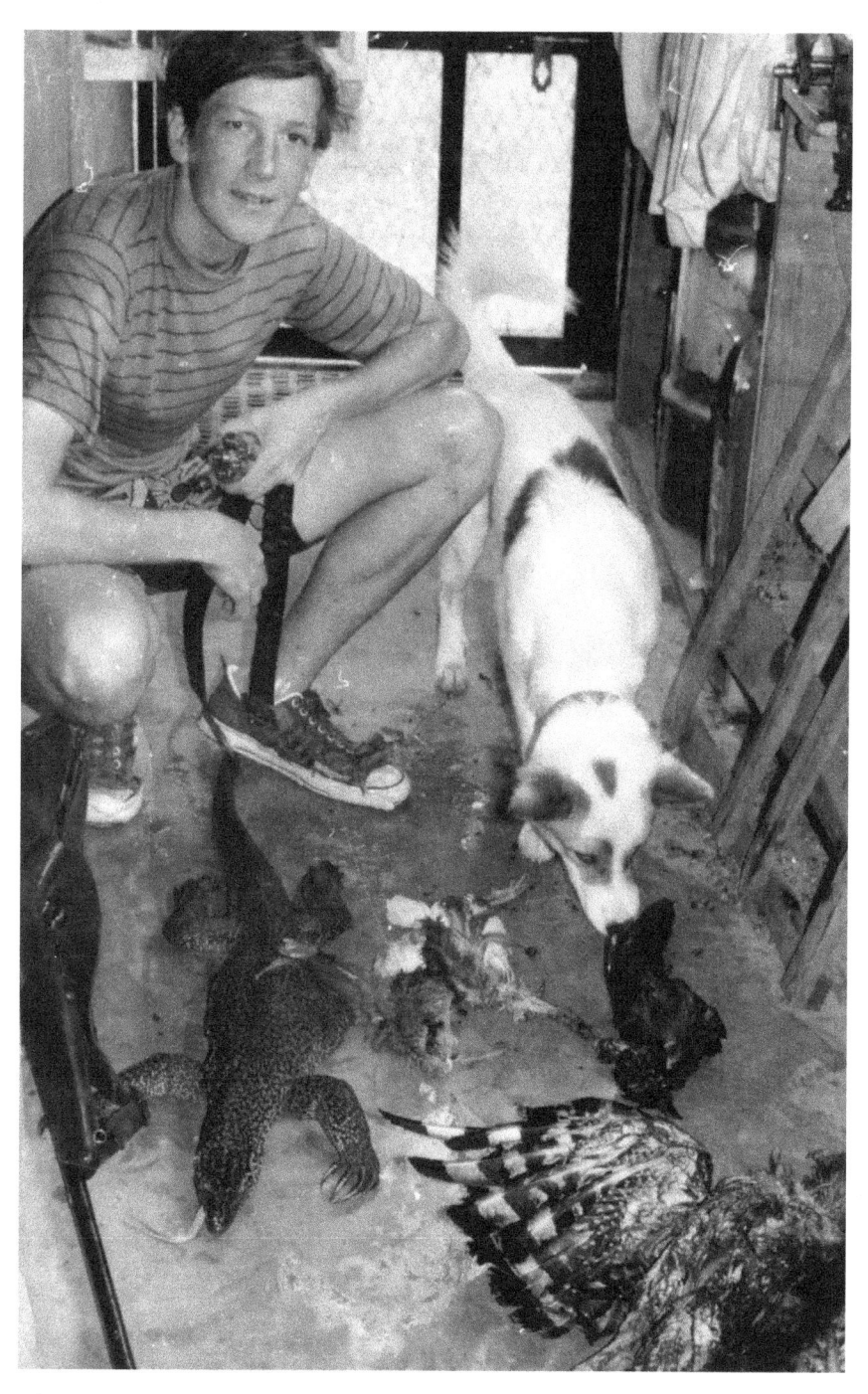

Above: David and our dog inspect their hunting quarry.

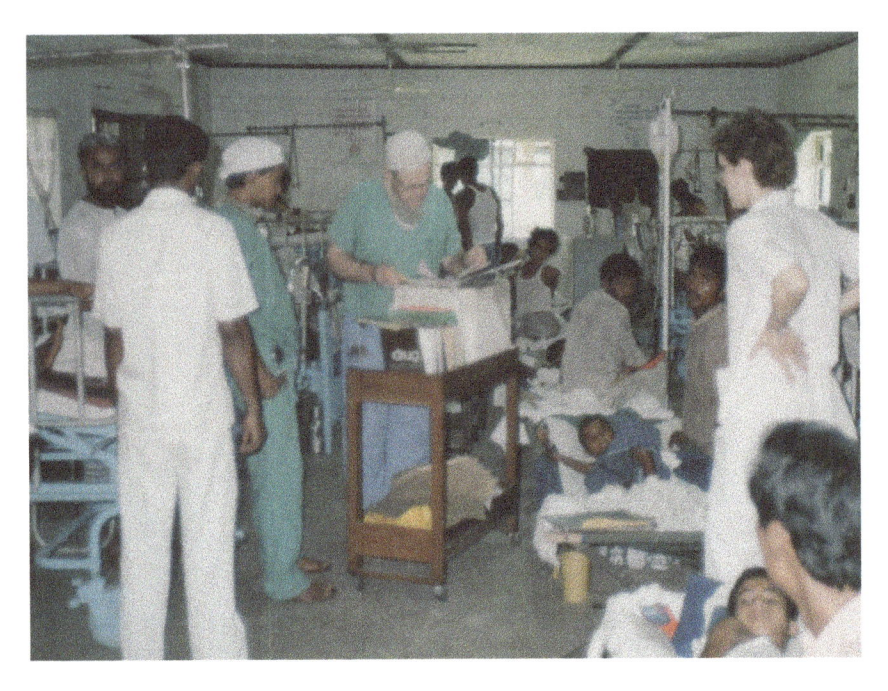

Above: Dr. Bullock makes rounds with his "Bullock Cart."

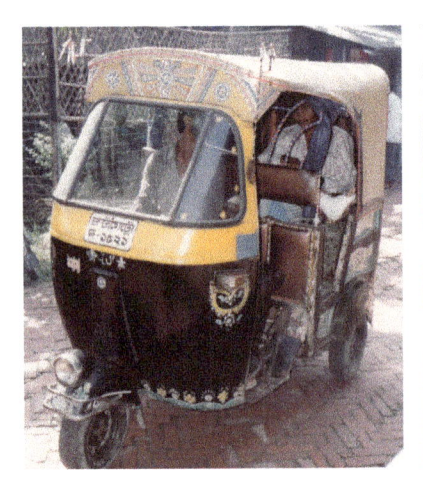

Left: Baby taxi brings patient to MCH.

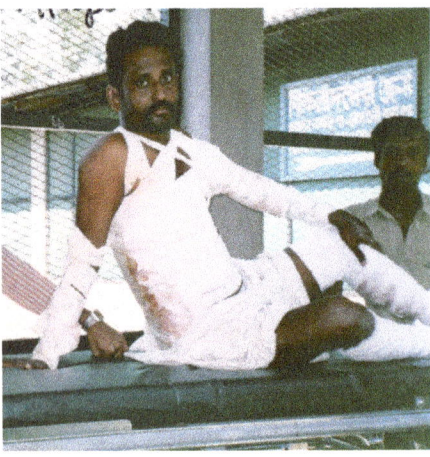

Right: Patient with rolled bandages sent from Women's Mite groups.

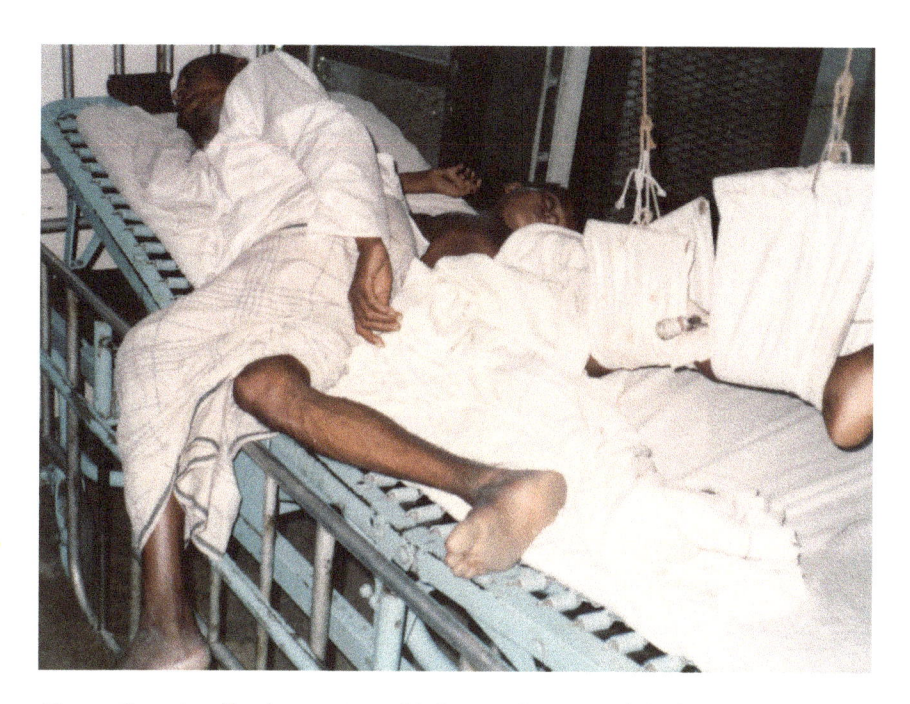

Above: Occasionally, the sangi would sleep in the patient's bed.

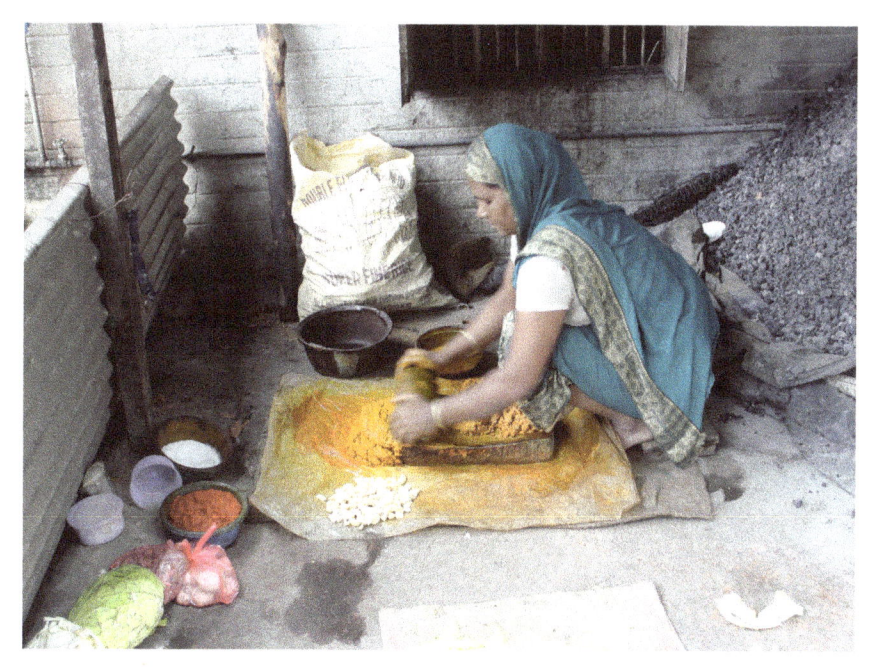

Above: A patient's sangi prepares meals for the patient and herself.

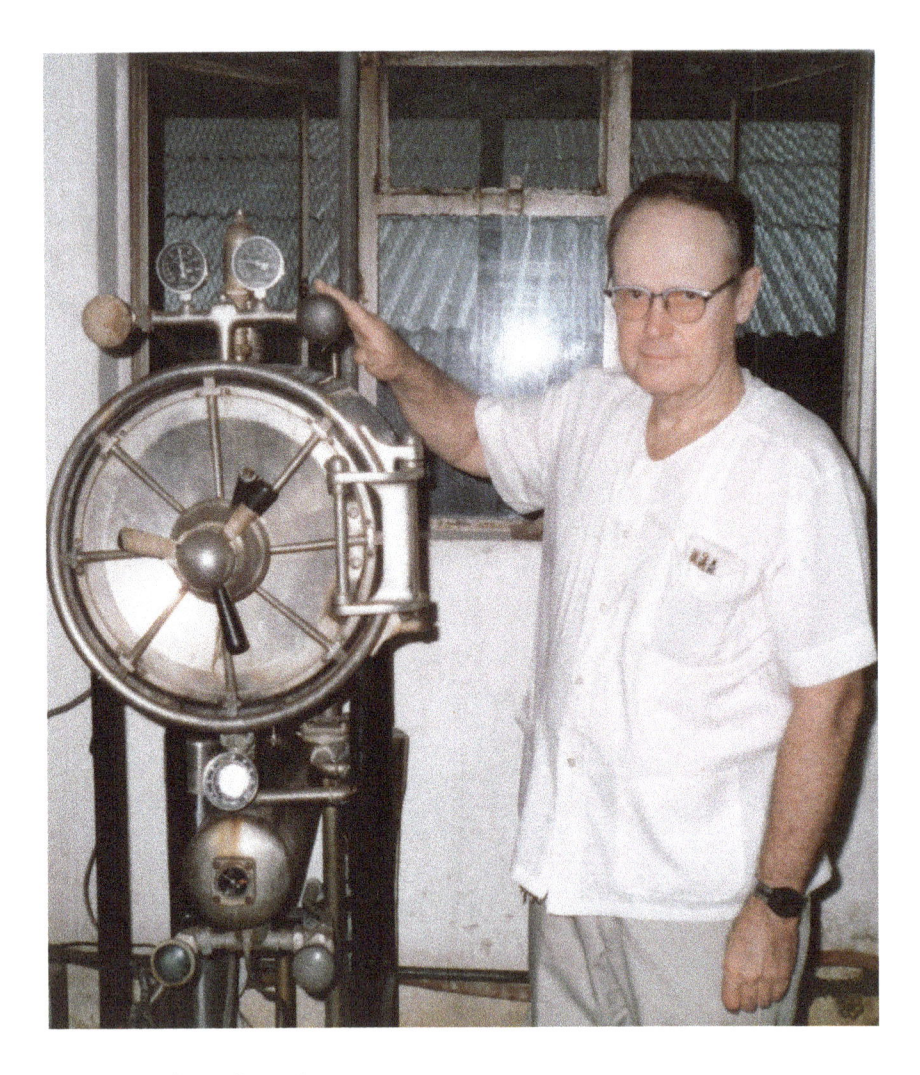

Above: Old "Noah" sterilizer unit.

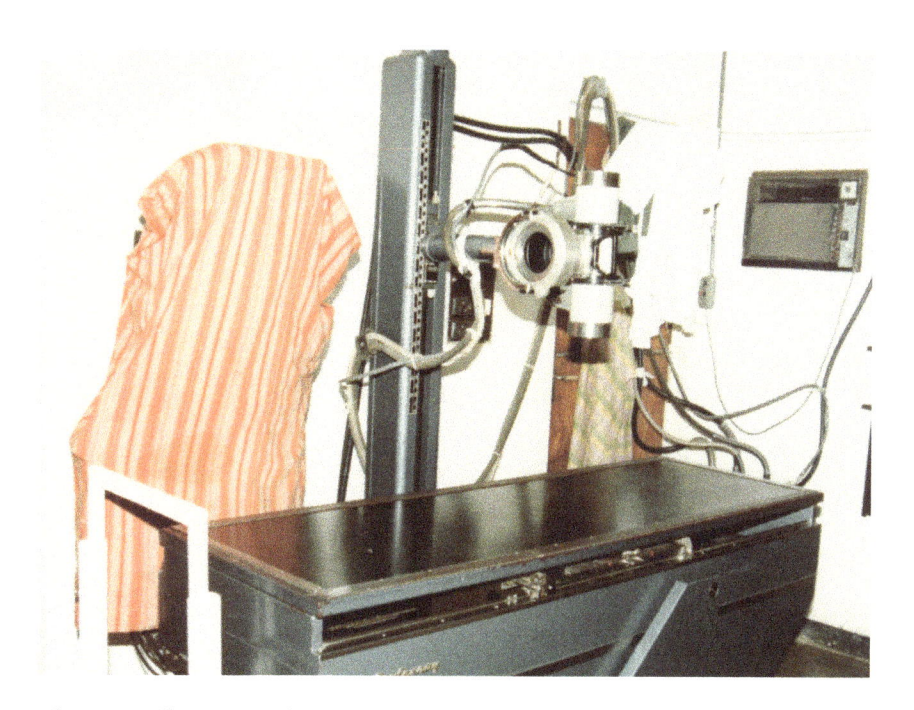

Above: Small X-ray machine.

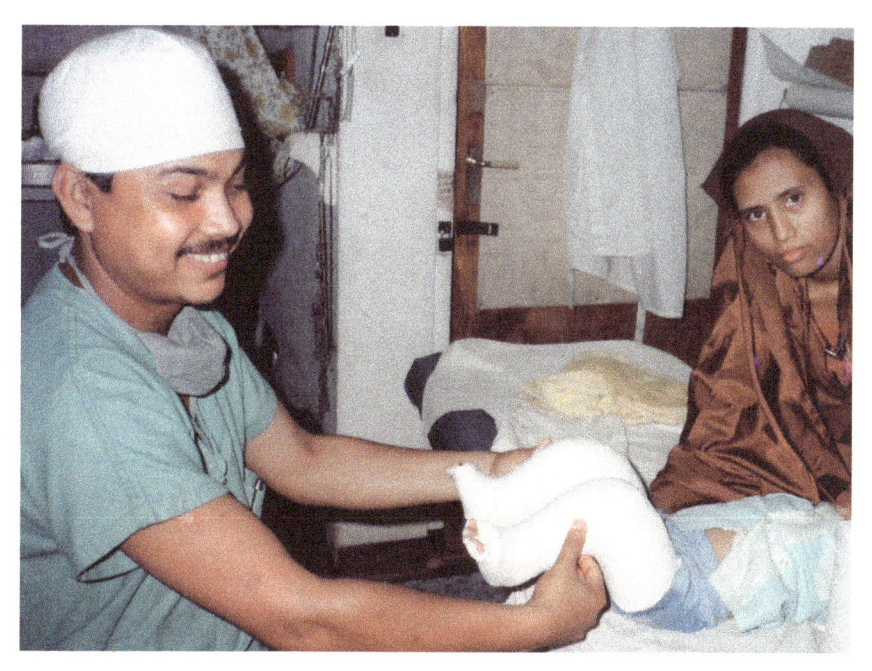

Above: Ortho tech applies casts to a baby with club feet.

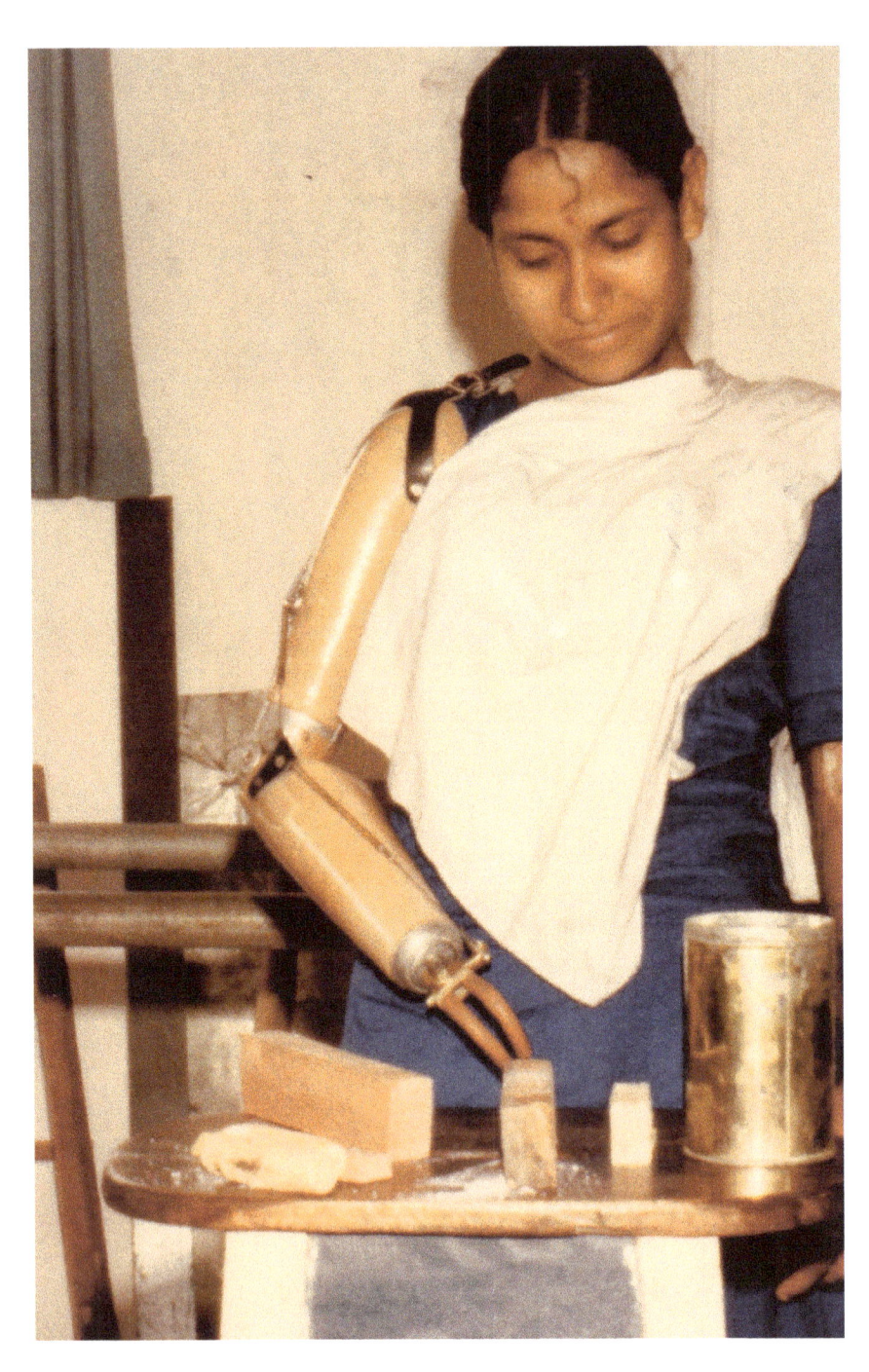

Above: Woman practices with a prosthetic arm and hook.

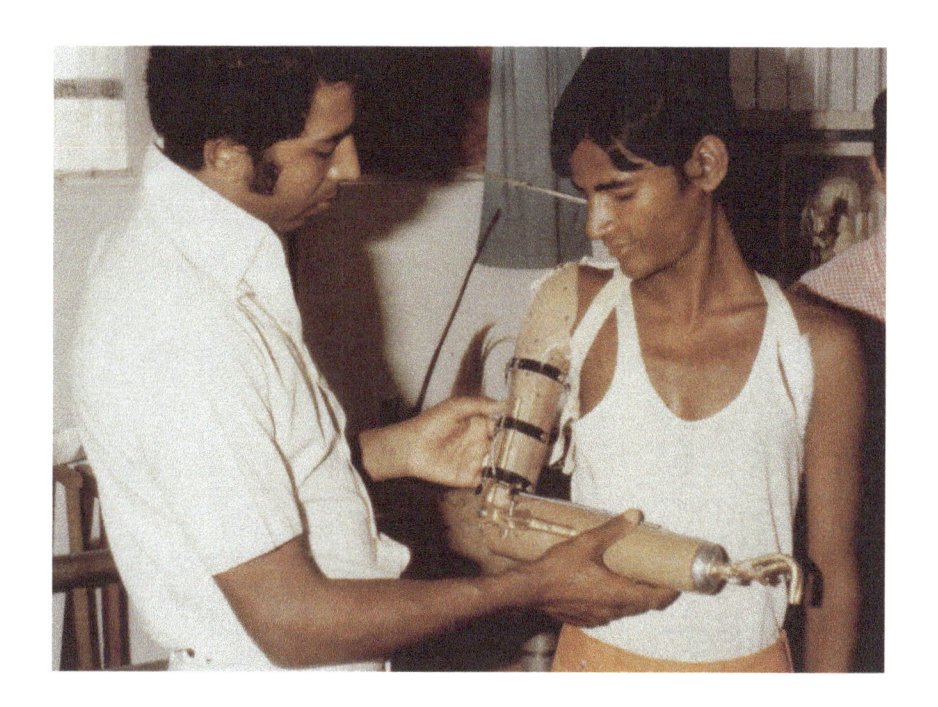

Above: Limb and Brace worker teaches man to use his prosthetic arm.

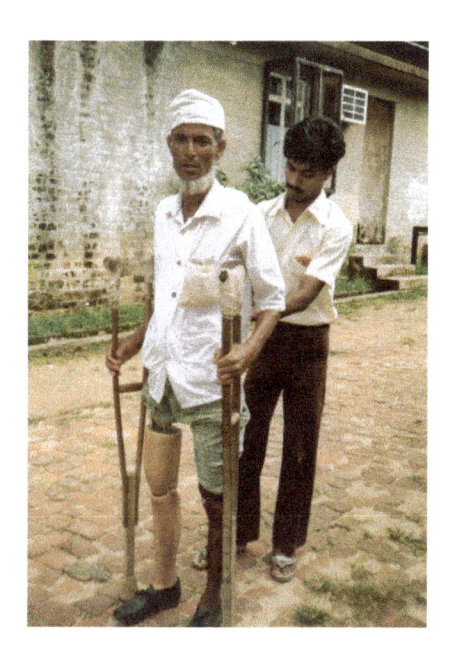

Left: HOPE Fund patient learning to use artificial leg.

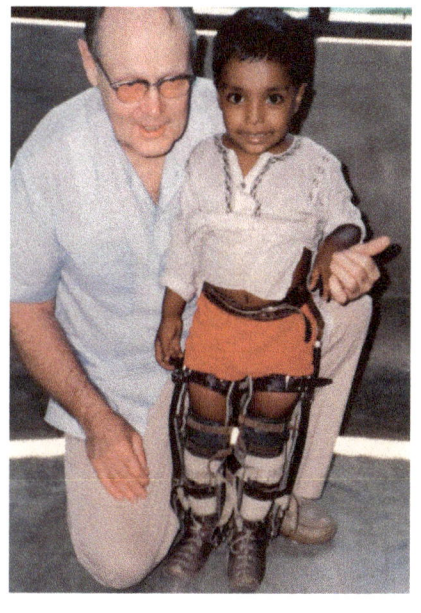

Right: Child with two artificial legs learns to walk with braces.

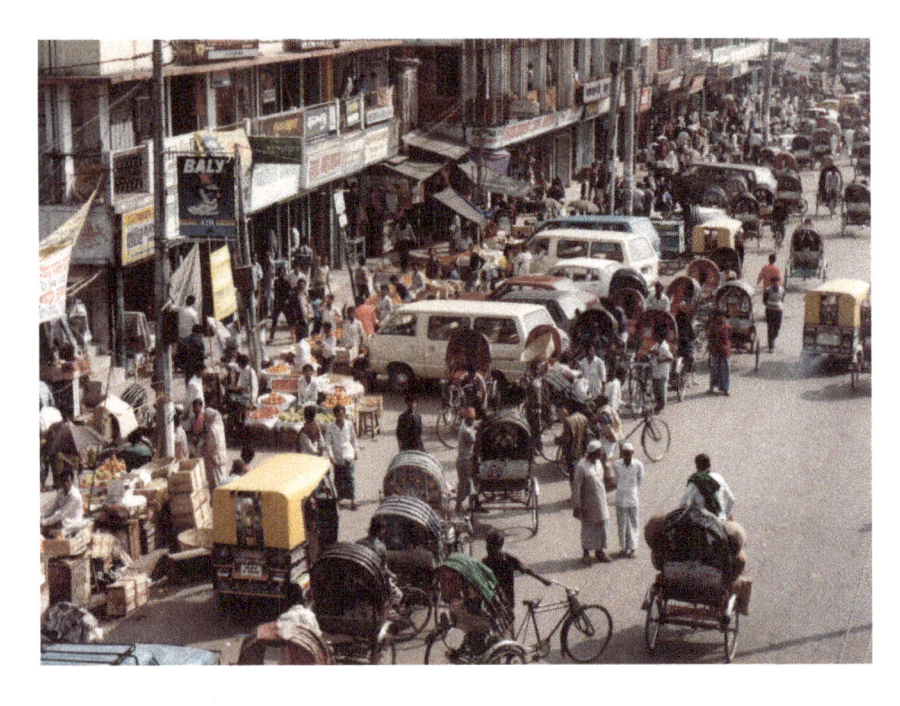

Above: Street vendors sell wares on crowded Chittagong street.

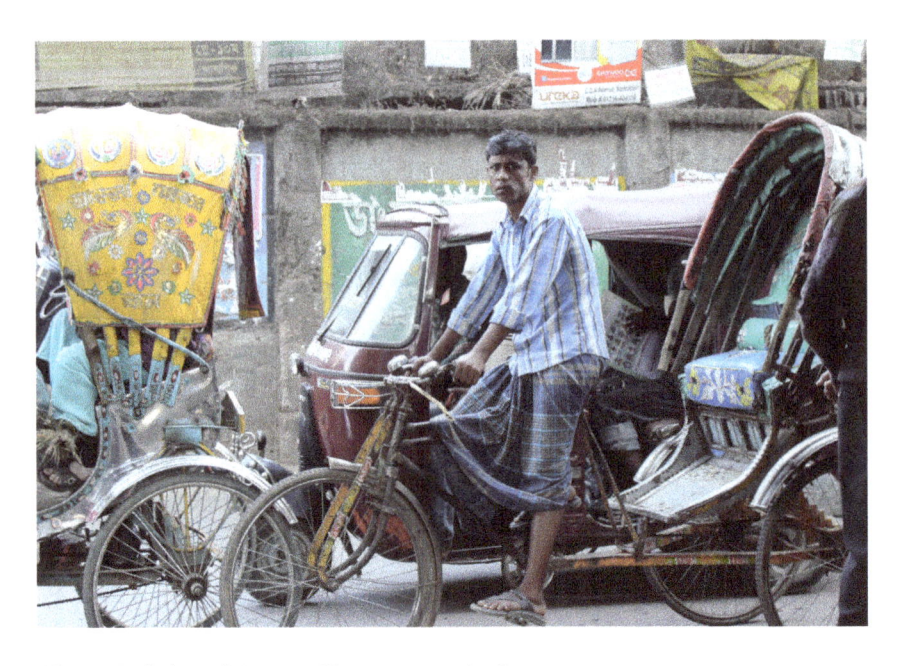

Above: Rickshaw driver in Chittagong waits for a passenger.

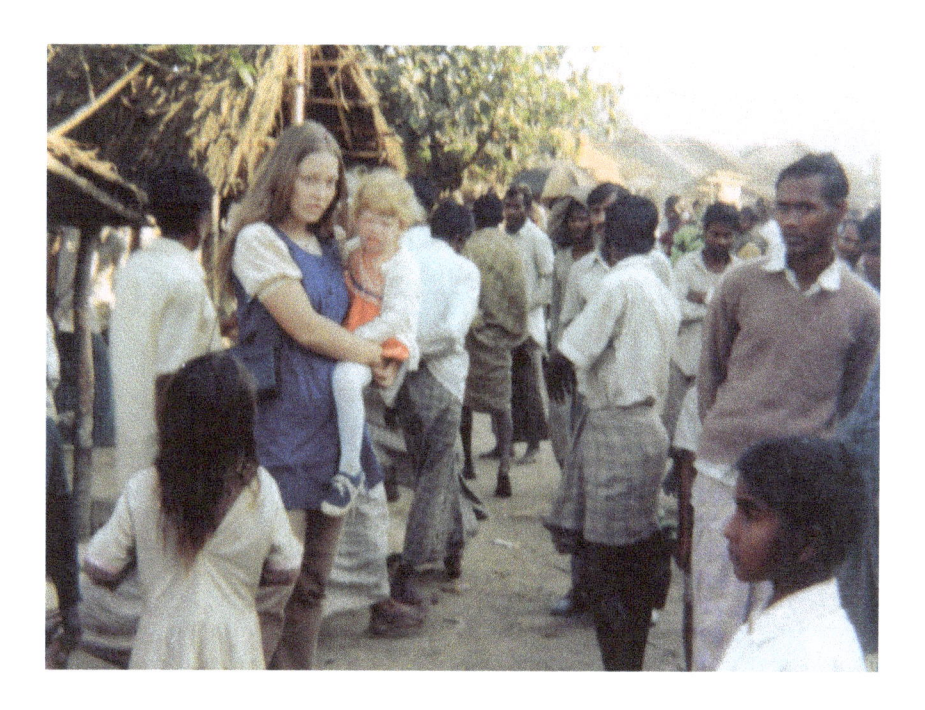

Above: Karen walks through Lama Bazaar in Hebron.

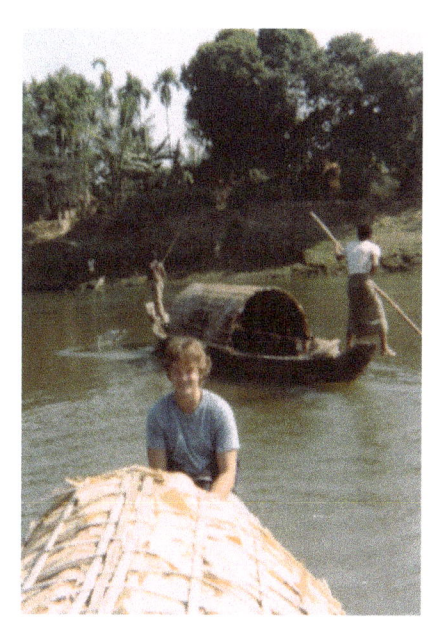

Left: Tense, Peter and Karen travel by sampan boat up the river to Hebron.

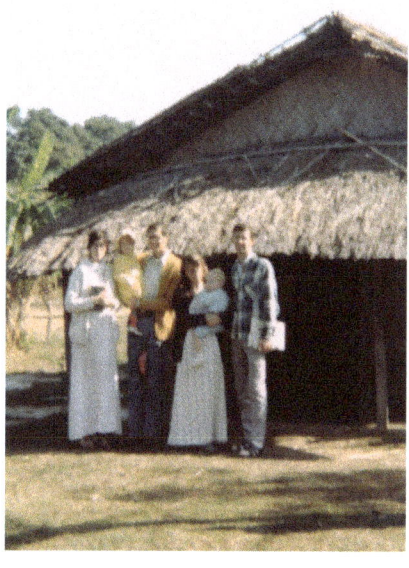

Right: Hebron team in front of the "Jesus House."

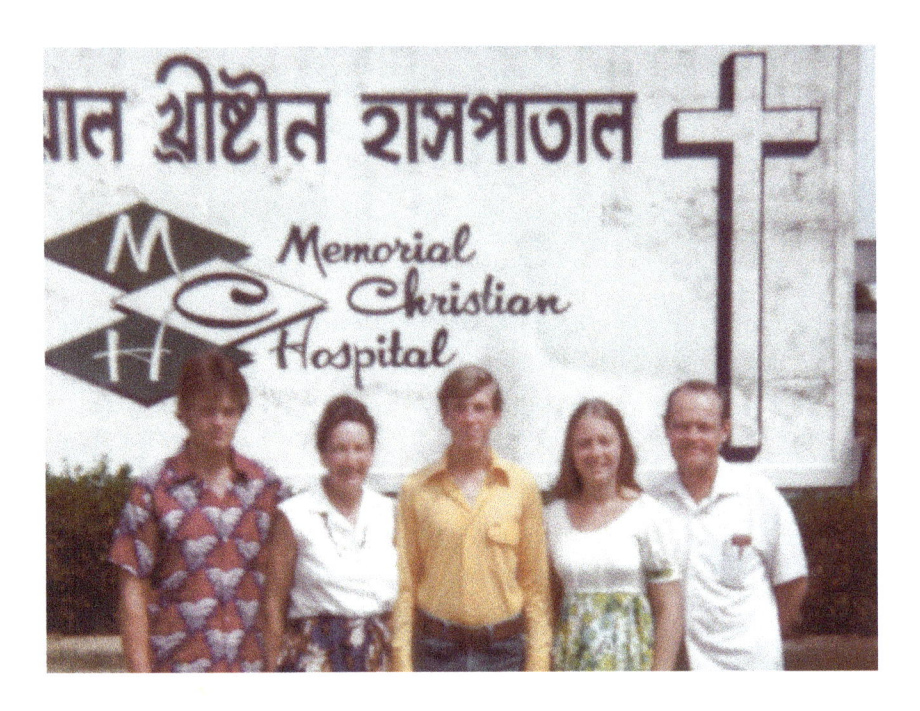

Above: Family visit at Malumghat.

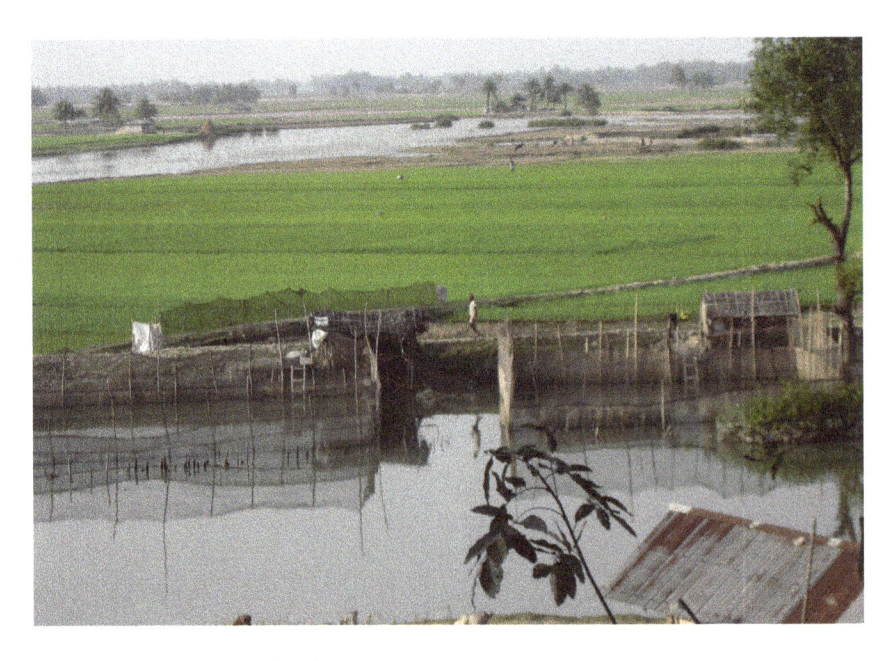

Above: Rice paddies behind MCH.

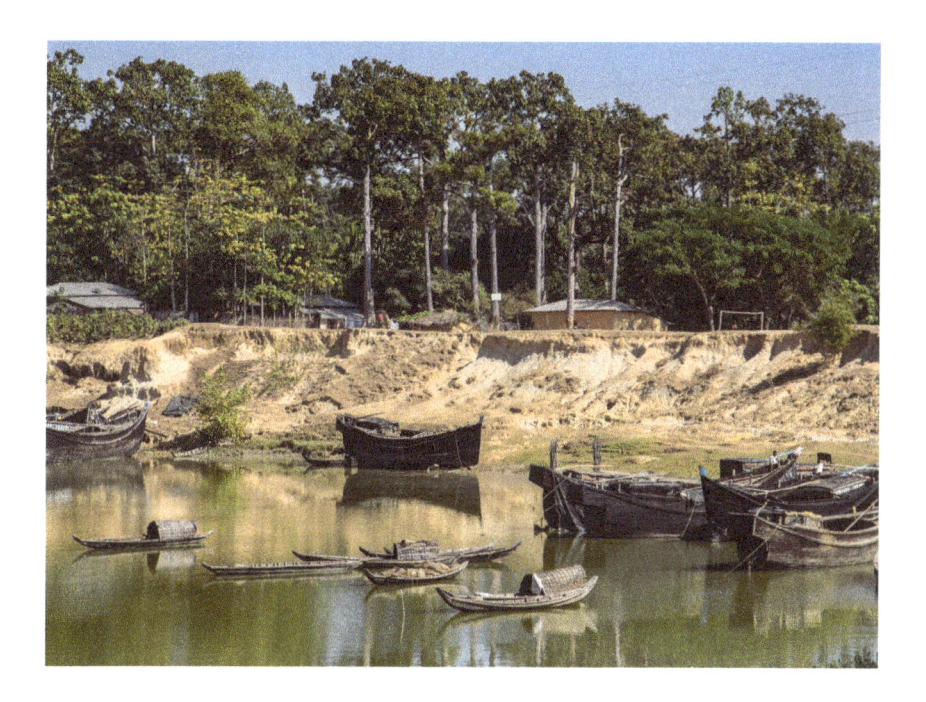

Above: Boat landing on the khal next to MCH property.

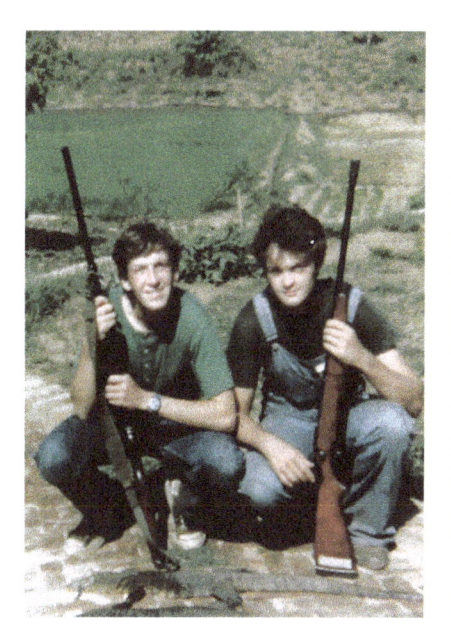

Left: David and Peter with lizards from a hunting trip in the jungle.

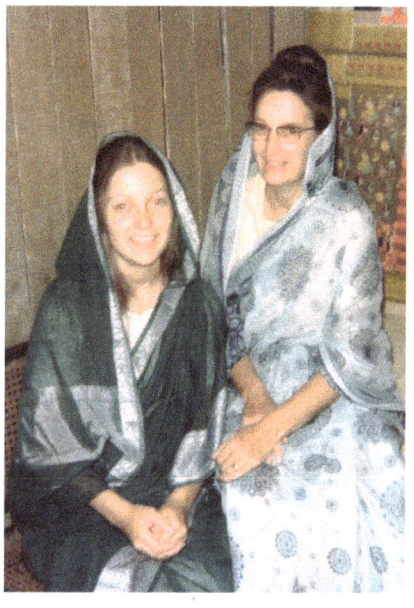

Right: Karen and Tense attend a Bangladeshi wedding.

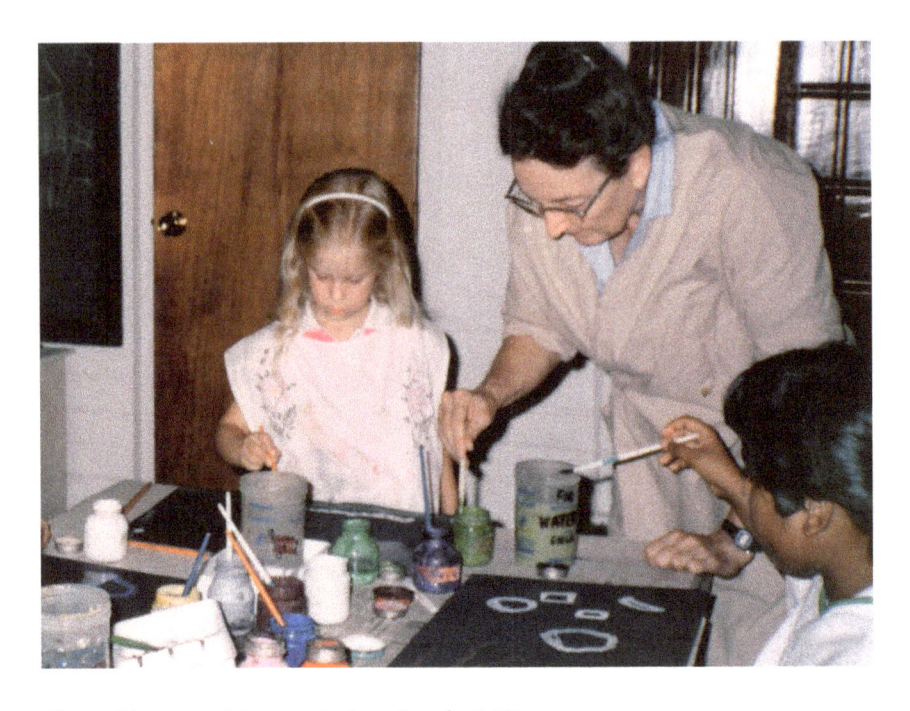

Above: Tense teaching a painting class for MKs.

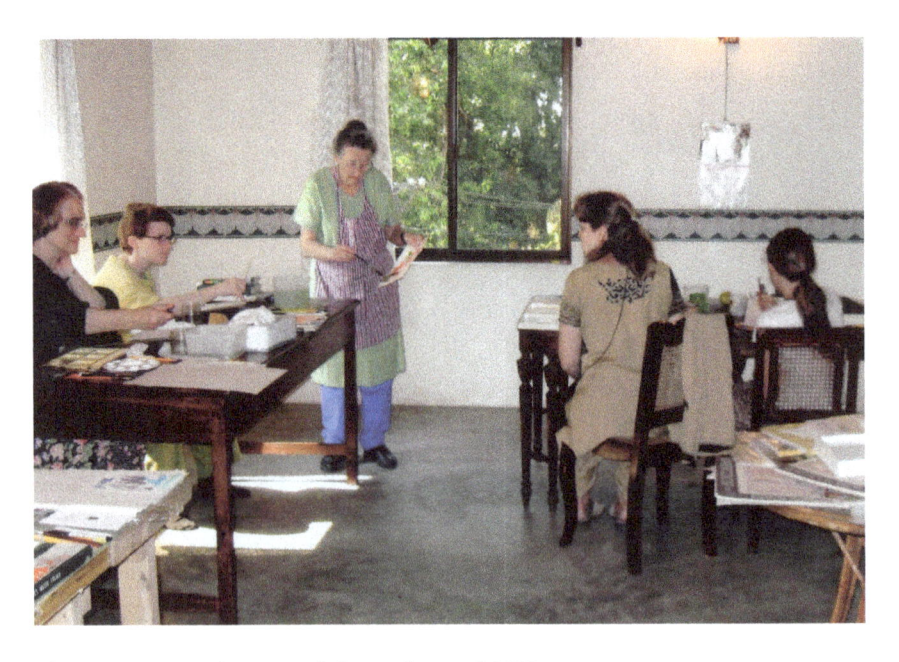

Above: Tense teaching an adult art class to MCH teammates.

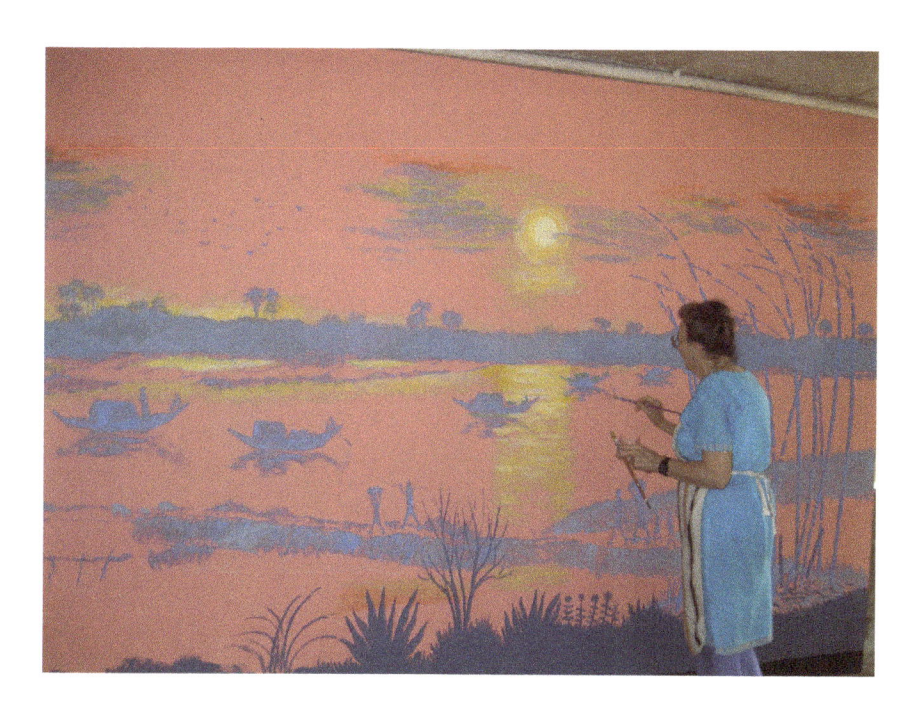

Above: Tense painted an 18' mural on the hospital wall.

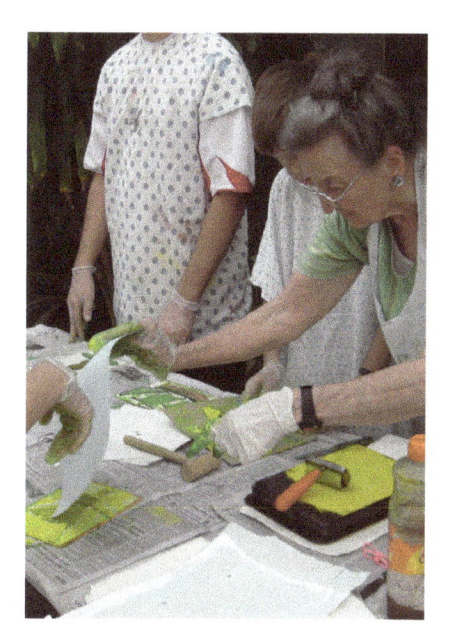

Left: Tense teaching printmaking to MKs.

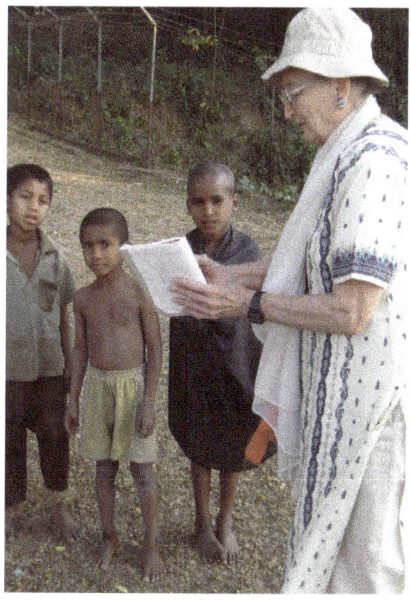

Right: Tense sketches as curious neighbor children watch.

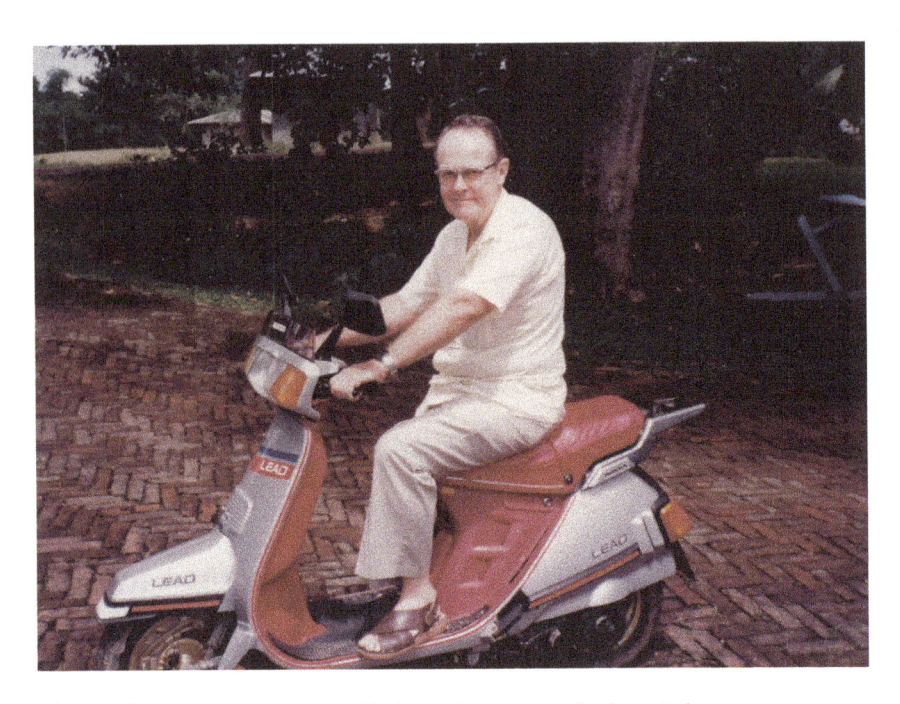

Above: The motor scooter provided quick access to the hospital.

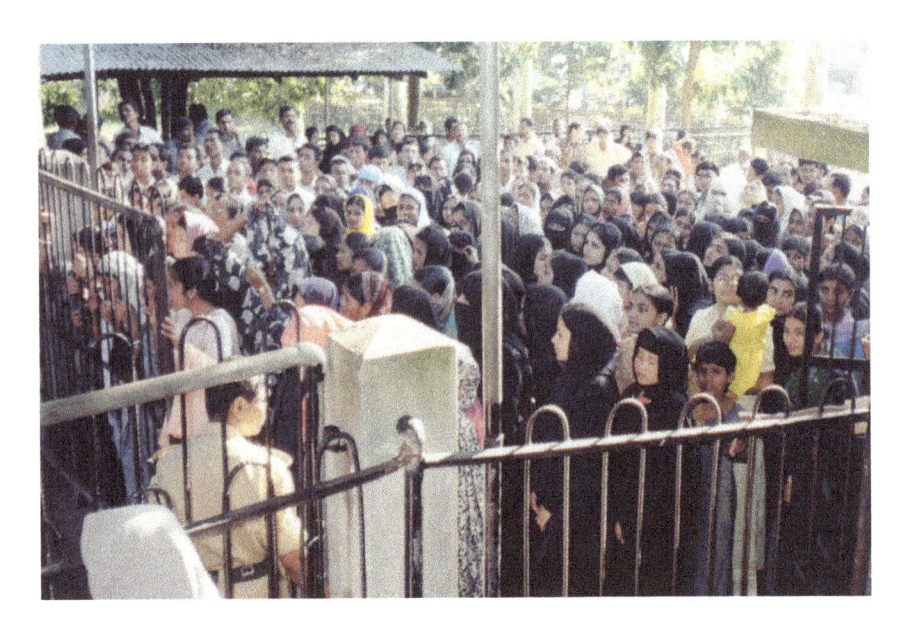

Above: Obstetric patients wait at the MCH gate to be allowed in for maternity care.

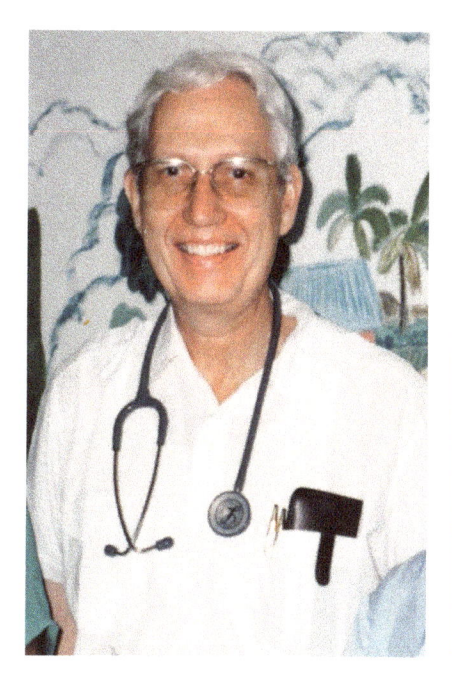

Left: Dr. Olsen, general surgeon, founded MCH in 1966.

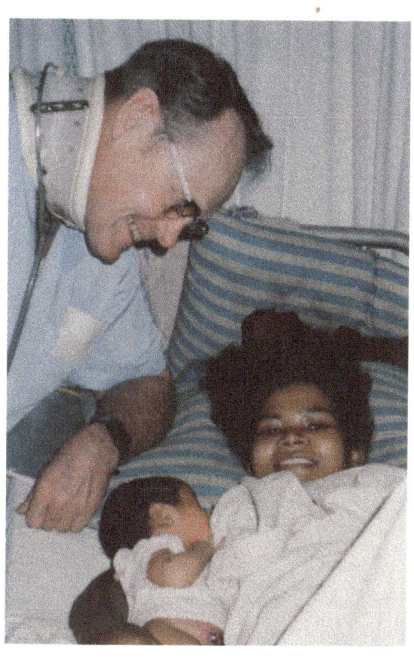

Right: John's new specialty —"Orthostetrics."

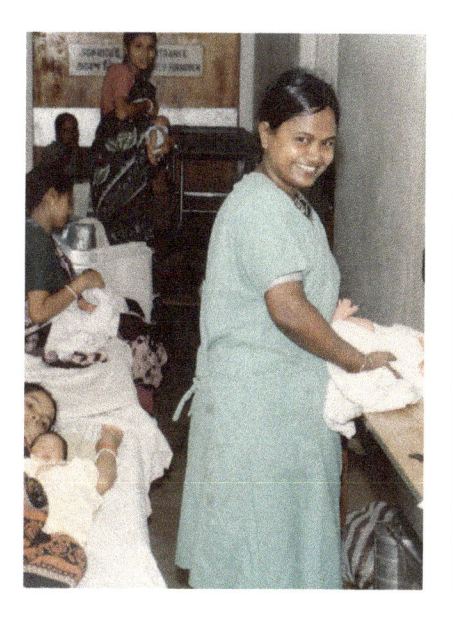

Left: Crowded OB Dept. with patients in the halls.

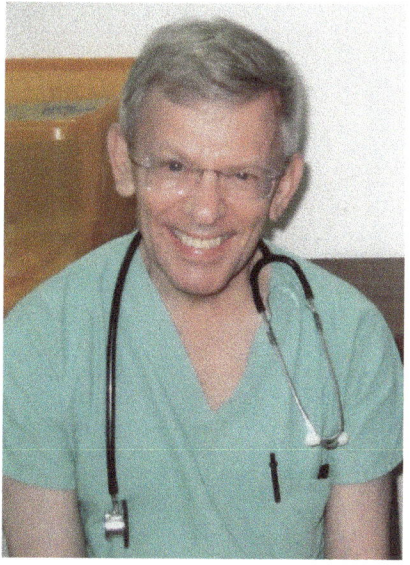

Right: Dr. Stagg and John were the only doctors at MCH during a three-month doctor shortage.

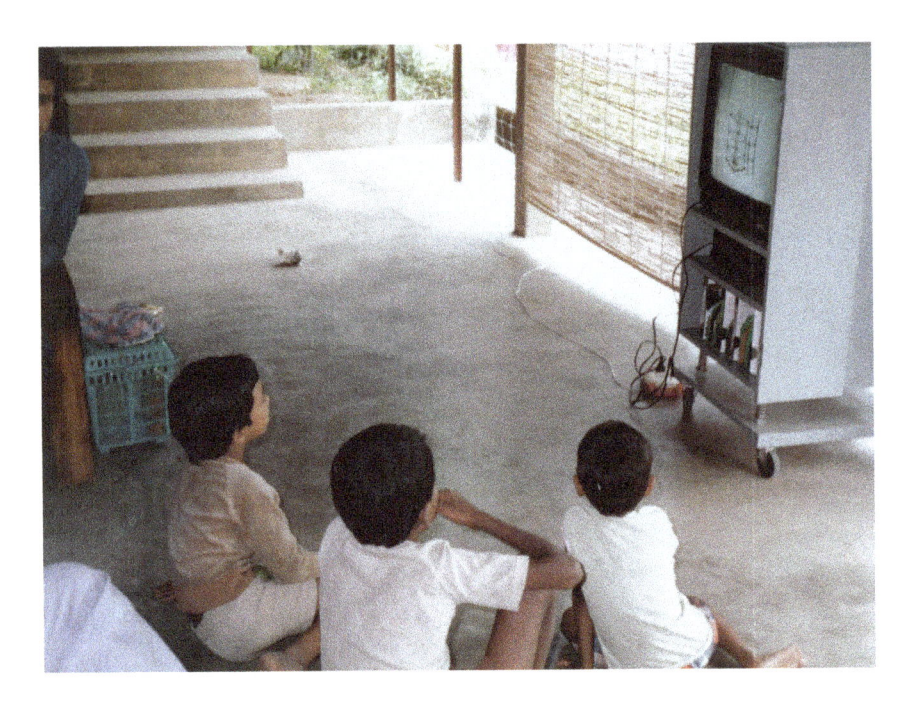

Above: Children watch health teaching video in OPD waiting room.

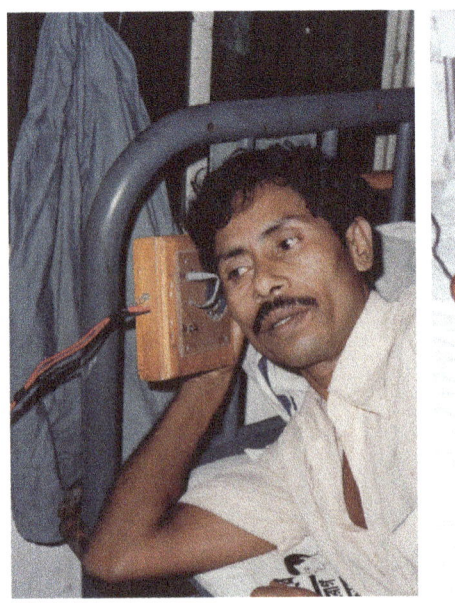

Left: Patient listens to Bible messages on a pillow speaker in the men's ward.

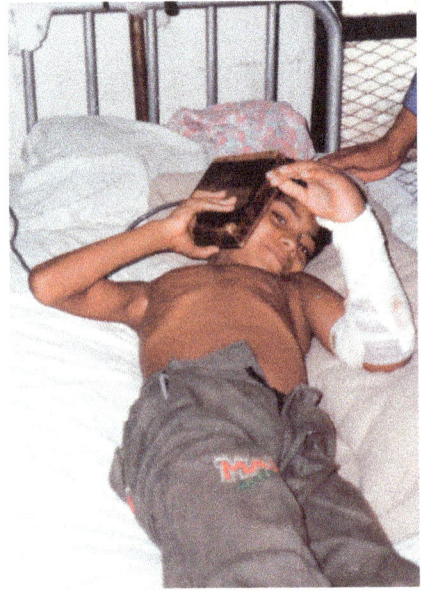

Right: Child listens to gospel message on pillow speaker.

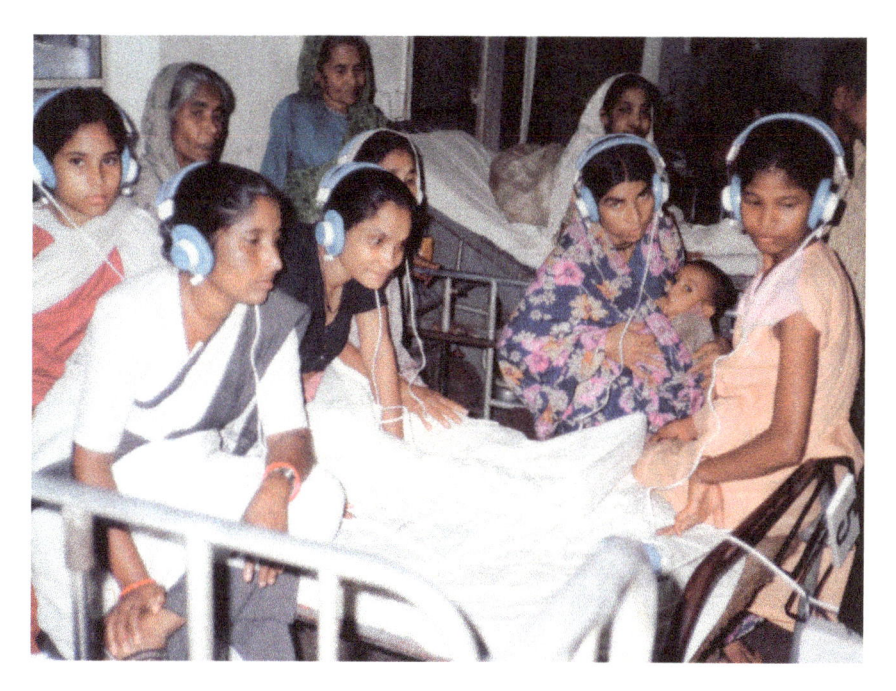

Above: Eager patients listen on headphones to God's Plan for Man Bible message in the women's ward.

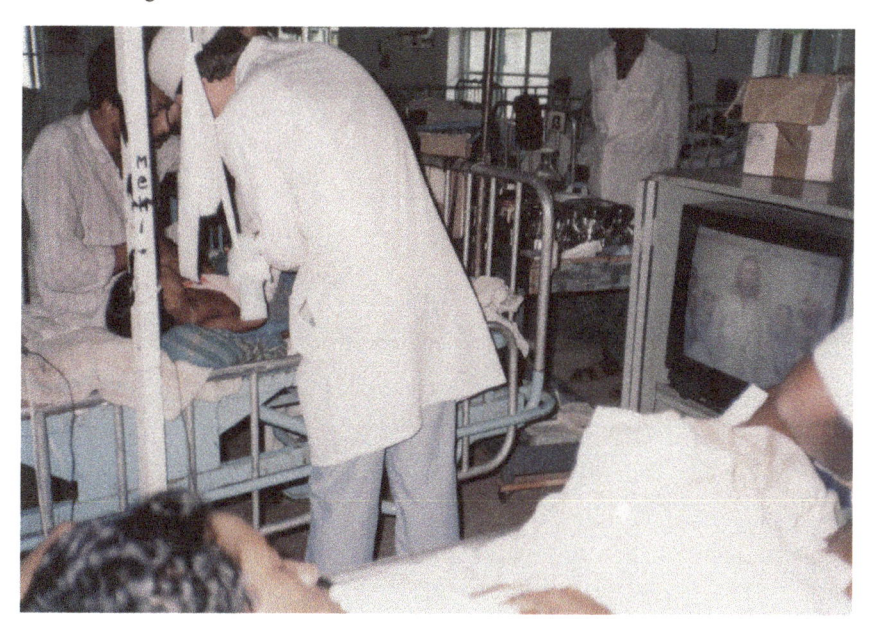

Above: Patient in men's ward watches *The Jesus Film* in a video cart.

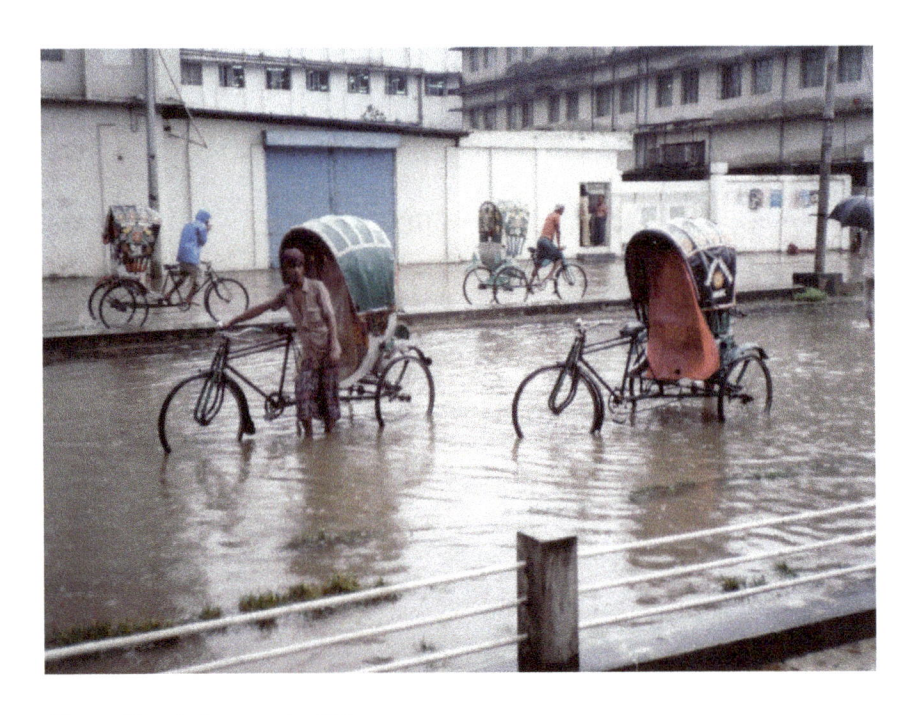

Above: Flooded streets in Chittagong.

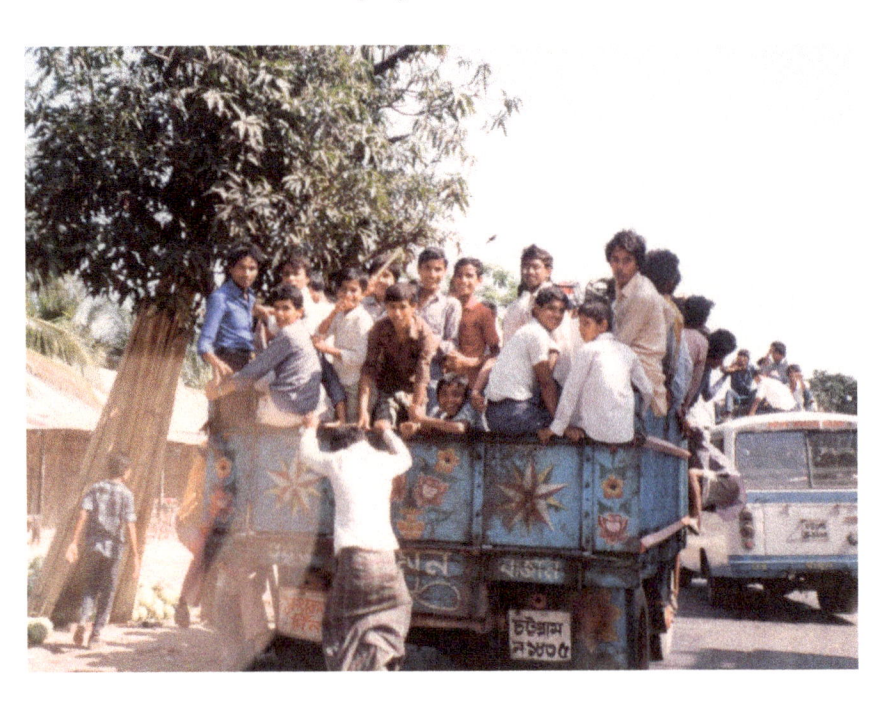

Above: Overloaded trucks often resulted in many casualties.

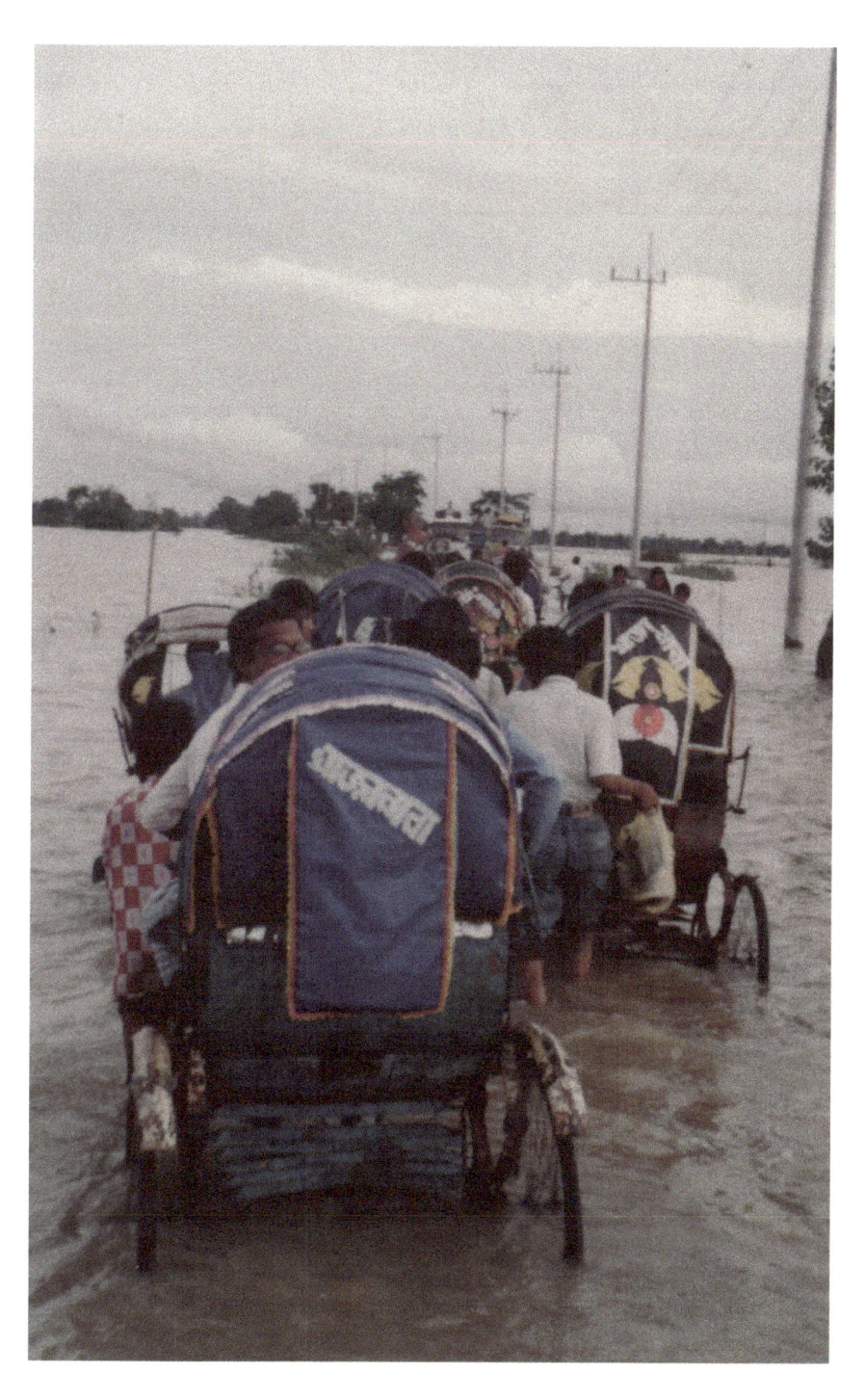

Above: Rickshaw drivers follow carefully on flooded road.

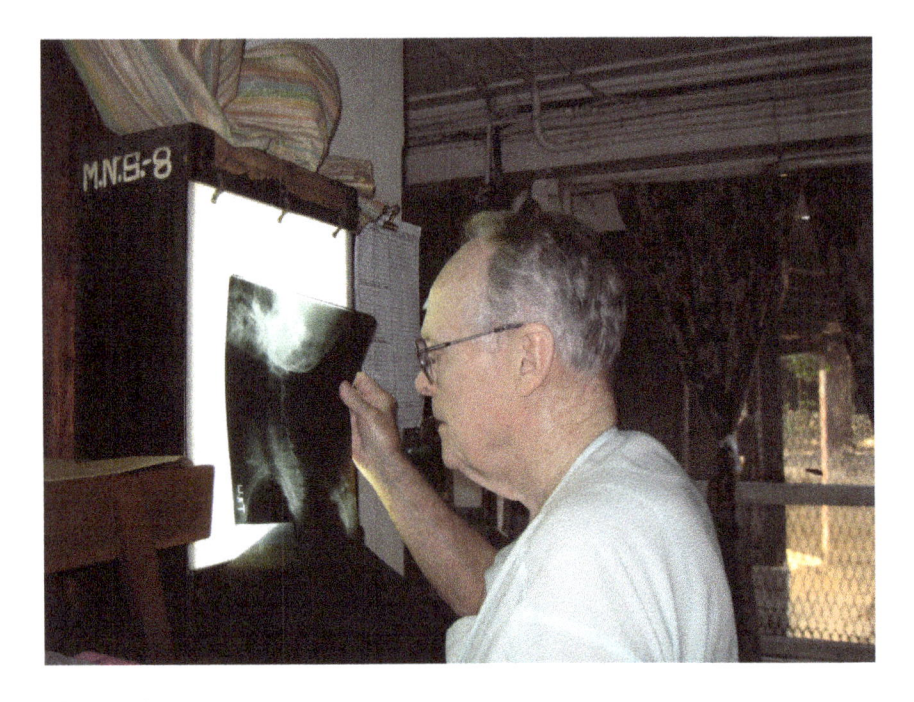

Above: John examines an X-ray.

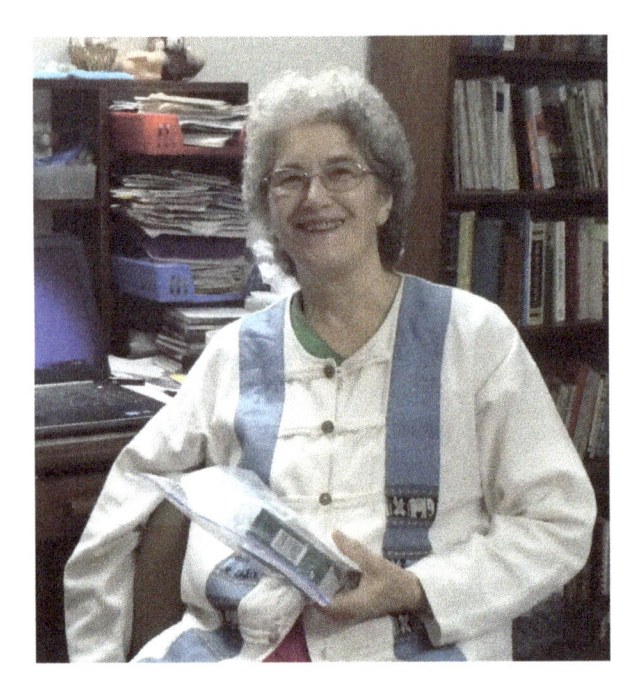

Left:
Nurse Nancie asks the usual question on a busy surgery day.

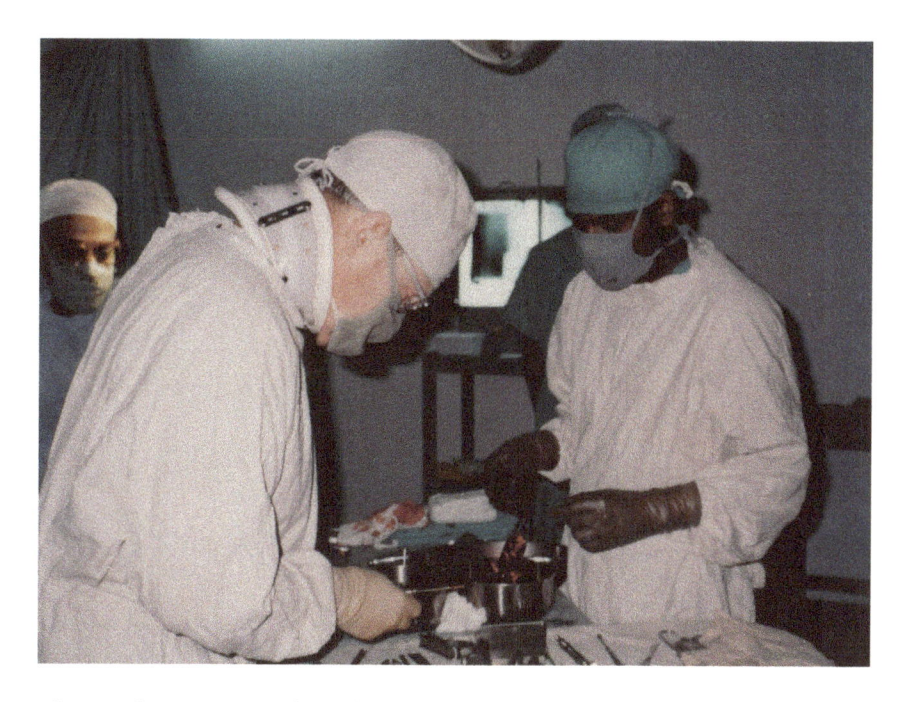

Above: John prepares orthopedic tools for surgery.

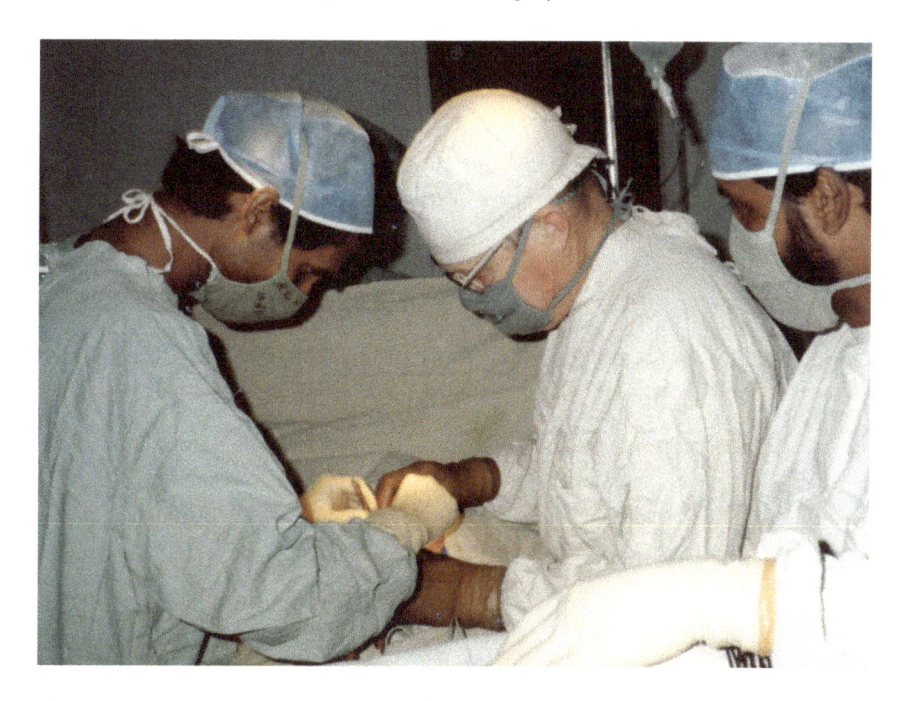

Above: John in surgery with ortho tech assisting.

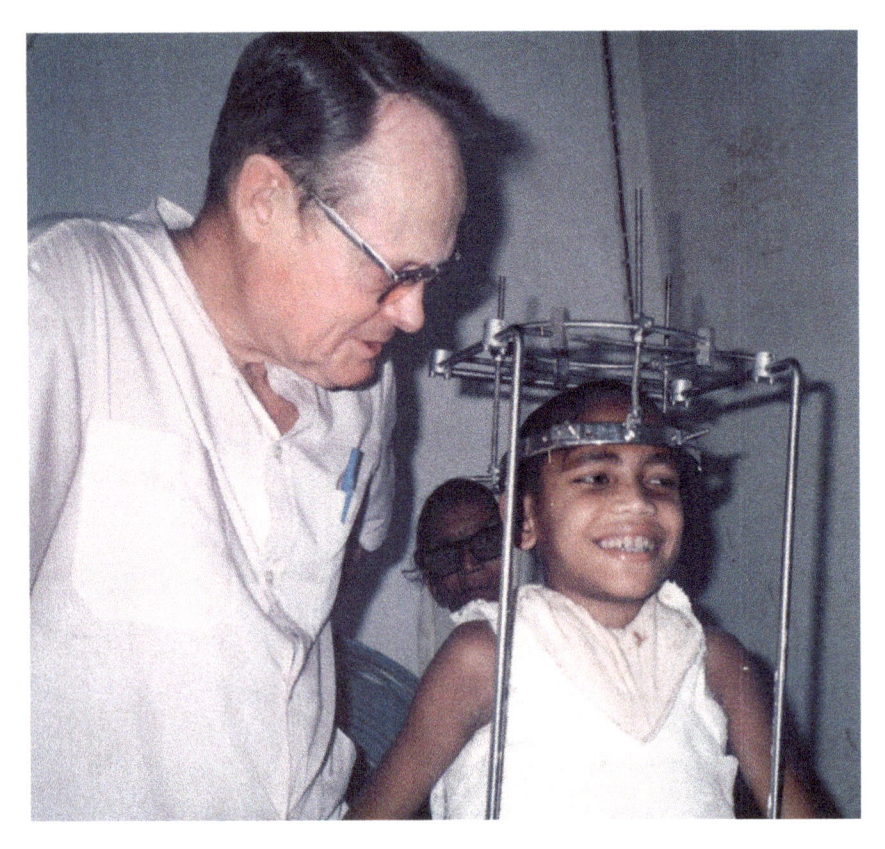

Above: My most challenging case—boy with a congenital vertebral problem.

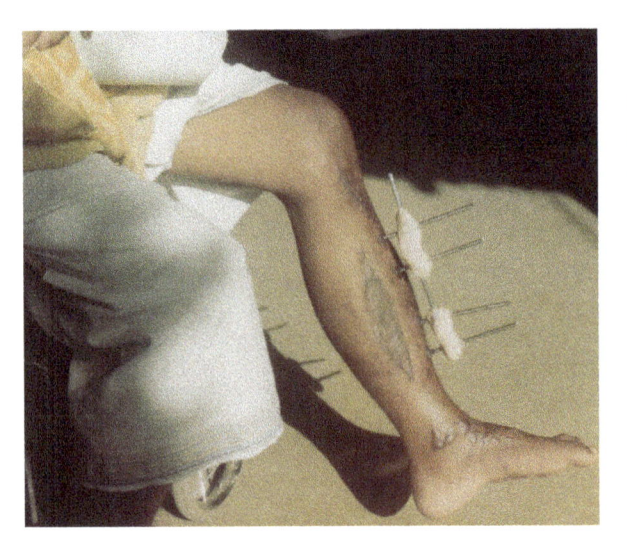

Left:
External fixation holds the deformed bone in the best alignment possible.

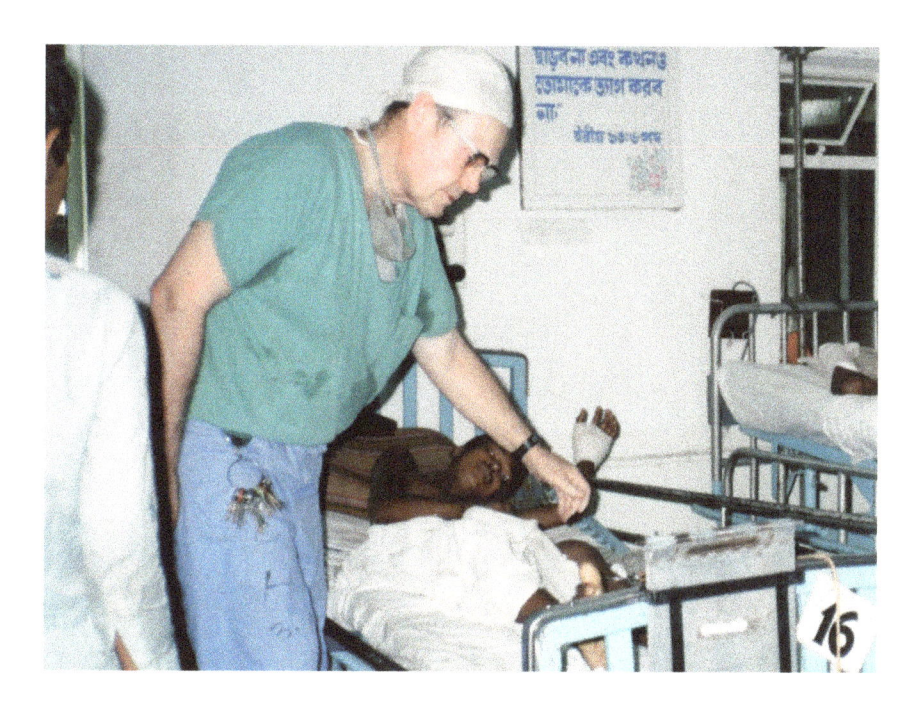

Above: John shows compassionate care to a Muslim patient.

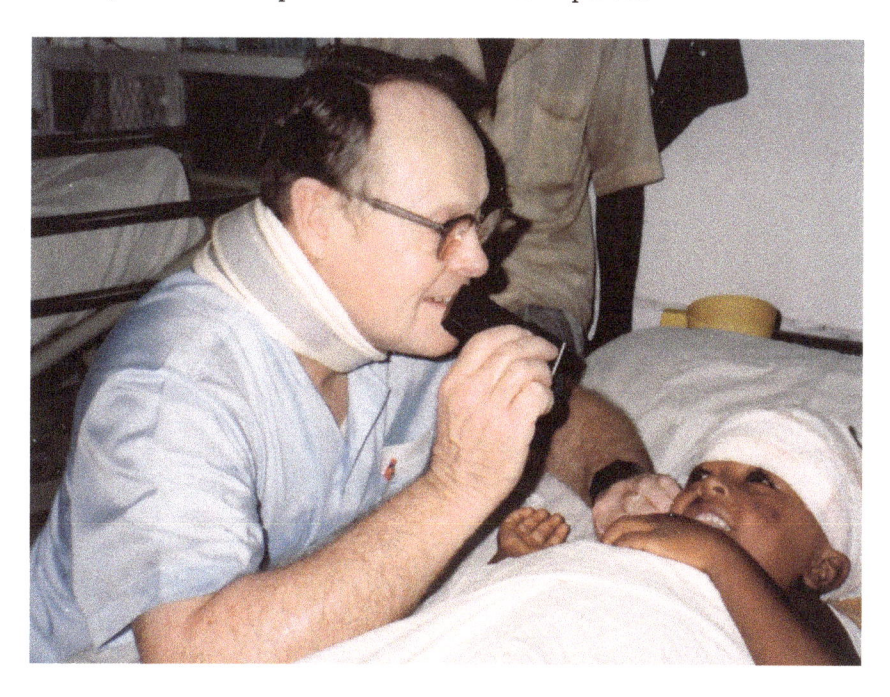

Above: Boy with head injury gets a toy yellow jeep.

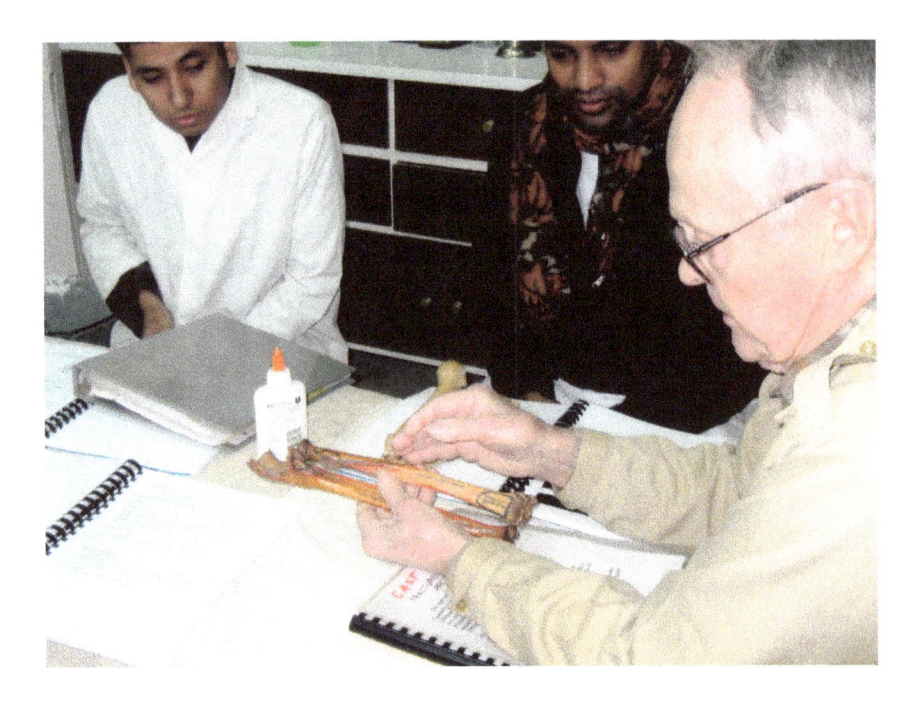

Above: Teaching orthopedic technicians.

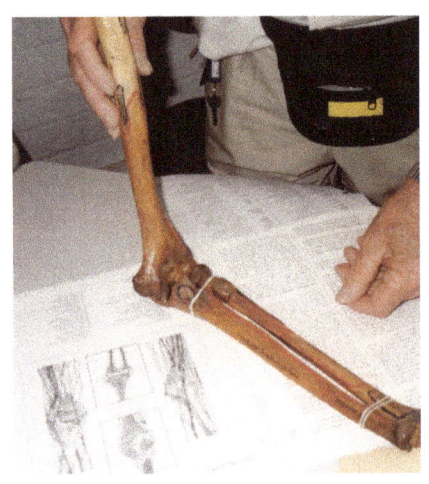

Left: The skeleton was valuable for teaching orthopedic procedures to technicians.

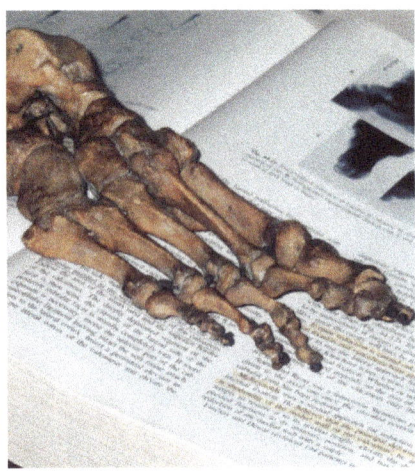

Right: Foot bones.

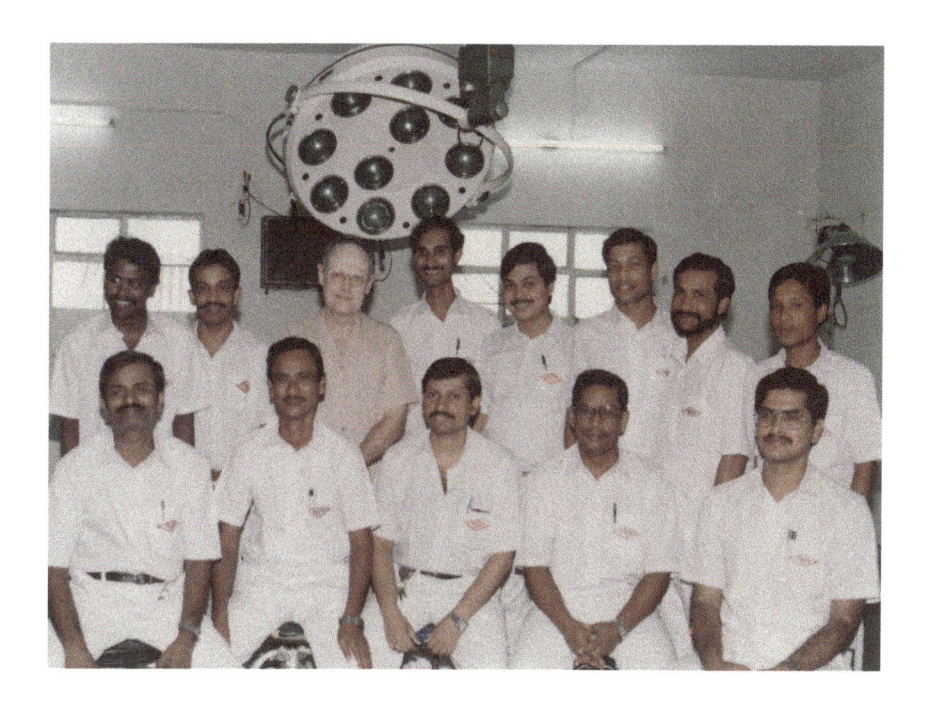

Above: John with ortho techs and OR staff.

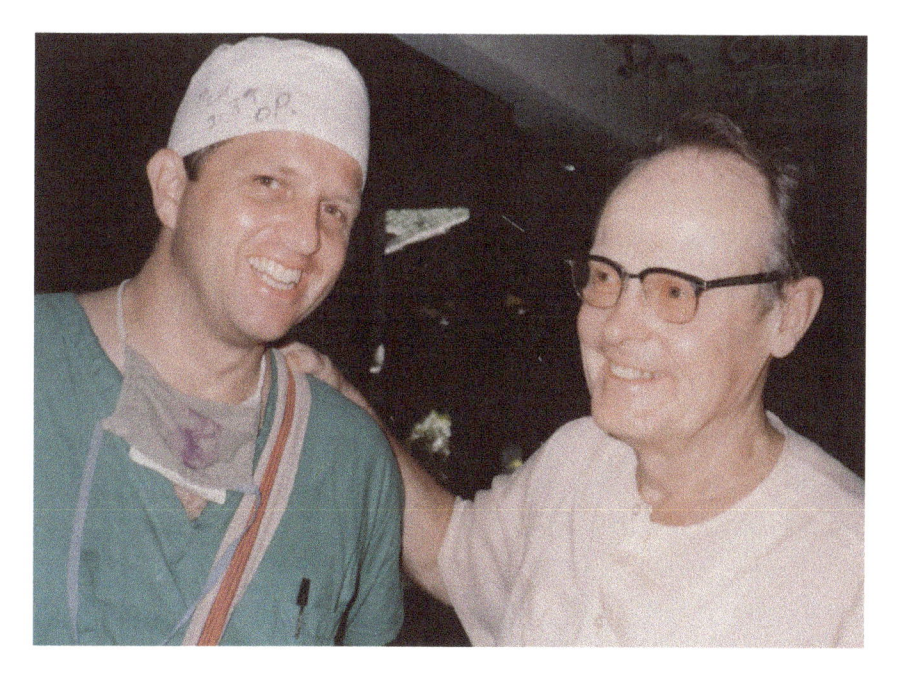

Above: John trained Dr. Goddard in orthopedic surgery.

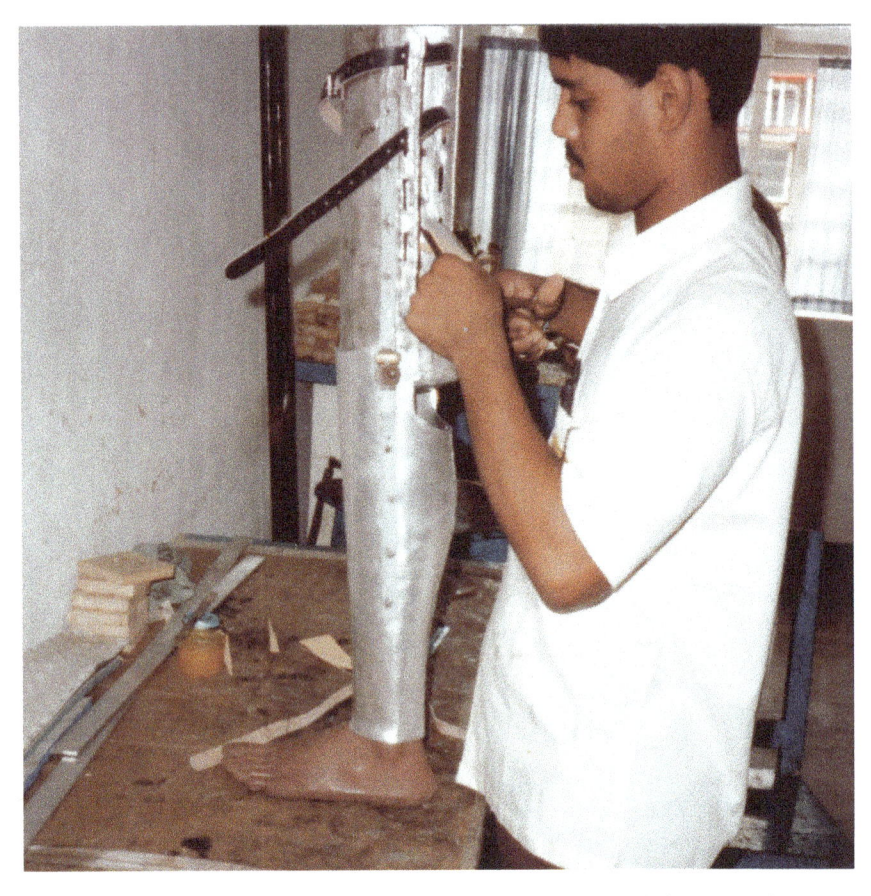

Above: Limb & Brace worker constructs aluminum leg shank for Jaipur foot.

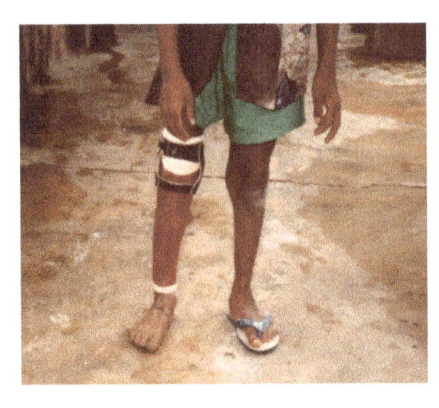

Left: Realistic Jaipur foot enables patients to walk barefoot.

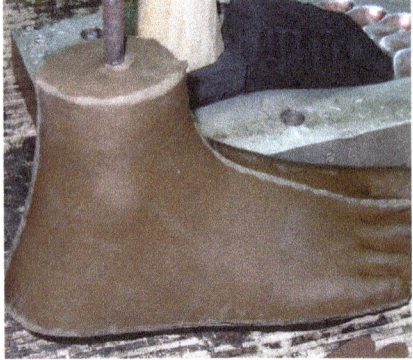

Right: Special molds were made to build the Jaipur foot at the Limb & Brace Shop.

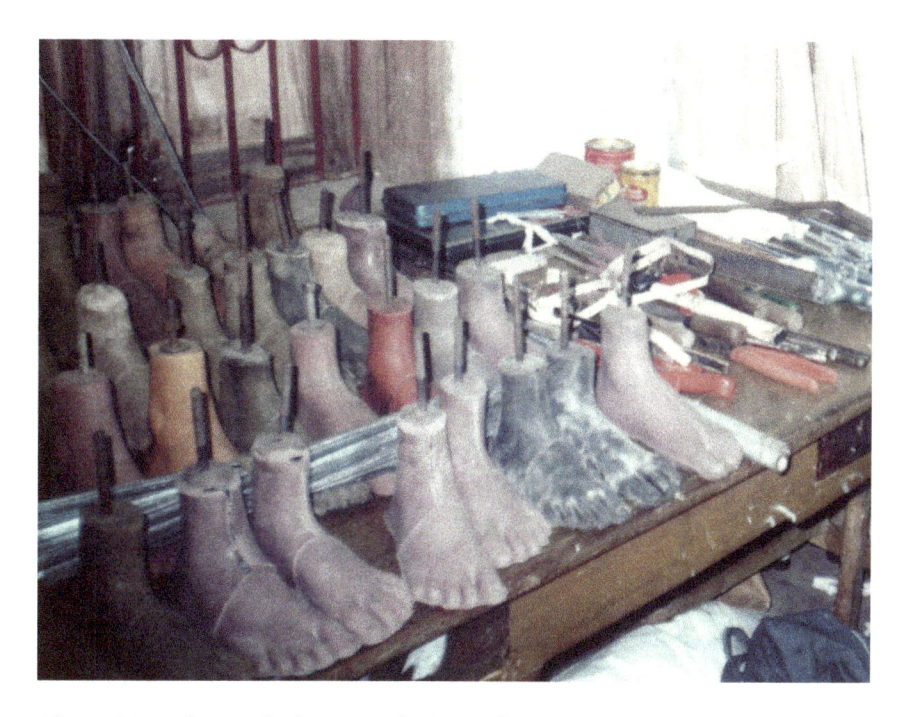

Above: Jaipur feet ready for use at the Jaipur foot camps.

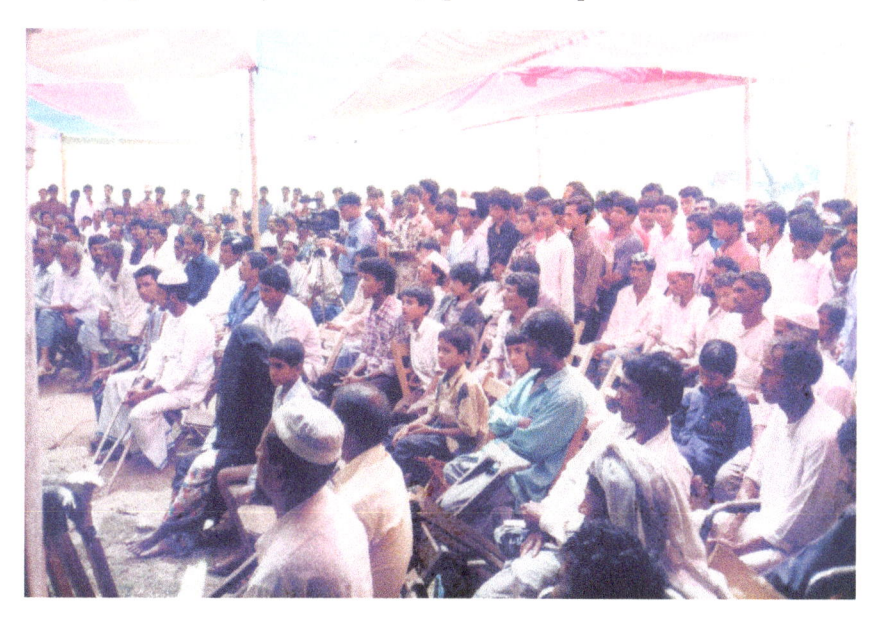

Above: Hundreds of hopeful amputees attended the Jaipur foot camps.

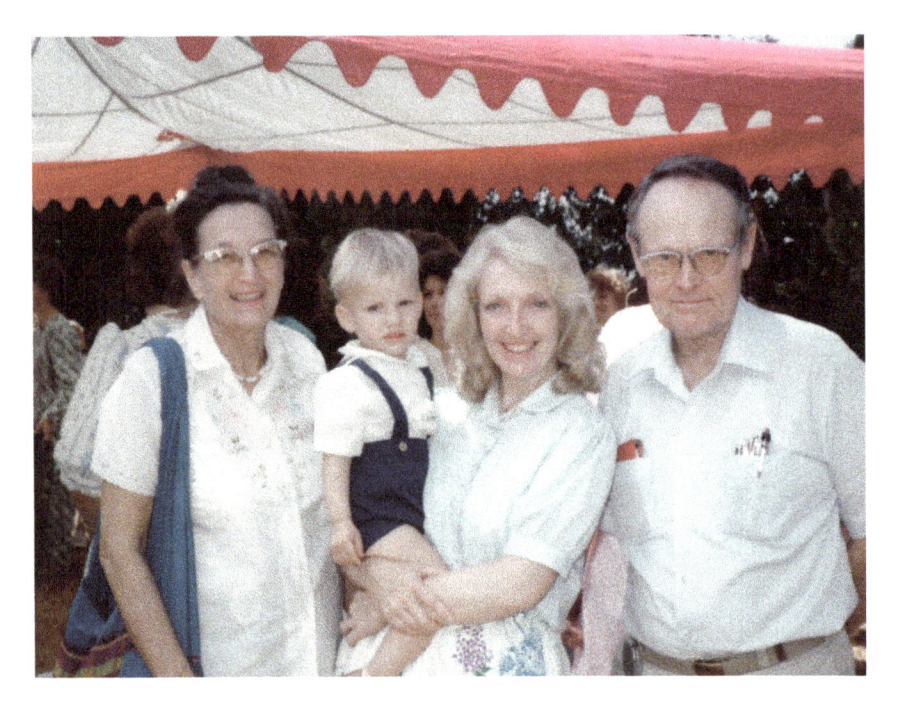

Above: Chrissa and our grandson came for a visit.

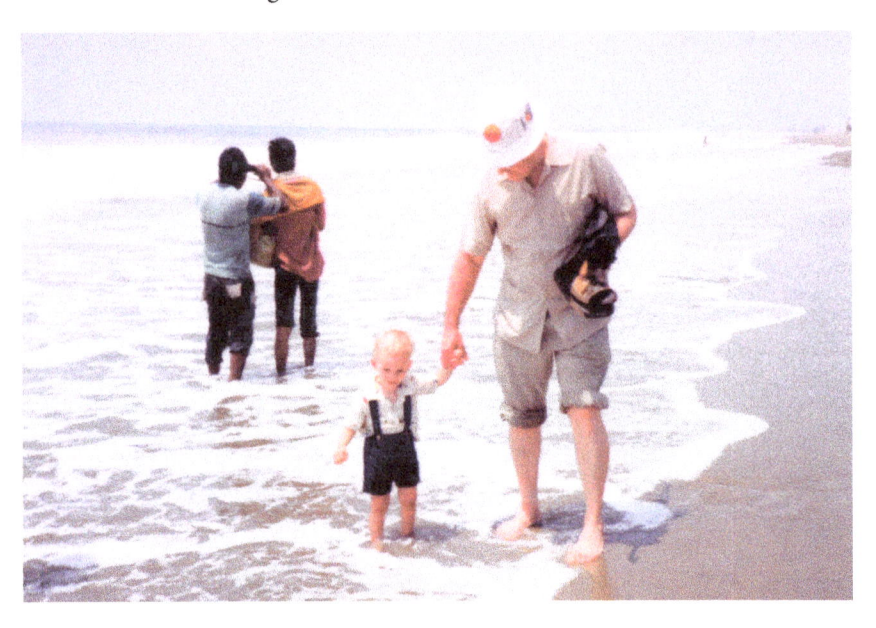

Above: John and grandson on the beach at Cox's Bazaar.

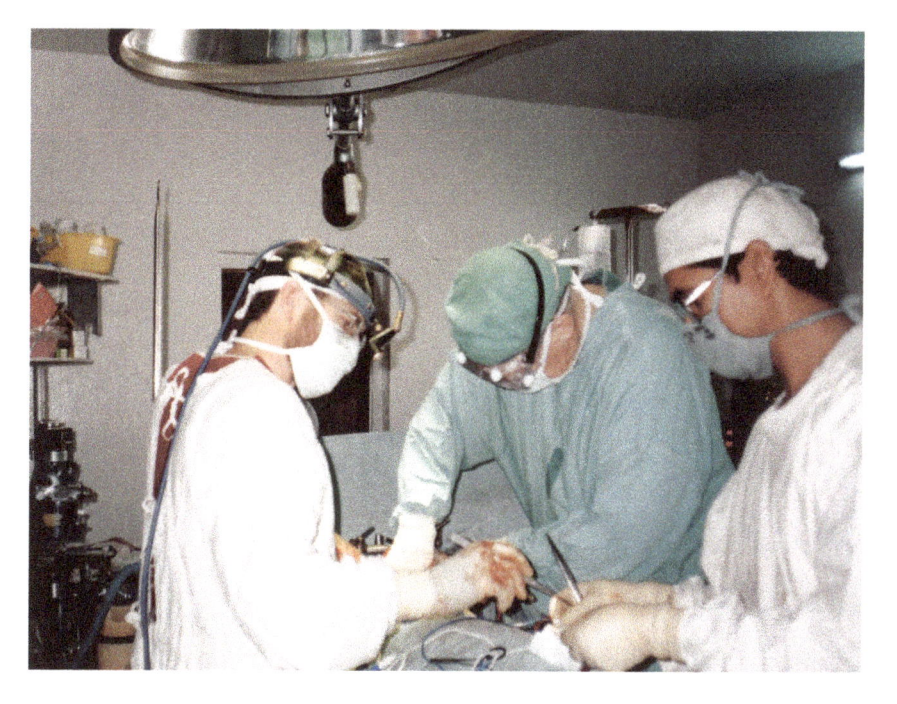

Above: John trained Dr. Steve Kelley in orthopedic surgery.

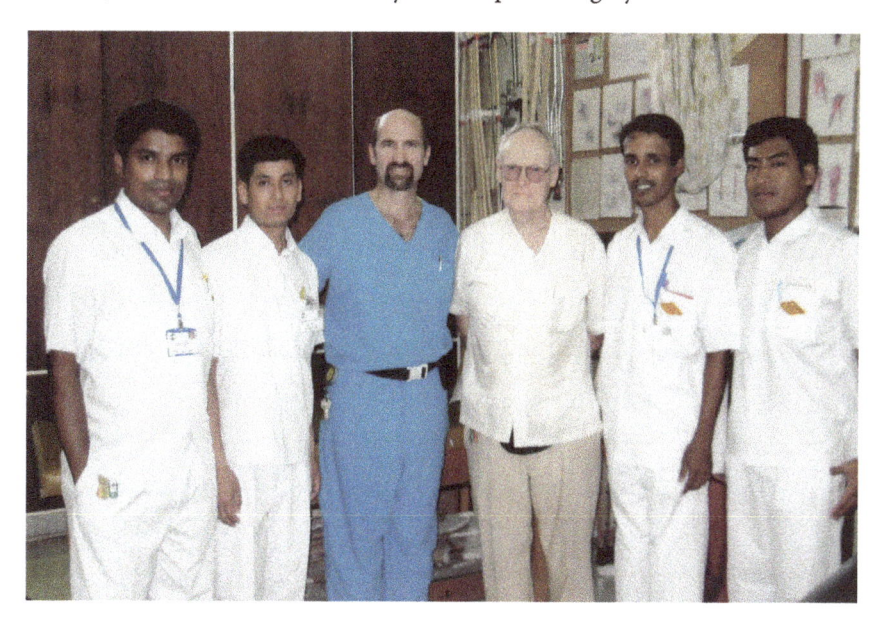

Above: Dr. Kelley, John, and ortho techs.

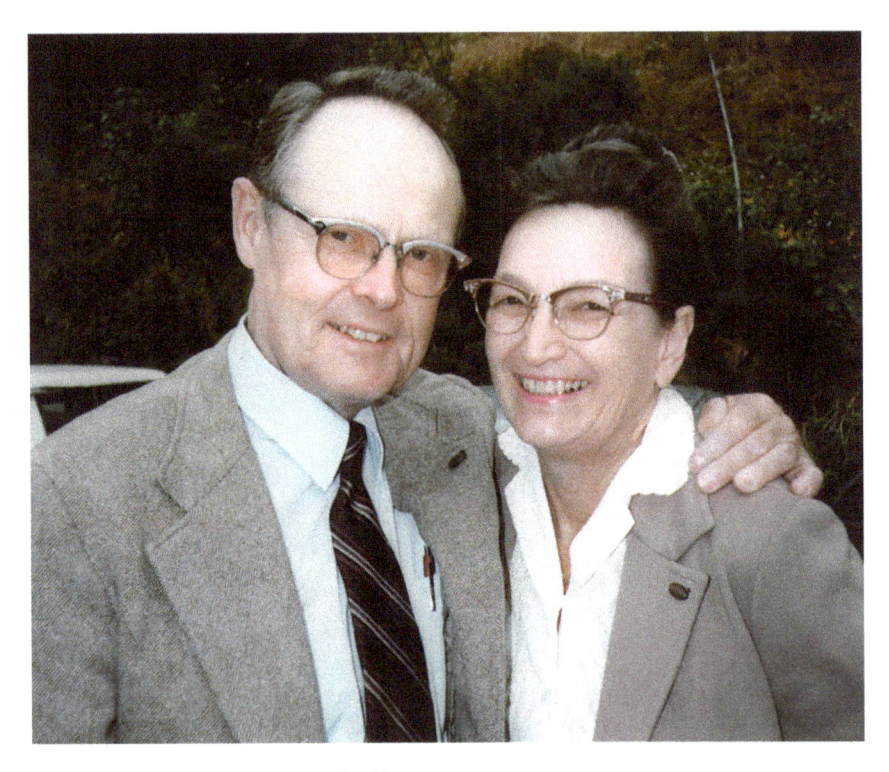

Above: Tense was my most valuable teammate.

Notes

FRONT MATTER

1 Helen Howarth Lemel, "Turn Your Eyes Upon Jesus," In *Majesty Hymns* (Greenville: Majesty Music, Inc., 1997), 639.

CHAPTER THREE—DECISIONS

2 Greg P. Hansen, "Beyond OMT: time for a new chapter in osteopathic medicine?" *Journal of Osteopathic Medicine* 106, no. 3 (March 2006), 114-116. https://www.degruyter.com/document/doi/10.7556/jom_2006_03.0005/html?srsltid=AfmBOorpJv2cE_fr-cwKFKEG1U3FL1imU3ygK1YtTi5OtqjYwksvPBEa.

3 Joel D. Howell, "The Paradox of Osteopathy." The New England Journal of Medicine 341, no. 19 (November 4, 1999): 1465. https://www.nejm.org/search?q=The+paradox+of+osteopathy+ (subscription required).

4 "Origins of Osteopathic Medicine," Tuscon Osteopathic Medical Foundation, https://www.tomf.org/osteopathic-medicine/origins-of-osteopathic-medicine.

5 "What is Osteopathic Medicine?" Philadelphia College of Osteopathic Medicine, https://www.pcom.edu/about/what-is-osteopathic-medicine.html.

6 Tuscon, "Origins," 1.

7 Tuscon, 1.

8 Howell, "Paradox," 1465.

9 Tuscon, "Origins," 1.

10 American Medical Association, "AOA and AMA stand against misrepresentation of osteopathic physicians," News release, Nov. 4, 2020, https://www.ama-assn.org/press-center/press-releases/aoa-and-ama-stand-against-misrepresentation-osteopathic-physicians.

11 Philadelphia, "What is Osteopathic Medicine?"

CHAPTER FIVE—PURSUIT OF ORTHOPEDIC TRAINING

12 Howell, "Paradox," 1466.

CHAPTER SIX—AN INTRIGUING CHALLENGE

13 J.B. Phillips, The New Testament in Modern English (New York: Macmillan Pub. Co., 1963).

14 Phillips, 512.

15 Phillips, 186.

16 Phillips, 249.

CHAPTER NINE—CHANGE OF COMMAND, CHANGE OF COURSE

17 R.B. Thieme, Jr., Christian at Ease! (Houston: R.B. Thieme, Jr., Bible Ministries), 21.

CHAPTER TEN—LETTING GO OF THE BRASS RING

18 "Rose Marie Durham," The Message 36, no. 12 (November/December 1971), 9.

19 Helen Howarth Lemmel, "Turn Your Eyes upon Jesus," In Majesty Hymns (Greenville: Majesty Music, Inc., 1997).

CHAPTER ELEVEN—THE ASSIGNMENT

20 Viggo B. Olsen, Daktar: Diplomat in Bangladesh (Chicago: Moody Press, 1973), 243-305.

CHAPTER FIFTEEN—ON WINGS OF EAGLES

21 Russel E. Ebersole and Nancy Goehring Ebersole, Interwoven (Harrisburg: ABWE Publishing, 2002), 201-241.

22 Viggo B. Olsen, Daktar II (Chicago: Moody Press, 1990), 182-183.

23 Jeannie Lockerbie, On Duty in Bangladesh (Grand Rapids: Zondervan Publishing House, 1973).

CHAPTER SIXTEEN—MEMORIAL CHRISTIAN HOSPITAL

24 Olsen, Daktar II, 192-194.

CHAPTER TWENTY-FIVE—A NEW AND STRANGE CULTURE

25 Olsen, Daktar.

CHAPTER THIRTY—PROVISION AND PROTECTION

26 Carolina W. Sandell Berg. "Day By Day," In Majesty Hymns (Greenville: Majesty Music, Inc., 1997), 448.

CONCLUSION—ONLY ONE LIFE

27 Charles Thomas Studd, "Only One Life." Cavaliers Only, https://www.cavaliersonly.com/poetry_by_christian_poets_of_the_past/poetry_by_missionary_ct_studd, lines 5-6.

Bibliography

ABWE. "Rose Marie Durham." The Message 36, no.12, November/December 1971.

American Medical Association. "AOA and AMA stand against misrepresentation of osteopathic physicians." News release, November 4, 2020. https://www.ama-assn.org/press-center/press-releases/aoa-and-ama-stand-against-misrepresentation-osteopathic-physicians.

Berg, Carolina W. Sandell. "Day By Day." In Majesty Hymns. Greenville: Majesty Music, Inc. 1997.

Ebersole, Russel E. and Nancy Goehring Ebersole. Interwoven. Harrisburg: ABWE Pub., 2002.

Hansen, Greg P. "Beyond OMT: time for a new chapter in osteopathic medicine?" Journal of Osteopathic Medicine 106, no. 3 (March 2006): 114-116. https://www.degruyter.com/document/doi/10.7556/jom_2006_03.0005/html?srsltid=AfmBOorpJv2cE_fr-cwKFKEG1U3FL1imU3ygK1YtTi5OtqjYwksvPBEa.

Howell, Joel D., MD, PhD. "The Paradox of Osteopathy." The New England Journal of Medicine 341, no. 19 (November 4, 1999): 1465-8. PMID: 10547412. https://www.nejm.org/search?q=The+paradox+of+osteopathy+.

Lemel, Helen Howarth. "Turn Your Eyes Upon Jesus." In Majesty Hymns. Greenville: Majesty Music, Inc., 1997.

Lockerbie, Jeannie. On Duty in Bangladesh. Grand Rapids: Zondervan Pub. House, 1973.

Olsen, Viggo B. Daktar: Diplomat in Bangladesh. Grand Rapids: Kregel Pub., 1996.

------. Daktar II. Chicago: Moody Press, 1990.

Philadelphia College of Osteopathic Medicine. "What is Osteopathic Medicine?" https://www.pcom.edu/about/what-is-osteopathic-medicine.html.

Phillips, J.B. The New Testament in Modern English. New York: Macmillan Pub. Co., 1958.

Studd, Charles Thomas. "Only One Life." Cavaliers Only: Poetry About Jesus and Salvation. https://www.cavaliersonly.com/poetry_by_christian_poets_of_the_past/only_one_life_twill_soon_be_past_-_poem_by_ct_studd.

Thieme, Jr., R.B. Christian at Ease! Houston: R.B. Thieme, Jr. Bible Ministries, 1963.

Tuscon Osteopathic Medical Foundation. "Origins of Osteopathic Medicine." https://www.tomf.org/osteopathic-medicine/origins-of-osteopathic-medicine.

Glossary

Arakan Road	The main road in Bangladesh, which runs south of Chittagong and connects to Burma (Myanmar) and the Arakan District.
AWANA	An acronym for "Approved Workmen Are Not Ashamed" (2 Timothy 2:15, KJV); the name of a children's Bible club.
Ayah	A nanny or child's nursemaid.
Banded Krait	Venomous snake in the cobra family in Asia; identified by a gold and black pattern on its back.
Bangladesh	South Asian country east of India, formerly called East Pakistan.
Baksheesh	A small amount of money given as a payment, bribe, or donation.
Bangladeshi	A citizen of Bangladesh.
Bengal	The region in South Asia that includes the country of Bangladesh and the West Bengal part of India.
Bengali	Language spoken in the Bengal part of India and Bangladesh.

Burka	A loose, full-length garment worn by Muslim women to cover the body in public, usually with a veiled opening for the eyes.
Canadian crutch	A forearm crutch with a cuff at the top that wraps around the forearm; also called an "elbow crutch."
Chittagong	A major port city in the Chittagong district 60 miles north of MCH.
Cox's Bazar	A popular tourist area and port city on the southeast coast of Bangladesh, famous for its 93-mile sandy beach.
Dacoit	An armed robber.
Dhaka	Capital city of Bangladesh.
Dhoti	A long piece of cotton fabric wrapped around the waist, worn with a Punjabi kurta (shirt).
Dokan	An open-air shop in the village market.
Expatriate	A citizen of one country living in another country.
Furlough	A time away from regular work when NGO workers travel to their home country to visit family members, report to supporting churches, rest, gather supplies, and prepare for the next term of service.
Godown	A warehouse or other facility for storing goods.
Gurjan tree	Tall trees with very hard wood and smooth, dark brown bark; sometimes planted in a row to form fence posts.
Khal	Water channel beside the hospital that feeds from the Bay of Bengal: used for shipping, fishing, and housing (in boats called sampans).
Khana	Meal or feast.
Kurta	Cotton, knee-length shirt; part of a Punjabi suit
Lungi	A multi-colored, cotton, men's skirt-like garment worn in South Asian countries; lungis are normally tied or wrapped around the waist and cover the legs down to the ankle.
Malumghat	A small town in the Cox's Bazar District of Bangladesh; the location of Memorial Christian Hospital.
Mishti doi	Traditional Bengali fermented sweet yogurt dessert.

MK	Missionary Kid; a child of NGO workers.
NGO	Non-governmental organization.
Peon	An unskilled person who does menial tasks or acts as a messenger.
Punjabi suit	Traditional clothing of Punjabi men; consists of a cotton knee-length long-sleeved shirt (kurta) with slits on the sides and worn with loose baggy pants, a lungi, or a dhoti.
Rickshaw	Three-wheeled cycle with a covered seat at the back for passengers; used as a taxi
Sangi	Caregiver (usually a family member) who accompanies the patient and provides food and personal care while the patient is in the hospital.
Saree	Elegant and traditional dress worn by South Asian women, consisting of five to seven yards of one piece of brightly colored silk, cotton, or synthetic cloth.
Taka	Basic unit of money in Bangladesh.
Typhoon	Severe tropical cyclone.

Bangladesh 1974

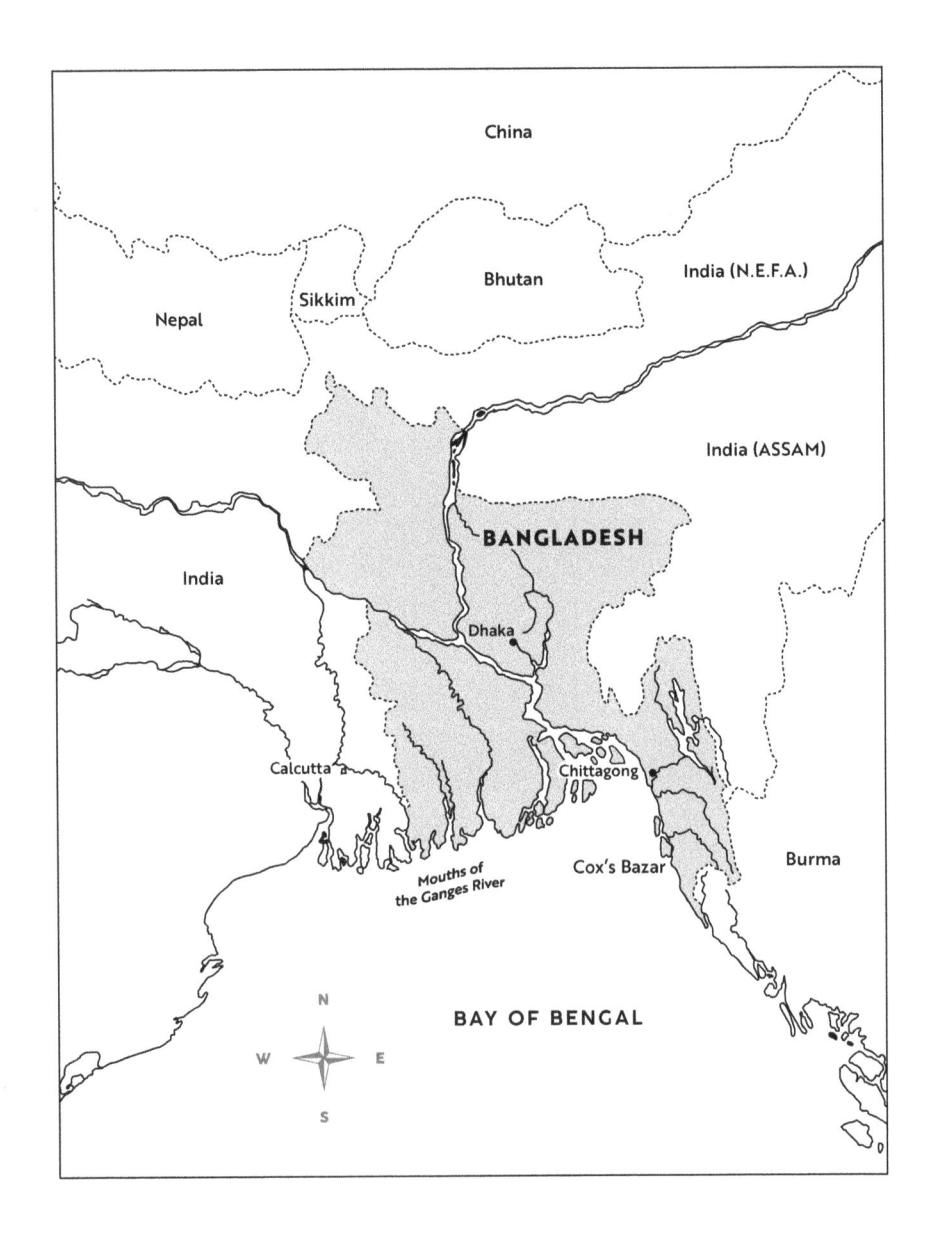

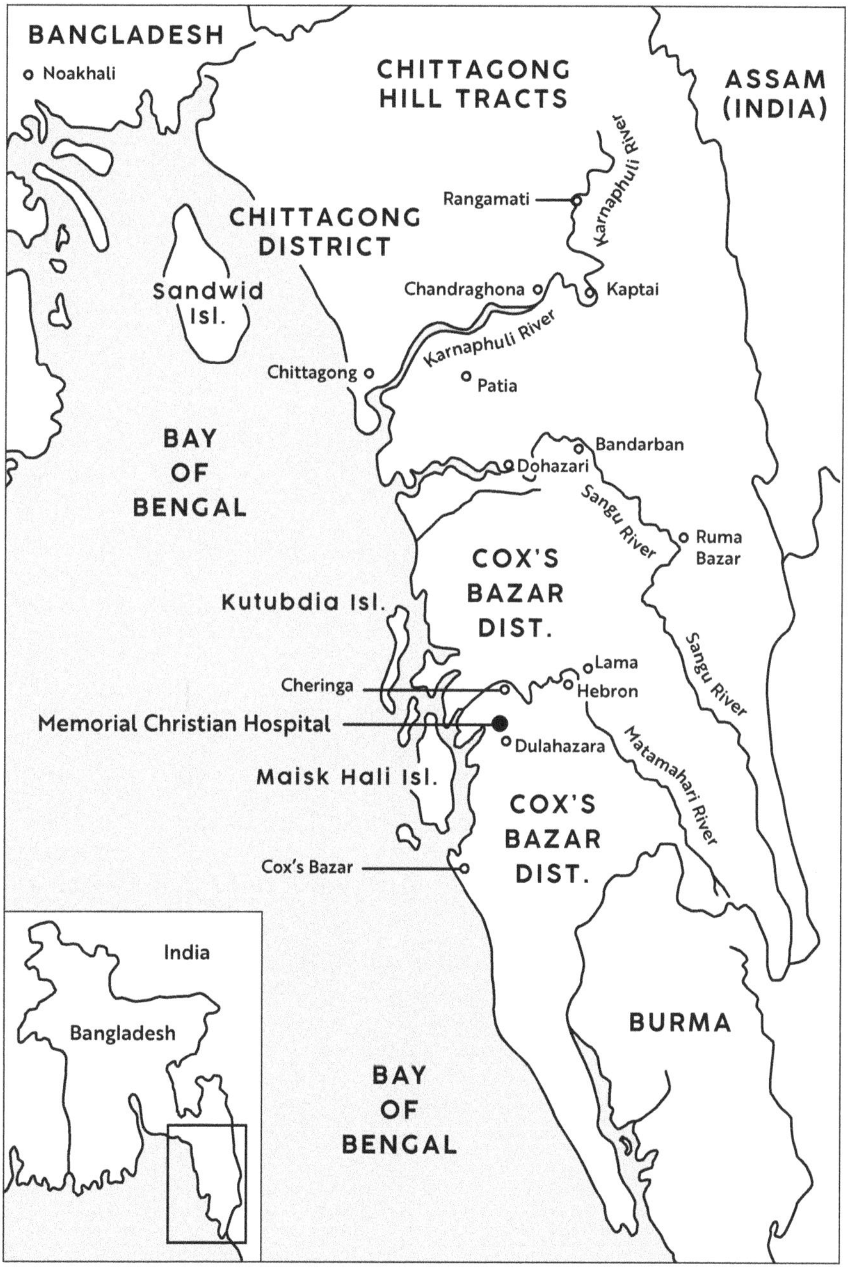
BANGLADESH
Noakhali
CHITTAGONG
HILL TRACTS
ASSAM
(INDIA)
Karnaphuli River
Rangamati
CHITTAGONG
DISTRICT
Sandwid
Isl.
Chandraghona
Kaptai
Karnaphuli River
Chittagong
Patia
BAY
OF
BENGAL
Bandarban
Dohazari
Sangu River
Ruma
Bazar
COX'S
BAZAR
DIST.
Kutubdia Isl.
Lama
Cheringa
Hebron
Sangu River
Memorial Christian Hospital
Dulahazara
Matamahari River
Maisk Hali Isl.
COX'S
BAZAR
DIST.
Cox's Bazar
India
Bangladesh
BURMA
BAY
OF
BENGAL

www.ingramcontent.com/pod-product-compliance
Lightning Source LLC
Chambersburg PA
CBHW051041180525
26716CB00026B/43